# Biosimilar Clinical Development

## Scientific Considerations and New Methodologies

# Chapman & Hall/CRC Biostatistics Series



## Published Titles

**Adaptive Design Methods in Clinical Trials, Second Edition**
Shein-Chung Chow and Mark Chang

**Adaptive Designs for Sequential Treatment Allocation**
Alessandro Baldi Antognini and Alessandra Giovagnoli

**Adaptive Design Theory and Implementation Using SAS and R, Second Edition**
Mark Chang

**Advanced Bayesian Methods for Medical Test Accuracy**
Lyle D. Broemeling

**Analyzing Longitudinal Clinical Trial Data: A Practical Guide**
Craig Mallinckrodt and Ilya Lipkovich

**Applied Biclustering Methods for Big and High-Dimensional Data Using R**
Adetayo Kasim, Ziv Shkedy, Sebastian Kaiser, Sepp Hochreiter, and Willem Talloen

**Applied Meta-Analysis with R**
Ding-Geng (Din) Chen and Karl E. Peace

**Basic Statistics and Pharmaceutical Statistical Applications, Second Edition**
James E. De Muth

**Bayesian Adaptive Methods for Clinical Trials**
Scott M. Berry, Bradley P. Carlin, J. Jack Lee, and Peter Muller

**Bayesian Analysis Made Simple: An Excel GUI for WinBUGS**
Phil Woodward

**Bayesian Designs for Phase I–II Clinical Trials**
Ying Yuan, Hoang Q. Nguyen, and Peter F. Thall

**Bayesian Methods for Measures of Agreement**
Lyle D. Broemeling

**Bayesian Methods for Repeated Measures**
Lyle D. Broemeling

**Bayesian Methods in Epidemiology**
Lyle D. Broemeling

**Bayesian Methods in Health Economics**
Gianluca Baio

**Bayesian Missing Data Problems: EM, Data Augmentation and Noniterative Computation**
Ming T. Tan, Guo-Liang Tian, and Kai Wang Ng

**Bayesian Modeling in Bioinformatics**
Dipak K. Dey, Samiran Ghosh, and Bani K. Mallick

**Benefit-Risk Assessment in Pharmaceutical Research and Development**
Andreas Sashegyi, James Felli, and Rebecca Noel

Published Titles

**Benefit-Risk Assessment Methods in Medical Product Development: Bridging Qualitative and Quantitative Assessments**
Qi Jiang and Weili He

**Bioequivalence and Statistics in Clinical Pharmacology, Second Edition**
Scott Patterson and Byron Jones

**Biosimilar Clinical Development: Scientific Considerations and New Methodologies**
Kerry B. Barker, Sandeep M. Menon, Ralph B. D'Agostino, Sr., Siyan Xu, and Bo Jin

**Biosimilars: Design and Analysis of Follow-on Biologics**
Shein-Chung Chow

**Biostatistics: A Computing Approach**
Stewart J. Anderson

**Cancer Clinical Trials: Current and Controversial Issues in Design and Analysis**
Stephen L. George, Xiaofei Wang, and Herbert Pang

**Causal Analysis in Biomedicine and Epidemiology: Based on Minimal Sufficient Causation**
Mikel Aickin

**Clinical and Statistical Considerations in Personalized Medicine**
Claudio Carini, Sandeep Menon, and Mark Chang

**Clinical Trial Data Analysis using R**
Ding-Geng (Din) Chen and Karl E. Peace

**Clinical Trial Methodology**
Karl E. Peace and Ding-Geng (Din) Chen

**Computational Methods in Biomedical Research**
Ravindra Khattree and Dayanand N. Naik

**Computational Pharmacokinetics**
Anders Källén

**Confidence Intervals for Proportions and Related Measures of Effect Size**
Robert G. Newcombe

**Controversial Statistical Issues in Clinical Trials**
Shein-Chung Chow

**Data Analysis with Competing Risks and Intermediate States**
Ronald B. Geskus

**Data and Safety Monitoring Committees in Clinical Trials**
Jay Herson

**Design and Analysis of Animal Studies in Pharmaceutical Development**
Shein-Chung Chow and Jen-pei Liu

**Design and Analysis of Bioavailability and Bioequivalence Studies, Third Edition**
Shein-Chung Chow and Jen-pei Liu

**Design and Analysis of Bridging Studies**
Jen-pei Liu, Shein-Chung Chow, and Chin-Fu Hsiao

**Design & Analysis of Clinical Trials for Economic Evaluation & Reimbursement: An Applied Approach Using SAS & STATA**
Iftekhar Khan

**Design and Analysis of Clinical Trials for Predictive Medicine**
Shigeyuki Matsui, Marc Buyse, and Richard Simon

**Design and Analysis of Clinical Trials with Time-to-Event Endpoints**
Karl E. Peace

**Design and Analysis of Non-Inferiority Trials**
Mark D. Rothmann, Brian L. Wiens, and Ivan S. F. Chan

**Difference Equations with Public Health Applications**
Lemuel A. Moyé and Asha Seth Kapadia

**DNA Methylation Microarrays: Experimental Design and Statistical Analysis**
Sun-Chong Wang and Arturas Petronis

**DNA Microarrays and Related Genomics Techniques: Design, Analysis, and Interpretation of Experiments**
David B. Allison, Grier P. Page, T. Mark Beasley, and Jode W. Edwards

**Dose Finding by the Continual Reassessment Method**
Ying Kuen Cheung

Published Titles

**Dynamical Biostatistical Models**
Daniel Commenges and
Hélène Jacqmin-Gadda

**Elementary Bayesian Biostatistics**
Lemuel A. Moyé

**Emerging Non-Clinical Biostatistics in Biopharmaceutical Development and Manufacturing**
Harry Yang

**Empirical Likelihood Method in Survival Analysis**
Mai Zhou

**Essentials of a Successful Biostatistical Collaboration**
Arul Earnest

**Exposure–Response Modeling: Methods and Practical Implementation**
Jixian Wang

**Frailty Models in Survival Analysis**
Andreas Wienke

**Fundamental Concepts for New Clinical Trialists**
Scott Evans and Naitee Ting

**Generalized Linear Models: A Bayesian Perspective**
Dipak K. Dey, Sujit K. Ghosh, and
Bani K. Mallick

**Handbook of Regression and Modeling: Applications for the Clinical and Pharmaceutical Industries**
Daryl S. Paulson

**Inference Principles for Biostatisticians**
Ian C. Marschner

**Interval-Censored Time-to-Event Data: Methods and Applications**
Ding-Geng (Din) Chen, Jianguo Sun,
and Karl E. Peace

**Introductory Adaptive Trial Designs: A Practical Guide with R**
Mark Chang

**Joint Models for Longitudinal and Time-to-Event Data: With Applications in R**
Dimitris Rizopoulos

**Measures of Interobserver Agreement and Reliability, Second Edition**
Mohamed M. Shoukri

**Medical Biostatistics, Third Edition**
A. Indrayan

**Meta-Analysis in Medicine and Health Policy**
Dalene Stangl and Donald A. Berry

**Mixed Effects Models for the Population Approach: Models, Tasks, Methods and Tools**
Marc Lavielle

**Modeling to Inform Infectious Disease Control**
Niels G. Becker

**Modern Adaptive Randomized Clinical Trials: Statistical and Practical Aspects**
Oleksandr Sverdlov

**Monte Carlo Simulation for the Pharmaceutical Industry: Concepts, Algorithms, and Case Studies**
Mark Chang

**Multiregional Clinical Trials for Simultaneous Global New Drug Development**
Joshua Chen and Hui Quan

**Multiple Testing Problems in Pharmaceutical Statistics**
Alex Dmitrienko, Ajit C. Tamhane,
and Frank Bretz

**Noninferiority Testing in Clinical Trials: Issues and Challenges**
Tie-Hua Ng

**Optimal Design for Nonlinear Response Models**
Valerii V. Fedorov and Sergei L. Leonov

**Patient-Reported Outcomes: Measurement, Implementation and Interpretation**
Joseph C. Cappelleri, Kelly H. Zou,
Andrew G. Bushmakin, Jose Ma. J. Alvir,
Demissie Alemayehu, and Tara Symonds

**Quantitative Evaluation of Safety in Drug Development: Design, Analysis and Reporting**
Qi Jiang and H. Amy Xia

**Quantitative Methods for Traditional Chinese Medicine Development**
Shein-Chung Chow

Published Titles

**Randomized Clinical Trials of Nonpharmacological Treatments**
Isabelle Boutron, Philippe Ravaud, and David Moher

**Randomized Phase II Cancer Clinical Trials**
Sin-Ho Jung

**Sample Size Calculations for Clustered and Longitudinal Outcomes in Clinical Research**
Chul Ahn, Moonseong Heo, and Song Zhang

**Sample Size Calculations in Clinical Research, Second Edition**
Shein-Chung Chow, Jun Shao, and Hansheng Wang

**Statistical Analysis of Human Growth and Development**
Yin Bun Cheung

**Statistical Design and Analysis of Clinical Trials: Principles and Methods**
Weichung Joe Shih and Joseph Aisner

**Statistical Design and Analysis of Stability Studies**
Shein-Chung Chow

**Statistical Evaluation of Diagnostic Performance: Topics in ROC Analysis**
Kelly H. Zou, Aiyi Liu, Andriy Bandos, Lucila Ohno-Machado, and Howard Rockette

**Statistical Methods for Clinical Trials**
Mark X. Norleans

**Statistical Methods for Drug Safety**
Robert D. Gibbons and Anup K. Amatya

**Statistical Methods for Healthcare Performance Monitoring**
Alex Bottle and Paul Aylin

**Statistical Methods for Immunogenicity Assessment**
Harry Yang, Jianchun Zhang, Binbing Yu, and Wei Zhao

**Statistical Methods in Drug Combination Studies**
Wei Zhao and Harry Yang

**Statistical Testing Strategies in the Health Sciences**
Albert Vexler, Alan D. Hutson, and Xiwei Chen

**Statistics in Drug Research: Methodologies and Recent Developments**
Shein-Chung Chow and Jun Shao

**Statistics in the Pharmaceutical Industry, Third Edition**
Ralph Buncher and Jia-Yeong Tsay

**Survival Analysis in Medicine and Genetics**
Jialiang Li and Shuangge Ma

**Theory of Drug Development**
Eric B. Holmgren

**Translational Medicine: Strategies and Statistical Methods**
Dennis Cosmatos and Shein-Chung Chow

Chapman & Hall/CRC Biostatistics Series

# Biosimilar Clinical Development

## Scientific Considerations and New Methodologies


Edited by

**Kerry B. Barker**
Pfizer, Cambridge, Massachusetts, USA

**Sandeep M. Menon**
Pfizer, Cambridge, Massachusetts, USA

**Ralph B. D'Agostino, Sr.**
Boston University, Massachusetts, USA

**Siyan Xu**
Novartis, Cambridge, Massachusetts, USA

**Bo Jin**
Pfizer, Cambridge, Massachusetts, USA



CRC Press
Taylor & Francis Group
Boca Raton London New York

CRC Press is an imprint of the
Taylor & Francis Group, an **informa** business
A CHAPMAN & HALL BOOK

CRC Press
Taylor & Francis Group
6000 Broken Sound Parkway NW, Suite 300
Boca Raton, FL 33487-2742



Printed and bound in India by Replika Press Pvt. Ltd.

Printed on acid-free paper
Version Date: 20161019

International Standard Book Number-13: 978-1-4822-3169-4 (Hardback)



**Library of Congress Cataloging-in-Publication Data**

Names: Barker, Kerry B., editor.
Title: Biosimilar clinical development : scientific considerations and new methodologies / editors, Kerry B. Barker [and four others].
Description: Boca Raton : Taylor & Francis, 2017. | Series: Chapman & Hall/CRC biostatistics series
Identifiers: LCCN 2016026606 | ISBN 9781482231694 (hardpack)
Subjects: LCSH: Biologicals. | Drug development--Methodology.
Classification: LCC RS162 .B5612 2017 | DDC 615.1/9--dc23
LC record available at https://lccn.loc.gov/2016026606

**Visit the Taylor & Francis Web site at**
**http://www.taylorandfrancis.com**

**and the CRC Press Web site at**
**http://www.crcpress.com**

# Contents

# Preface

This book is a handbook for clinical developers working on biosimilars. It presents state-of-the-art scientific considerations and new methodologies in biosimilar clinical development. It also provides open research problems, questions, and considerations in the area of clinical sciences, statistics, and regulatory sciences.

Biological drug development is on an upward trajectory and a rapidly growing segment in the pharmaceutical industry. On the one hand, biological products have delivered exceptional clinical results, but on the other hand they have introduced high costs to patients and the health care system in the past decade. As a number of top-selling biologic brands are on the verge of losing product patent protection over the next few years, the demand for development and marketing of biosimilars has grown exponentially worldwide. The regulatory, clinical, and statistical research has attracted much attention to the literature in the past few years, and numerous regulatory guidance and scientific papers have been published on biosimilar clinical development. However, very few books are devoted solely to the scientific considerations and methodologies in biosimilar clinical development and this book is designed and constructed to fill this void.

Chapter 1 presents an overview of the development of biosimilars. The evolution of legal and regulatory requirements on the development of biosimilars is presented in this chapter. The differences in the developmental requirements for generic, biosimilar, and innovator products are illustrated. The stepwise approach to demonstrate biosimilarity and assessment of biosimilarity based on totality of the evidence are summarized. General scientific considerations for biosimilar clinical development are also discussed.

Following Chapter 1, the book presents a number of important scientific considerations on biosimilar clinical development, and also describes some new methodologies for design and analysis of biosimilar clinical trials. Chapter 2 illustrates the scientific considerations for the discovery of therapeutic targets and biomarkers, a topic that is rarely detailed in biosimilar literature. Clinical trials are usually tested on pre-defined therapeutic targets and biomarkers, without disclosing much on how they are identified. This chapter provides a thorough introduction to the discovery of therapeutic targets and biomarkers using a systems biology approach. It includes "omics" technology, molecular pathway, regulatory network, multiomics data, and modeling strategies.

Chapter 3 describes the development of immunogenic response toward biologics and the strategies to reduce immunogenicity. Immunogenicity to biologics represents a major reason for treatment discontinuation. Biologic drugs, including biosimilars, have the potential to elicit an immunogenic response, which are generally assessed by measuring antidrug antibodies (ADA). This chapter reveals the mechanism of ADA generation, the impact of ADA on the safety/efficacy profile of a drug, the factors that influence the immunogenicity, and the ways to measure immunogenicity of biosimilars.

Chapter 4 discusses the topic of interchangeability. Biosimilarity does not automatically imply interchangeability. For a biosimilar to be considered interchangeable with a reference product, it has to be shown by sponsors and approved by health regulatory authorities that the biosimilar produces the same clinical result as the reference product in any given patient, and repeated switching or alternating between the biosimilar and the reference product presents no greater safety or efficacy risk than continued use of the reference product. While these requirements for interchangeability have been made clear by the Biologics Price Competition and Innovation Act (BPCIA) of 2009, there remain many challenging and unsolved problems on how to demonstrate interchangeability in a scientific, clinically meaningful, and practically feasible way. This chapter presents scientific considerations and new methodologies to evaluate interchangeability between a biosimilar and its corresponding reference product. Specifically, clinical trial study designs and statistical analyses on interchangeability as well as interchangeability among several biosimilars and their reference products and its impact on drug pharmacovigilance are discussed.

Chapter 5 builds a framework of metrics to measure similarity. Biosimilar interchangeability with a reference product requires "similar" or "highly similar" characteristics. But unfortunately, it is still quite challenging to answer questions of "what is highly similar?" and "how to measure the similarity?" The difficulties, which result from manufacturing complexity and large variability of biologics, are well-recognized by the scientific community. This chapter introduces two scientific principles that can be used to establish the threshold for similarity in each metric. The first principle is that a biosimilarity criterion should be determined in a way that it allows the reference product to claim similarity to itself with a high probability. And the second is that all commercial lots of the reference product should meet a pre-set lot-consistency criterion with a high probability. Following the proposed metrics and established thresholds, the corresponding statistical approaches are described.

Many new statistical methods and their applications in biosimilar clinical trials have been covered in this book in the succeeding chapters (Chapters 6 through 11).

Chapter 6 will discuss six frequentist analysis strategies when accounting for covariate effects to demonstrate noninferiority in biosimilar clinical trials, including fixed margin (FM) method; synthesis (Syn) method; modified covariate adjustment fixed margin (CovFM) method; modified covariate-adjustment, synthesis method (CovSyn); two-stage covariate-adjustment fixed margin (2sFM) method; and two-stage covariate-adjustment synthesis

(2sSyn) method. Statistical operating characteristics among these six methods are compared.

Chapter 7 presents a novel method in inference of equivalence. A likelihood approach is proposed that retains the unspecified variances in the model and partitions the likelihood function into two components: F-statistic function for variances and t-statistic function for the ratio of two means. By incorporating unspecified variances, the proposed method can help identify numeric range of variances, where equivalence is more likely to be achieved, which cannot be accomplished by traditional analysis methods.

Chapter 8 discusses two multiplicity adjustment strategies in testing for bio-equivalence (BE) including a closed-test procedure that controls family-wise error rate (FWER) by treating the two metrics as a co-primary endpoint problem, and an alpha-adaptive sequential testing (AAST) that controls FWER by pre-specifying the significance level ($\alpha_1$) on area under the concentration–time curve (AUC) and obtaining it for $C_{max}$ ($\alpha_2$) adaptively after testing of AUC.

Chapter 10 discusses three major issues with the current practice of margin specifications: the subjectivity in the process of determining the margin, the data variability not considered or only implicitly expressed, and the concern of bio-creep controversy. An average inferiority measure (AIM) is introduced as a tool for specification of margins to address these issues and the standardized margins derived from AIM reflect naturally the variability of data. The applications of AIM are presented for the normal, binary, and the survival data.

Both Chapters 9 and 11 illustrate application of Bayesian methods in biosimilar clinical trials. Chapter 9 provides two case studies to demonstrate application of the Bayesian paradigm. The first case study is the application onto an interim analysis (IA) of a pharmokinetic (PK) similarity trial to determine probability of success. The second case is the application of deriving an equivalence margin to demonstrate equivalence in the efficacy of a biosimilar versus its reference product for the treatment of rheumatoid arthritis disease.

Chapter 11 presents a framework of the design and analysis of biosimilar clinical trials using Bayesian methods. Bayesian approach, appropriate for any scientific investigation as an iterative process of integrating and accumulating information, is a natural alternative to the classical approach for investigating biosimilars where comparisons are made against products that have already been licensed, thus presenting the current investigation with a wealth of historical data. In such settings, investigators can assess the current state of knowledge regarding the risk and benefit of an investigational product, gather new data from additional trials to address remaining questions, and then update and refine their hypotheses to incorporate both new and historical data. Both fully Bayesian approach and hybrid Bayesian approaches are described. The advantages and disadvantages of both approaches are discussed as well.

We are very grateful to all the contributors to this book, including Claudio Carini, Candida Fratazzi, Steven Ye Hua, Mani Lakshminarayanan, Gang Li, Jianjun (David) Li, Shujie Li, Shan Mei Liao, Ronald G. Menton, Fanni Natanegara, Attila A. Seyhan, Weichung Joe Shih, and Jin Xu. Special thanks also go to our executive editor, John Kimmel, project manager, Balasubramanian Shanmugam, and project editor, Iris Fahrer, for their patience and assistance with the publication of the book.

**Kerry B. Barker**
**Sandeep M. Menon**
**Ralph B. D'Agostino**
**Siyan Xu**
**Bo Jin**

# *Editors*

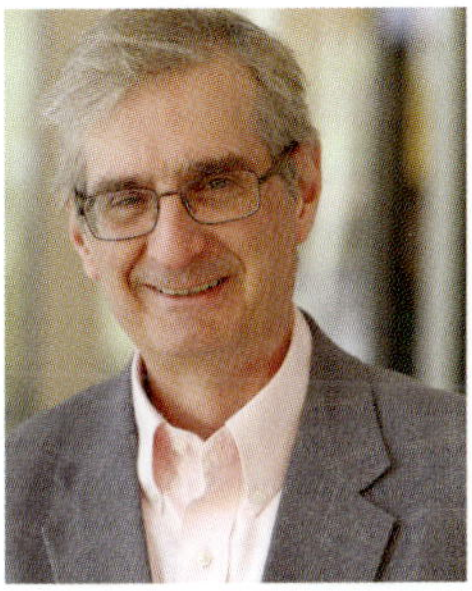

**Kerry B. Barker, PhD**, is currently the vice president of the statistics group in Early Oncology Development and Clinical Research at Pfizer Inc. He earned his doctoral degree in statistics from the University of Kentucky. From 2010 to 2015, he led the entire statistical clinical program for all biosimilars at Pfizer. He led the effort to design and analyze the phase I and phase III programs for both oncological biosimilars and inflammatory biosimilars. He interacted extensively with all regulatory agencies throughout the world, including the U.S. Food and Drug Administration (FDA), Committee for Medicinal Products for Human Use (CHMP), and Pharmaceuticals and Medical Devices Agency (PMDA). He has given talks on biosimilars at statistical meetings and Drug Information Association (DIA), as well as coauthoring papers on biosimilars, often with others contributing to the book. Overall, Dr. Barker has spent more than 28 years working in pharmaceutical and medical device companies. He has designed and analyzed clinical studies for over 24 approved drugs. He was the head of the Corporate R&D Statistical group at Baxter for 6 years. While at Baxter, he supported manufacturing; chemistry, manufacturing, and controls (CMC); medication delivery; and clinical trials. He spent most of his career in research and development but did work 2 years in marketing and 1 year as a clinical project team leader. He has worked in all phases of development in wide range of therapeutic areas including oncology, cardiovascular system, gastrointestinal (GI), vaccines, and dermatology.

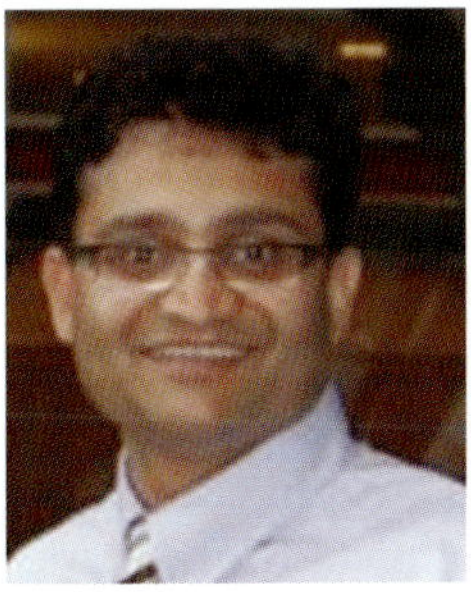

**Sandeep M. Menon, PhD**, is currently the vice president and head of Statistical Research and Consulting Center at Pfizer Inc. and also holds adjunct faculty positions at Boston University and Tufts University School of Medicine. His group, located at different Pfizer sites globally, provides scientific and statistical leadership and provides consultation to the Global Head of Statistics, senior Pfizer management in Discovery, Clinical Development, Legal, Commercial, and Marketing. His responsibilities also include providing a strong presence for Pfizer in regulatory and professional circles to influence content of regulatory guidelines and their interpretation in practice. Previously, he held positions of increased responsibility and leadership where he was in charge of all the biostatistics activities for the entire portfolio in his unit, spanning from discovery (target) through proof-of-concept studies for supporting immunology and autoimmune disease, inflammation and remodeling, rare diseases, cardiovascular and metabolism, and center of therapeutic innovation. He was responsible for overseeing biostatistical aspects of more than 40 clinical trials, over 25 compounds, and 20 indications. He is a core member of the Pfizer Global Clinical Triad (Biostatistics, Clinical, and Clinical Pharmacology) Leadership team. He has been in the industry for over a decade and prior to joining Pfizer he worked at Biogen Idec and Aptiv Solutions. Dr. Menon is passionate about teaching and has been teaching part-time over a decade. He has taught introductory, intermediate, and advanced courses in biostatistics including adaptive designs in clinical trials. He has taught short courses internationally and is a regular invited speaker and panelist in academic, U.S. Food and Drug Administration (FDA)/industry forums and business management schools. His research interests are in adaptive designs and personalized medicine. He has several publications in top-tier journals and recently coauthored and coedited books titled *Clinical and Statistical Considerations in Personalized Medicine* and *Modern Approaches to Clinical Trials Using SAS: Classical, Adaptive, and Bayesian Methods*. He is an active member of the Biopharmaceutical Section of the American Statistical Association (ASA), serving as an associate editor of ASA journal—*Statistics in Biopharmaceutical Research* (SBR)—and as a core member of the ASA Samuel S. Wilks Memorial Medal Committee. He is the vice-chair of the cross-industry Drug Information Association (DIA)-sponsored Adaptive Design Scientific Working Group (ADSWG), member of biomarker identification sub team formed under the currently existing multiplicity working group sponsored by the Society for Clinical trials and an invited program committee member at Biopharmaceutical Applied Statistics Symposium (BASS). He is on the editorial board for *Journal of Medical Statistics and Informatics* and on the advisory board for the MS in Biostatistics program at Boston University. Sandeep earned his medical degree from the University of Bangalore (formerly Karnataka University), India, and later completed his master's and doctoral degrees in biostatistics at Boston University and was a research fellow at Harvard Clinical Research Institute. He has received several awards for academic and research excellence.

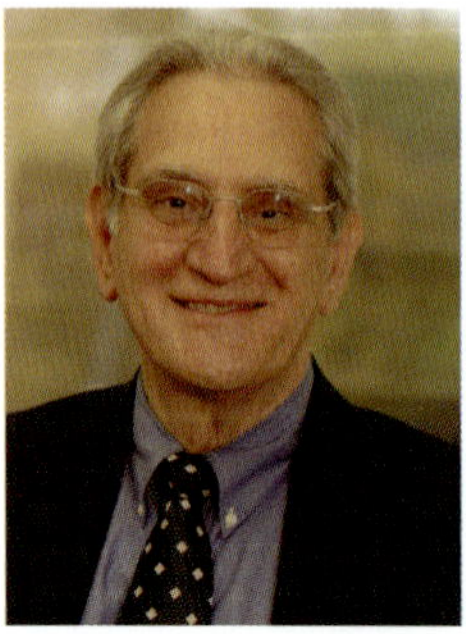

**Ralph B. D'Agostino, Sr., PhD**, serves as a professor of Mathematics/Statistics, Biostatistics and Epidemiology at Boston University. He earned his postdoctoral degree in 1968 from Harvard University. His major fields of research are clinical trials, epidemiology, prognostics models, longitudinal analysis, multivariate analysis, robustness, and outcomes/effectiveness research. Thomson Reuters announced that he is in the top 1% of the Most Cited Authors in Clinical Medicine (2014) and in World's Most

Influential Minds in Clinical Medicine (2015). He has extensive experience since the 1980s in developing cardiovascular risk prediction models, which have been used in Treatment Guidelines sponsored by the National Institutes of Health (NIH) and American Heart Association, and web-based models for general consumer use. He is a fellow of the American Statistical Association and the American Heart Association. Dr. D'Agostino has been with the Framingham Heart Study since 1981 and was co-principal investigator of the Core contract and director of Data Management and Statistical Analysis for the study for more than 30 years. He is also the director of the Statistics and Consulting Unit and the executive director of the MA/PhD Program in Biostatistics. He is a special government employee (SGE) of the U.S. Food and Drug Administration (FDA). He has been affiliated with the FDA's Center for Drugs Evaluation and Research (CDER) since 1974 as an expert consultant to the Biometrics Division, the Over-the-Counter Drugs Division, the Oncology Drugs Division, the Cardiovascular-Renal Drugs Division, and the Gastrointestinal Drugs Division. He is also a consultant to the Device Division. Further, he has served on a number of advisory committees and was the chair of the Nonprescription Drugs Advisory Committee (NDAC). He has twice been the recipient of the FDA's Commissioner's Special Citation (1981 and 1995). In December 2015, he served as an acting chair on the Psychopharmacologic Drugs Advisory Committee (PDAC). He has over 700 publications in peer-reviewed journals and is coauthor/editor of 10 books, including *Factor Analysis: An Applied Approach, Goodness-of-Fit Techniques, Mathematical Models in Health Services Research, Practical Engineering Statistics, Tutorials in Biostatistics* (two volumes), *Introductory Applied Biostatistics, Pharmaceutical Statistics Using SAS: A Practical Guide, Managing Cardiovascular Risk, Therapeutic Strategies in Cardiovascular Risk,* and *Missing Data in Clinical Trials.* Currently, Dr. D'Agostino is an editor of *Statistics in Medicine,* statistical consultant on the editorial board of the *New England Journal of Medicine,* and statistical consultant on the editorial board of *Current Therapeutic Research.* He is also an editor of the *Wiley Encyclopedia of Clinical Trials* and an associate editor of the *Encyclopedia of Biostatistics.* He has served on the editorial boards of the *American Statistician, Journal of the American Statistical Association, Biostatistica,* and *Health Services and Outcomes Research Methodology.*

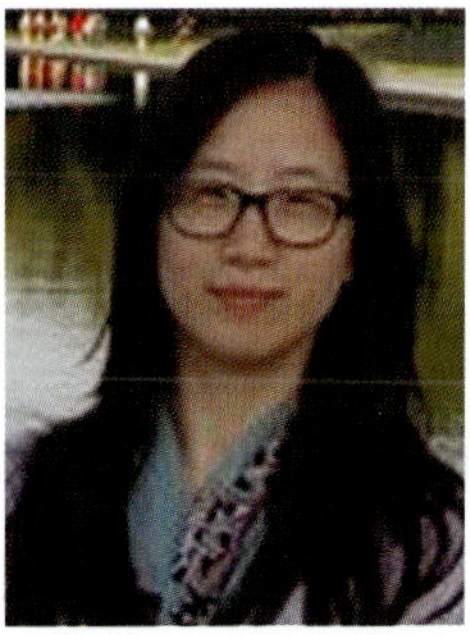

**Siyan Xu, PhD,** is a senior principal biostatistician at Novartis Pharmaceuticals, Oncology Business Unit. She earned her postdoctoral degree from Boston University in 2013. Before joining Novartis, she participated in a Pfizer research project in biosimilars. She is an outstanding researcher in the field of biostatistics. Her research interests include but not limited to multiplicity, noninferiority, bioequivalence, and dose finding in clinical trials. She has served as a critical member for a number of clinical trial teams for compounds including Zykadia and ribociclib. Currently Dr. Xu holds a lead statistician role with a number of project teams performing exposure–response analyses to enable dose and regimen selection for compounds in early stages of clinical development, and contributes to drug development in lymphoma, solid tumor, hematological tumor, multiple myeloma, and immune oncology. She has demonstrated strong competencies in using creative statistical methods to solve practical problems in clinical trials. She has been the leader to create a wiki platform, which is a user-friendly, easy-to-read access programming code warehouse. She codeveloped a novel methodology to incorporate exposure into dose selection in real time and is currently trying to implement first in human oncology trials. She is a core member in developing a Shiny Application and R package for various dose–exposure–response models. She has been a leading author of several methodology papers published in top international scientific journals. The noninferiority methodology has been endorsed by U.S. Food and Drug Administration (FDA), European regulatory agencies, and Japanese regulatory agencies, and is directly applicable in biosimilar studies at Pfizer, Inc. The publications on bioequivalence and equivalence is highly impactful to the clinical trial design and marketing of the product. It potentially minimizes the number of patients exposed to experimental treatment and reduces the cost of drug development. In addition, she participated in the Framingham Heart Study and contributed in identifying novel atrial fibrillation loci, as well as having been a statistical consultant in various projects in hip arthroscopy. She has been an invited speaker in national and internal conferences and an invited reviewer for several scholarly journals.

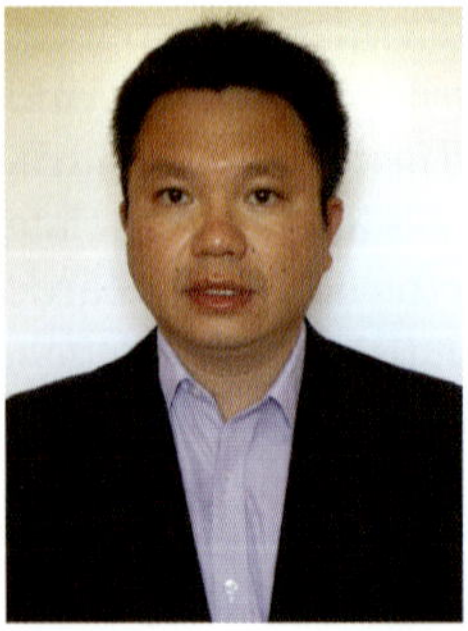

**Bo Jin, PhD**, is currently a director of biostatistics at the Department of Early Oncology Development and Clinical Research in Pfizer Inc. He earned his doctoral degree in statistics from Virginia Tech in 2004. He worked as a biostatistician at Merck & Co. from 2004 to 2010 and has been with Pfizer since 2010. His research focuses on design and analysis of noninferiority and equivalence clinical trials, and applications of statistical modeling and simulation in clinical trials. Dr. Jin has authored/coauthored more than 20 articles in in peer-reviewed scientific journals in both medical and statistical research areas and also has made many presentations at international conferences.

# *Contributors*

**Kerry B. Barker**
Pfizer Inc.
Cambridge, Massachusetts

**Claudio Carini**
Pfizer Inc.
Cambridge, Massachusetts

**Ralph B. D'Agostino, Sr.**
Epidemiology and Biostatistics
Boston University
Boston, Massachusetts

**Candida Fratazzi**
Boston Biotech Clinical Research
Cambridge, Massachusetts

**Steven Ye Hua**
Pfizer Worldwide Research—
Clinical Biostatistics
San Diego, California

**Bo Jin**
Pfizer Inc.
Cambridge, Massachusetts

**Mani Lakshminarayanan**
Pfizer Inc.
Collegeville, Pennsylvania

**Gang Li**
Statistics & Decision Sciences
Janssen R&D US
Titusville, New Jersey

**Jianjun (David) Li**
GPD Statistics
Pfizer Inc.
Collegeville, Pennsylvania

**Shujie Li**
Pfizer (China) Research &
Development Center
Shanghai, PR China

**Shan Mei Liao**
Pfizer (China) Research &
Development Center
Shanghai, China

**Sandeep M. Menon**
Pfizer Inc.
Cambridge, Massachusetts
Boston University
Boston, Massachusetts
Tufts University
Boston, Massachusetts

**Ronald Menton**
Novartis Institutes for Biomedical
Research
Cambridge, Massachusetts

**Fanni Natanegara**
Eli Lilly and Company
Indianapolis, Indiana

**Weichung Joe Shih**
Department of Biostatistics
Rutgers School of Public Health
Rutgers University
Piscataway, New Jersey

**Attila A. Seyhan**
Translational Research Institute for Metabolism and Diabetes
Florida Hospital
Orlando, Florida

and

MIT Research Affiliate
Department of Chemical Engineering
Massachusetts Institute of Technology
Cambridge, Massachusetts

**Jin Xu**
BARDS
Merck Research Labs
North Wales, Pennsylvania

**Siyan Xu**
Novartis Institutes for Biomedical Research
Cambridge, Massachusetts

# 1

# *Biosimilars for Drug Development: The Time Is Now!*

**Bo Jin, Sandeep M. Menon, Kerry B. Barker, and Ralph B. D'Agostino**

**CONTENTS**

**ABSTRACT** Biological drugs have taken a fast-growing segment in the pharmaceutical industry. At the same time, a number of top-selling biologic brands are attributable to lose product patent protection over the next few years, opening a wealth of opportunities for the development of biosimilar products. In fact, legal and regulatory pathways have been established in the past decade in many countries throughout the world, which allow the development of biosimilar products for the global market. This chapter presents an overview of the development of biosimilar products. Among others, the evolution of legal and regulatory requirements on the development of biosimilar products is presented in this chapter. The differences among the development requirements for generic, biosimilar, and innovator products are illustrated. The stepwise approach to demonstrate biosimilarity and assessment of biosimilarity based on totality of the evidence are described. General scientific considerations in the clinical program for a biosimilar development are discussed in detail. At the end of this chapter, an overview of the topics to be covered by this book is provided.

## 1.1 Background

With the rapid development of modern biological technology, biologic drug products have played more and more import roles in treating many life-threatening and chronic diseases. Consequently, biologic drugs are a fast-growing segment in the pharmaceutical industry. A report by Visiongain predicts that the world market for biologic drugs will reach US$270 billion in 2019 [1]. At the same time, a number of top-selling biologic brands in various therapeutic areas such as oncology, rheumatoid arthritis, and diabetes is attributable to lose product patent protection over the next few years, opening a wealth of opportunities for biosimilar players. IMS Health estimates that US$67 billion in global sales will be off-patent by 2019.

In the past decade, legal and regulatory pathways have been established in many countries throughout the world, which allow development of biosimilar products for the global market. The European Union (EU) is the first region in the world to have set a legal framework and a regulatory pathway for biosimilars. The "concept of similar biological medicinal product" was adopted in the EU legislation in 2004 and came into effect in 2005 (Directive 2001/83/EC, as amended by Directive 2003/63/EC and Directive 2004/27/EC) (European Commission, 2001). Thereafter, European Medicines Agency (EMA) has developed overarching and product-specific scientific guidelines providing a robust regulatory process in which to be able to grant marketing authorization for biosimilar medicinal products. These guidelines, both overarching and product specific, are revised on a regular basis to reflect the experience gained with biosimilar applications and approvals and to take into account evolving science and technology. The most recent revisions in 2014 on three overall guidelines: the overarching guideline [2], quality issues guideline [3], and nonclinical and clinical issues guidelines [4] outlined the general principles on biosimilar development, introduced the possibility of using a non-EU reference product throughout the comparability program, and addressed some issues for biosimilars on the extrapolation of efficacy and safety from one therapeutic indication to other.

Many other regions and/or countries have followed and adopted the EU standard. The Japanese Ministry of Health, Labor, and Welfare (MHLW) published a guideline for quality, safety, and efficacy of biosimilars in 2009 [5], which followed the similarity concept outlined by the EMA. Other regulators, including some Asian countries or regions such as South Korea, Malaysia, Singapore, Taiwan, and Sir Lanka, have also followed and developed local guidelines to reflect the EMA guidelines. The World Health Organization (WHO) published guidelines on biosimilar [6] in 2009, which share much common ground with the EU guidelines in terms of the requirements for proven similarity, clinical immunogenicity, indication extrapolation, risk management, and pharmacovigilance plan. The Canadian guidelines issued by the federal regulatory authority Health Canada (Guidance for Sponsors: Information and Submission Requirements for Subsequent Entry Biologics (SEBs); Health Canada, 2010) [7] shares comparable concepts and principles of both the EMA and WHO guidelines. The emerging markets such as Brazil, Russia, China, and India largely recognize the WHO biosimilars guidelines although they have some country-specific requirements.

The legislative route for biosimilars in the United States started with the enacted health care reform law, the Patient Protection and Affordable Care Act (PPAC Act) (2010), which was signed into law in March 2010. Among others, the PPAC Act amends the Public Health Service (PHS) Act to create an abbreviated approval pathway for biological products that are demonstrated to be "highly similar" (biosimilar) to or "interchangeable" with a

Food and Drug Administration (FDA)-approved biological product. These statutory provisions are also referred to as the Biologics Price Competition and Innovation Act of 2009 (BPCI Act) (Title VII, 2010) [8]. After a few years following the BPCI Act, FDA have developed several guidance for the pharmaceutical industry on the submissions of biosimilar product applications. Most recently, the FDA guidance in 2015 on scientific considerations in demonstrating biosimilarity to a reference product [9] recommends that sponsors use a stepwise approach in their development of biosimilar products and indicates that FDA considers the totality of the evidence provided by a sponsor to support a demonstration of biosimilarity. General scientific principles are discussed in the guidance on conducting comparative structural and functional analysis, animal testing, human pharmacokinetic (PK) and pharmacodynamic (PD) studies, clinical immunogenicity assessment, and clinical safety and effectiveness studies. The other FDA guidance in 2015 on quality considerations [10] provides some recommendations on the scientific and technical information of the chemistry, manufacturing, and controls (CMC) section of a marketing applicant for a proposed biosimilar product. The FDA 2014 draft guidance on clinical pharmacology data to support a demonstration of biosimilarity to a reference product [11] discusses some concepts related to clinical pharmacology testing for biosimilar products, the approaches for developing the appropriate clinical pharmacology database, and the utility of modeling and simulation for designing clinical trials.

## 1.2 Definitions of Biosimilar

According to the EMA guidelines [2], biosimilar is a biological medicinal product that contains a version of the active substance of an already authorized original biological medicinal product (reference medicinal product) in European Economic Area (EEA). Similarity to the reference medicinal product in terms of quality characteristics, biological activity, safety, and efficacy based on a comprehensive comparability exercise needs to be established. The U.S. FDA guidance [9] defines a biosimilar as the biological product that is highly similar to the reference product notwithstanding minor differences in clinically inactive components, and that there are no clinically meaningful differences between the biological product and the reference product in terms of the safety, purity, and potency.

Biosimilar products are also referred to as follow-on biologics (FOBs) by the U.S. FDA, similar biotherapeutic products (SBPs) by WHO, and SEBs by Health Canada. WHO defines SBP as a biotherapeutic product, which is similar in terms of quality, safety, and efficacy to an already licensed reference biotherapeutic product [6]. Health Canada defines SEB as a biological drug that enters the market subsequent to a version previously authorized in Canada and with demonstrated similarity to a reference biologic drug [7]. Table 1.1 presents various definitions of biosimilar products. Although the definitions vary by different regulatory agencies, there are three necessary conditions to be met to be considered a biosimilar: (1) the biosimilar is a biological product, (2) the reference is already licensed at a certain country/region, and (3) the biosimilar has demonstrated similarity in terms of quality, safety, and efficacy to the reference product.

**TABLE 1.1**

Definitions of Biosimilar

| Term | Regulatory Agency | Definition |
|---|---|---|
| Biosimilar | EMA | A biological medicinal product that contains a version of the active substance of an already authorized original biological medicinal product (reference medicinal product) by the EEA. Similarity to the reference medicinal product in terms of quality characteristics, biological activity, safety, and efficacy based on a comprehensive comparability exercise needs to be established. |
| Biosimilar/FOB | FDA | A biological product that is highly similar to the reference product notwithstanding minor differences in clinically inactive components. There are no clinically meaningful differences between the biological product and the reference product in terms of the safety, purity, and potency. |
| SBP | WHO | A biotherapeutic product, which is similar in terms of quality, safety, and efficacy to an already licensed reference biotherapeutic product. |
| SEB | Canada | A biological drug that enters the market subsequent to a version previously authorized in Canada and with demonstrated similarity to a reference biologic drug. |
| FOB | Japan | A biotechnological drug product developed to be comparable in regard to quality, safety, and efficacy to an already approved biotechnology-derived product of a different company. |
| Biosimilar | Korean | A biological product that demonstrated its equivalence to an already approved reference product with regard to quality, safety, and efficacy [12]. |
| Biosimilar | South Africa | A biological medicine that is manufactured to be similar to registered originator medicines. An appropriate comparability exercise is required to demonstrate that whether the biosimilar and the reference medicinal products have similar profiles in terms of physicochemical properties, quality, safety, and efficacy [13]. |

*Notes:* EEA, European Economic Area; EMA, European Medicines Agency; FDA, Food and Drug Administration; FOB, follow-on biologic; SBP, similar biotherapeutic product; SEB, subsequent entry biologic; WHO, World Health Organization.

## 1.3 Different Development Requirements for Generic, Biosimilar, and Innovator Products

The development pathways for innovator, generic, and biosimilar products have some fundamental differences. An innovator (brand name) product, before its approval by regulatory agencies onto market, needs to go through stand-alone comprehensive quality, preclinical, and clinical exercise. In clinical stage, all-phase (Phase I to Phase IV) clinical trials are usually necessary.

When an innovator small-molecule product's patent expires, pharmaceutical companies may file an abbreviated new drug application for the approval of the generic copies of the innovator drug product. Although the generic drug still needs to address its own quality issues, for clinical exercise worldwide, regulatory agencies have established one-size-fits-all criterion for the approval of generic drug products, which requires the evidence of average bioavailability to be provided through the conduction of a bioequivalence (BE) study. For small-molecule drug products, the assessment of BE serves as a surrogate for the evaluation of drug safety and effectiveness, which is based on the assumption that if the generic product and the reference are shown to be bioequivalent in average bioavailability, they will have the same therapeutic effect and hence can be used interchangeably.

Unlike small molecular drugs with clearly and well-defined composition and structure (e.g., a statin weighs about 400 Da), biological compounds are derived from living cells, often through recombinant DNA technology; are significantly larger (e.g., 5,000–300,000 Da); are complex structures; present challenges to characterize with existing scientific methods; and are difficult to reproduce. Furthermore, biological compounds have stronger immunogenic properties than small-molecule drugs, potentially leaving patients irreparably harmed by an adverse immune response. Consequently, there is general consensus that the assessment methodology of BE for small molecules is not appropriate and sufficient for the assessment of biosimilarity. Table 1.2 provides a brief comparison on the development requirements for generic, biosimilar, and innovator products.

As shown in Table 1.2, the focuses of a biosimilar product differ from that of an innovator product. On the quality assessment, a biosimilar does not only need to have its own stand-alone program but also needs to have very comprehensive comparison with reference product. The quality assessment requirements are probably even higher for a biosimilar than those for an innovator product. On the other hand, the development for a biosimilar may not need a comprehensive preclinical assessment. Phase 2 dose finding studies are not needed for a biosimilar program, and Phase 3 study is usually in one representative indication. Figure 1.1 presents a closer comparison between the development of a biosimilar and that of an innovator product.

**TABLE 1.2**

Comparison on the Development Requirements for Generic, Biosimilar, and Innovator Products

| | Innovator | Generic | Biosimilar |
|---|---|---|---|
| Quality | Stand-alone program | Stand-alone program plus comparison with reference product | Stand-alone program plus very comprehensive comparison with reference product |
| Preclinical | Full preclinical program | Usually no data required | Usually abbreviated program, depending on complexity of molecule |
| Clinical | Full clinical program<br>• Phase 1<br>• Phase 2<br>• Phase 3 in all indications to be licensed<br>• Postapproval follow-up | • BE study<br>• No other clinical studies | • Phase I PK and PD studies<br>• No Phase 2 studies required<br>• Phase 3 study in one adequately sensitive indication<br>• Postapproval follow-up |

*Notes:* BE, bioequivalence; PD, pharmacodynamic; PK, pharmacokinetic.

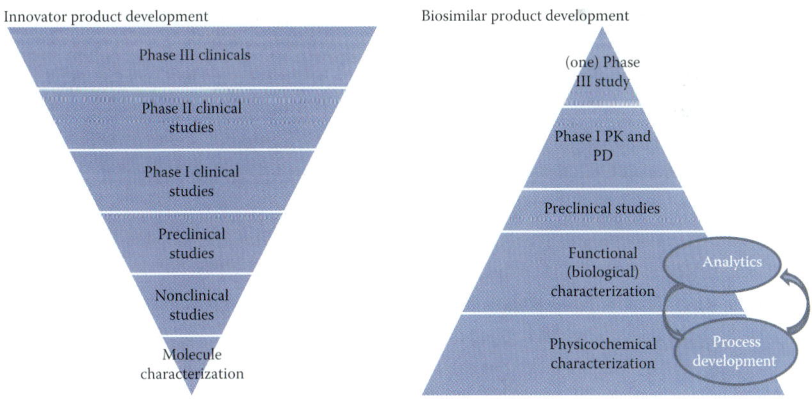


**FIGURE 1.1**
Comparison between the development of a biosimilar and that of an innovator product.

## 1.4 Stepwise Approach to Demonstrate Biosimilarity and Assessment of Biosimilarity Based on Totality of the Evidence

The objective of a biosimilar development program is not to independently establish the safety and effectiveness of the biosimilar. Instead, it is to establish similarity between the biosimilar and the reference product by the best possible means, ensuring that the previously proven safety and efficacy of the reference medicinal product also applies to the biosimilar. Following this objective, a stepwise approach is recommended by both EMA guidelines [3] and FDA guidance [9] for the development of any biosimilars. First, the sponsors should start with a comprehensive physicochemical and biological characterization of a biosimilar candidate. The extent and nature of the subsequent nonclinical *in vivo* studies and clinical studies to be performed depend on the level of evidence obtained in the previous step(s), including the robustness of the physicochemical, biological, and nonclinical *in vitro* data. In other words, the development program should remove residual uncertainties on biosimilarity step by step, with the ultimate goal of excluding any relevant differences between the biosimilar and the reference products.

FDA guidance also brings in the concept of totality of the evidence for the assessment of biosimilarity. That is, when reviewing an application package of a biosimilar by a sponsor, the FDA will consider the totality of the data and information submitted in the application package, including structural and functional characterization, nonclinical evaluation, human PK and PD data, clinical immunogenicity data, and comparative clinical study data. The FDA intends to use a risk-based approach to evaluate all available data and information submitted in support of the biosimilarity of the proposed product.

Clinical data may not be sufficient to justify substantial differences in quality attributes according to the concept of totality of the evidence. On the other hand, a sponsor may be able to demonstrate biosimilarity even though there are formulation or minor structural differences, provided that the sponsor provides sufficient data and information demonstrating that the differences are not relevant and clinically meaningful and the proposed product otherwise meets the statutory criteria for biosimilarity. For example, differences in certain posttranslational modifications or differences in certain excipients (e.g., human serum albumin) might not preclude a finding of biosimilarity if data and information provided by the sponsor show that the proposed product is highly similar to the reference product notwithstanding minor differences in clinically inactive components and that there are no clinically meaningful differences between the products in terms of safety, purity, and potency [9].

On March 6, 2015, the U.S. FDA approved Sandoz's Zarxio (filgrastim-sndz), the first biosimilar product approved in the United States. The FDA's approval of Zarxio is based on the review of evidence that included structural and functional characterization, animal study data, human PK and PD data, clinical immunogenicity data, and other clinical safety and effectiveness data that demonstrate Zarxio is biosimilar to Neupogen. The rationale (essentially totality of the evidence) of the approval of Zarxio was in line with the FDA's current thinking on key scientific and regulatory factors involved in submitting applications for biosimilar products, which are reflected in the FDA current guidance documents.

## 1.5 Nonclinical Program for a Biosimilar Development

Similarity comparison in terms of protein structure and the functional characterization of protein pharmacologic activity is the first step and serves as the foundation in the demonstration of biosimilarity. It is expected that the expression construct for a proposed product will encode the same primary amino acid sequence as its reference product. However, minor modifications such as N- or C-terminal truncations that are not expected to change the product performance may be justified. Other relevant characteristics of the protein products, such as the primary, secondary, tertiary, quaternary structure, posttranslational modifications, and biological activities, should also be considered and compared so as to demonstrate that the proposed product is highly similar to the reference product notwithstanding minor differences in clinically inactive components. In fact, the similarity exercise in comparative structural and functional characterization may also provide the scientific justification for a selective and targeted approach to subsequent animal and/or clinical studies to demonstrate biosimilarity. A nonclinical program for a biosimilar development is not the focus of this book. Readers may refer to the EMA guidelines and the FDA guidance on the detailed scientific considerations for analytical comparison in protein structure and the functional characterization of protein pharmacologic activity of *in vitro* and *in vivo* studies.

## 1.6 Clinical Program for a Biosimilar Development

Once the similarity in protein structure and the functional characterization of protein pharmacologic activity has been established between a biosimilar candidate and its reference product, the clinical program for the biosimilar will start. The objective of the clinical program is to demonstrate that there are no clinically meaningful differences between the proposed biosimilar and the reference product in terms of the safety, purity, and potency of the product. As mentioned in Sections 1.4 and 1.5, the nature and scope of the clinical program will depend on the nature and extent of residual uncertainty about biosimilarity after conducting structural and functional characterization and, where relevant, animal studies.

The clinical biosimilar comparability exercise also follows a stepwise procedure that starts with PK and, if feasible, PD studies, followed by a comparative clinical efficacy and safety trial. In the following context, we discuss some scientific considerations of the clinical program of a biosimilar development.

1. Pharmacokinetic and Pharmacodynamic Studies
2. Comparative Efficacy and Safety Studies

### 1.6.2 Comparative Efficacy and Safety Studies

As mentioned in Section 1.6.1.4, a comparative efficacy and safety study is necessary to support the demonstration of biosimilarity when there is residual uncertainty on any clinically meaningful differences between the proposed biosimilar and the reference product in previously conducted nonclinical studies and clinical studies. We discuss the scientific factors to consider in a comparative efficacy and safety study in Sections 1.6.2.1 through 1.6.2.8.

#### 1.6.2.1 Selection of Population and Dose

The choice of study population should allow for an assessment of clinically meaningful differences between the proposed biosimilar and the reference product. The population should be adequately sensitive to allow for the detection of the differences in PK and PD profiles. Usually the study population should be the same as that studied for the licensure of the reference product for the same indication. However, there are cases where a study population could be different from that in the clinical studies that supported the licensure of the reference product. For example, if the reference product has been applied in a certain patient population based on postapproval clinical trial results, although the population was not the one the drug originally licensed and the patient population may be more sensitive to detecting the differences between the proposed biosimilar and the reference product in terms of efficacy, safety, and/or immunogenicity, this population may be considered in the comparative efficacy and safety study. The dose studied in the comparative efficacy and safety study is usually the one in the licensure of the reference product for the same patient population.

#### 1.6.2.2 Study Endpoint and Similarity Assessment Metrics

A sponsor should use efficacy endpoint as the primary endpoint that can assess clinically meaningful differences between the proposed product and the reference product in a comparative clinical study, and the endpoint should be appropriately sensitive to detect the difference between the proposed biosimilar and the reference product. In some scenarios, the primary endpoint can be the same as the one that was used in the studies for the licensure of the reference product, e.g., ACR20 response rate or DAS28 change from baseline in the studies for patients with rheumatoid arthritis; in other scenarios such as in oncology trials, the primary endpoint in the comparative study is usually objective response rate (ORR), not the overall survival (OS) or progress-free survival (PFS). Although OS and/or PFS are commonly used in the studies for the licensure of the reference product, ORR is considered to be a more sensitive endpoint for the detection of the differences between the proposed biosimilar and the reference product, and thus is more appropriate to be the primary endpoint in the comparative study [3].

The similarity assessment metrics in the primary endpoint have two common options as well: the absolute difference in the primary endpoint between treatment groups, e.g., the ORR difference between the proposed biosimilar and the reference product, and the ratio in primary endpoint between treatment groups, e.g., the ORR ratio between the proposed biosimilar and the reference product. The metrics of ratio may be less affected by variability in the event rates in reference group that would occur in a future study, as an example provided in the FDA noninferiority (NI) guidance [15]. That being said, it seems to use ratio to assess similarity if there were relatively large variability in the treatment effect for the reference product. FDA NI guidance suggests that the selection of the metrics should be "based upon clinical interpretation, medical context, and previous experience with the behavior of the rates of the outcome." In fact, both metrics of difference and ratio have been seen in biosimilar comparative studies.

#### *1.6.2.3 Study Design: Equivalence versus Noninferiority*

In general, an equivalence design should be used in a comparative study. In the equivalence trial, the proposed biosimilar needs to be shown neither inferior to nor superior to the reference product. In some cases, an NI design may be considered. The EMA guidelines [3] suggest that the use of NI design should be "justified on the basis of a strong scientific rationale and taking into consideration the characteristics of the reference product, e.g. safety profile/tolerability, dose range, dose-response relationship." The FDA guidance [9] provides more specific rationales when an NI design may be considered. It says, "depending on the study population and endpoint(s), ruling out only inferiority may be adequate to establish that there are no clinically meaningful differences between the proposed product and the reference product. For example, if it is well established that doses of a reference product pharmacodynamically saturate the target at the clinical dose level and it would be unethical to use lower than clinically approved doses, an NI design may be sufficient."

The objective of the comparative study is always to rule out clinically meaningful differences between the proposed product and the reference product, regardless whether an equivalence trial or NI trial is used. When the possibility of significant and clinically relevant increase in efficacy can be excluded on scientific and mechanistic grounds, such as the scenarios that FDA guidance describes (saturated PD effect at the clinical dose level and it being unethical to use lower than the clinically approved dose), an NI design may be considered in the comparative study.

#### *1.6.2.4 Equivalence Hypothesis Test and Equivalence Margins*

To establish equivalence is to demonstrate both NI and nonsuperiority at the same time. Statistically, this objective is translated into the following hypothesis test:

Null hypothesis: $H_0$: $\mu \leq \theta_L$ or $\mu \geq \theta_U$ (the treatment difference is outside the equivalence margin),

Alternative hypothesis: $H_1$: $\theta_L < \mu < \theta_U$ (the treatment difference is within the margins),

where μ is the metrics to assess similarity in primary endpoint, which can be difference or ratio as we discussed in previous context, and $\theta_L$ and $\theta_U$ are equivalence margins ($\theta_L$ and $\theta_U$ may also be considered as NI and nonsuperiority margins, respectively). Note that this hypothesis test is equivalent to the simultaneous tests for two sets of hypotheses (NI test: $H_{a0}$: $\mu \leq \theta_L$ versus $H_{a1}$: $\mu > \theta_L$ and nonsuperiority test: $H_{b0}$ $\mu \geq \theta_U$ versus $H_{b1}$ $\mu < \theta_U$).

Typically symmetric equivalence margins are used in the comparative study, which means that $\theta_U = -\theta_L$ when the assessment metric is difference and $\log(\theta_U) = -\log(\theta_L)$ when the assessment metric is ratio. When the equivalence margins are symmetric, we may use the same rational as specified in the guidance for NI clinical trials [15] to determine the NI margin first and then nonsuperiority margin is determined automatically.

Symmetric margins would be reasonable when, for example, there are dose-related toxicities. If the dose used in the comparative study is near the plateau of the dose–response curve and there is little likelihood of dose-related toxicities, asymmetric equivalence margins could be considered with a larger upper bound to rule out superiority rather than lower bound to rule out inferiority [9]. Li et al. [16] proposed a trial design for the evaluation of biosimilarity, which involves an NI margin and an asymmetrical nonsuperiority margin. The use of asymmetric margins could lead to a smaller sample size than that would be needed with symmetric margins and thus increase the operational feasibility of the comparative study. On the other hand, if there is observed clear superiority in such design setup, an additional study data and further investigations may not be unavoidable before biosimilarity can be concluded [9].

#### *1.6.2.5 Statistical Analysis for Primary Endpoint*

The *two one-sided tests* (TOSTs) method is the simplest and most widely used approach to test equivalence. This is done using two simultaneous one-sided tests (NI and nonsuperiority) with type I error of α for each test [17,18]. Alternatively, the $(1 - 2\alpha) \times 100\%$ CI of μ is constructed, and the equivalence is established (the alternative hypothesis is favored) when the CI is contained completely within the range $(\theta_L, \theta_U)$.

There seems to be no consensus yet globally on what should be the type I error of α. WHO guidance [6] indicates that α may be considered to be 0.025.

There is no explicit statement of $\alpha$ in the EMA guidelines and the FDA guidance, while $\alpha = 0.05$ was used in FDA briefing document [19] to the advisory committee meeting for Sandoz's proposed biosimilar to Neupogen® (later approved as Zarxio in 2015).

Analysis population for the primary endpoint needs to be carefully considered as well. The intent-to-treat (ITT) population includes every subject who is randomized and does not remove patients with noncompliance, protocol deviations, withdrawal, or anything that happens after randomization from the analysis [20]. Although considered as a conservative analysis in the superiority trial setting and therefore appropriate for the primary analysis for primary endpoints, the ITT population is not conservative in equivalence and NI trials due to a tendency for biasing the results toward equivalence (or NI) [15]. On the other hand, the per-protocol (PP) population, which excludes data from patients with major protocol violations, can also bias results [20,21].

Sanchez and Chen [22], employing simulations in analyzing continuous outcome data, found that "... the conservatism or anticonservatism of the PP or ITT analysis depends on many factors, including the type of protocol deviation and missingness, the treatment trajectory (for longitudinal study) and the method of handling missing data in ITT population. The test for NI is usually anticonservative in the presence of noncompliance. An analysis based on the PP population is generally deficient in the presence of nontrivial missingness, such as dropout due to lack of efficacy, and leads to anticonservative results. The performance of ITT analysis is sensitive to the imputation method employed ... ."

The regulatory agencies currently require that NI and equivalence should be assessed in both populations. In fact, the CPMP Points to Consider [23] document states that "... In an NI trial, the full analysis set and the PP analysis set have equal importance and their use should lead to similar conclusions for a robust interpretation ...". And FDA NI guidance [15] states that "... It is therefore important to conduct both ITT and as-treated analyses in NI studies. Differences in results using the two analyses will need close examination...." Consequently, sponsors should monitor clinical trials closely to minimize attrition and noncompliance in the trial and expect that the ITT population and the PP population in this trial are close to each other and should also closely examine any differences (if they arise) between the results by the two populations.

#### *1.6.2.6 Sample Size and Duration of Study*

The size of a comparative study should have adequate statistical power for the equivalence hypothesis test on the primary efficacy endpoint. The sample size and duration of the comparative clinical study should also be adequate to allow for the detection of clinically meaningful differences between the two products in terms of safety and immunogenicity.

#### *1.6.2.7 Safety and Immunogenicity Data*

The comparative study is also to assess the similarity in the long-term safety and immunogenicity profiles between the proposed biosimilar and the reference product. Care should be given to compare the type, severity, and frequency of the adverse reactions between the biosimilar and the reference product, particularly on those specific safety issues that have been noticed for the reference product, as well as the possible safety concerns that may result from a manufacturing process different from that of the reference product, especially those related to infusion-related reactions and immunogenicity. The overall immunogenicity assessment should consider the nature of the immune response (e.g., anaphylaxis, neutralizing antibody [Nab], etc.), the clinical relevance (on both efficacy and safety) and severity of consequences (e.g., loss of efficacy and other adverse effects), the incidence of immune responses, etc.

#### *1.6.2.8 Meeting the Requirements by Different Regulatory Agencies*

Comparative studies are usually global clinical trials, and at the end the trial results may serve as pivotal study results in the submissions of the proposed biosimilars to various regulatory agencies. There is no global harmonized regulatory guidance on comparative studies for biosimilars yet, and different regulatory agencies may have different views on designs of comparative studies, such as patient population, primary endpoint, similarity assessment metrics, equivalence margins, and statistical analysis issues. It is important for sponsors to get agreement with all regulatory agencies on the study designs for the comparative studies. In case when there are different requirements for the same comparative studies, for example, different equivalence margins and/or different type I errors for different regulatory filings, the study protocols should specify the requirements agreed with different regulatory filings before the study is conducted.

## 1.7 Extrapolation from One Indication to Other Indications

Usually the comparative efficacy and safety study is conducted in only one indication that has been licensed for the reference product. However, when biosimilarity has been concluded at the end of the comparative efficacy study, sponsors may seek the approval for the proposed biosimilar in all the indications for the reference product, and justifications for the extrapolation of clinical data from one indication to other indications of the reference product become the key to that objective. It should be noted that by end of the comparative efficacy and safety study, it is expected that the safety and efficacy can be extrapolated when biosimilar comparability has been demonstrated by thorough physicochemical and structural analyses as well as by *in vitro* functional tests complemented with clinical data (efficacy and safety and/or PK/PD data) in one therapeutic indication [9].

As the FDA guidance [9] suggests, specific scientific factors to consider for extrapolation include:

1. The MOA(s) in each condition of use for which licensure is sought; this may include:
   a. The target/receptor(s) for each relevant activity/function of the product.
   b. The binding, dose/concentration response, and pattern of molecular signaling upon engagement of target/receptor(s).
   c. The relationships between product structure and target/receptor interactions.
   d. The location and expression of the target/receptor(s).
2. The PK and biodistribution of the product in different patient populations. (Relevant PD measures may also provide important information on the MOA.)
3. The immunogenicity of the product in different patient populations.
4. Differences in expected toxicities in each condition of use and patient population (including whether expected toxicities are related to the pharmacological activity of the product or to off-target activities).
5. Any other factor that may affect the safety or efficacy of the product in each condition of use and patient population for which licensure is sought.

If the conditions of use with respective to the factors as above are same or similar across indications, then the extrapolation of data across indications may be acceptable. Otherwise, additional data may be needed to justify indication extrapolations.

## 1.8 Postapproval Safety Monitoring

Preapproval clinical safety data of biosimilars are usually limited in that (1) usually there are clinical data in one tested patient population while there are no data for the biosimilar in other indications that the reference product may have been licensed; (2) the data and the duration of studies are usually insufficient to identify rare adverse effects. Therefore, clinical safety of biosimilars must be monitored closely on an ongoing basis during the postapproval phase including continued benefit–risk assessment.

EMA requires sponsors to have a risk management plan in accordance with current EU legislation and pharmacovigilance guidelines. And FDA also requires postapproval safety monitoring for biosimilars. Readers may refer to the EMA guidelines [3] and the FDA guidance [9] for the requirements of postapproval safety monitoring for biosimilars.

## 1.9 Topics in the Book

So far we have reviewed the concept of biosimilar, the overall regulatory requirements, nonclinical and clinical studies for biosimilar development, and general scientific considerations for the clinical studies for biosimilar development. In the following chapters of the book, we will present some topics on scientific considerations for biosimilar clinical development and some new methodologies that have been applied in biosimilar clinical development.

### 1.9.1 Systems Biology Approach for the Discovery of Therapeutic Targets and Biomarkers

The discovery of therapeutic targets and biomarkers plays an important role in both nonclinical and clinical studies for biologics and biosimilars. Chapter 2 will discuss systems biology as a holistic approach to obtain, integrate, and analyze complex datasets from multiple experimental sources using interdisciplinary tools and review examples of modeling strategies to build cellular models on the basis of detailed multiparametric datasets.

### 1.9.2 Understanding Immunogenicity to Biologics and Biosimilars

Chapter 3 will provide an in-depth understanding of the cellular and molecular mechanism sustaining the immunogenic response that will likely ameliorate the safety profile of biologics/biosimilars. The chapter will address the mechanistic basis of ADA generation to biologics/biosimilars, the importance of patient populations in generating an immunogenic response, the impact of ADA and Nab on the safety profile of a drug, and the importance of pursuing the appropriate assays to measure immunogenicity in patients treated with biologics and biosimilars and the potential differences between reference products and biosimilars. Of course, the ultimate goal will be the identification of specific factors that influence the immunogenic response and consequently, the management of immunogenicity to biologics and biosimilars.

### 1.9.3 Interchangeability

Chapter 4 will discuss the interchangeability of biosimilars. Interchangeability needs to be shown through comparability clinical studies by sponsors. The definitions of the two aspects of interchangeability, switching and alternating, will be presented in the chapter. The chapter will also discuss study designs and statistical analysis on interchangeability, as well as interchangeability among several biosimilars and their reference products, and the interchangeability impact on drug pharmacovigilance.

### 1.9.4 Metrics to Measure Similarity

A biosimilar FOB should be "highly similar" to its reference product. But how similar is highly similar? How do we measure the similarity? These are hard questions and there has been no consensus on how to address these questions. Chapter 5 will present some metrics to measure the similarity and propose two scientific principles, which can be used to establish the threshold for similarity in each metric. The first principle is that a biosimilar criterion should be determined in a way that it allows the reference product to claim similarity to itself with a high probability. And the second is that all commercial lots of the reference product should meet a preset lot consistency criterion with a high probability. Following the proposed metrics and established thresholds, the corresponding statistical approaches are proposed for evaluating the similarity.

### 1.9.5 Average Inferiority Measure and Standardized Margins

Chapter 10 will discuss three major issues with the current practice of margin specifications: The subjectivity in the process of determining the margin, the data variability not considered or only implicitly expressed, and the concern of biocreep controversy. An average inferiority measure (AIM) is introduced as a tool for specification of margins to address these issues and the standardized margins derived from AIM reflect naturally the variability of data. The applications of AIM will be presented for the normal, binary, and the survival data.

### 1.9.6 Design and Analysis of Noninferiority Trials

Chapters 6 and 11 will discuss some new methods for design and analysis of NI trials. Chapter 11 will present the design and analysis of clinical trials involving biosimilar products using Bayesian methods. Both fully Bayesian approach and hybrid Bayesian approaches will be described. And the advantages and disadvantages by both approaches will be discussed as well.

Chapter 6 will discuss six frequentist-way analysis strategies, including fixed margin (FM) method, synthesis (Syn) method, modified covariate-adjustment fixed margin (CovFM) method, modified covariate-adjustment synthesis (CovSyn) method, two-stage covariate-adjustment fixed margin (2sFM) method, and two-stage covariate-adjustment synthesis (2sSyn) method. Statistical operating characteristics among these six methods will be compared.

### 1.9.7 Novel Method in Inference of Equivalence

Chapter 7 will present a novel method in inference of equivalence. A likelihood approach will be proposed that retains the unspecified variances in the model and partitions the likelihood function into two components: *F*-statistic function for variances and *t*-statistic function for the ratio of two means. By incorporating unspecified variances, the proposed method can help identify numeric range of variances, where equivalence is more likely to be achieved, which cannot be accomplished by traditional analysis methods.

### 1.9.8 Multiplicity Adjustments in Testing for Bioequivalence

Clinical PK and PD studies for biosimilars often involve the BE test for the proposed biosimilar and the reference product. The BE is usually demonstrated by rejecting two one-sided null hypotheses using the TOSTs for the primary metrics: AUC and $C_{max}$. The decision rule for BE often requires equivalence to be achieved on both metrics that contain four one-sided null hypotheses together, without adjusting for multiplicity, the family-wise error rate (FWER) could rise above the nominal type I error rate $\alpha$. Chapter 8 will discuss two multiplicity adjustments strategies in testing for BE including a closed-test procedure that controls FWER by treating the two metrics as a co-primary endpoint problem, and an alpha-adaptive sequential testing (AAST) that controls FWER by prespecifying the significance level on AUC ($\alpha_1$) and obtaining it for $C_{max}$ ($\alpha_2$) adaptively after testing of AUC.

### 1.9.9 Case Studies on the Applications of Bayesian Methods

Chapter 9 will present two case studies to demonstrate application of the Bayesian paradigm. The first case study is the application onto an interim analysis (IA) of a PK similarity trial to determine probability of success. The second case is the application on deriving an equivalence margin to demonstrate equivalence in efficacy of a biosimilar drug versus innovative (original) biologic drug for the treatment of rheumatoid arthritis disease.

## References

1. Global Biologics Market, Industry and R&D: Forecasts 2015–2025. https://www.visiongain.com/Report/1485/Global-Biologics-Market-Industry-and-R-D-Forecasts-2015-2025 (Accessed 8 May, 2015).
2. EMA Guideline on similar biological medicinal products, October 2014. http://www.ema.europa.eu/docs/en_GB/document_library/Scientific_guideline/2014/10/WC500176768.pdf.

3. EMA Guideline on similar biological medicinal products containing biotechnology-derived proteins as active substance: Non-clinical and clinical issues, December 2014. http://www.ema.europa.eu/docs/en_GB/document_library/Scientific_guideline/2015/01/WC500180219.pdf.
4. EMA Guideline on similar biological medicinal products containing biotechnology-derived proteins as active substance – Quality issues, 22 May 2014. http://www.ema.europa.eu/docs/en_GB/document_library/Scientific_guideline/2014/06/WC500167838.pdf.
5. MHLW Guideline for Ensuring Quality, Safety and Efficacy of Biosimilar Products, 4 March 2009. http://www.pmda.go.jp/files/000153851.pdf.
6. WHO Guidelines on evaluation of similar Biotherapeutic Products (SBPs), ECBS, 19–23 October 2009. http://www.who.int/biologicals/publications/trs/areas/biological_therapeutics/TRS_977_Annex_2.pdf?ua=1.
7. Health Canada Guidance for Sponsors: Information and Submission Requirements for Subsequent Entry Biologics (SEBs), 5 March 2010. http://www.hc-sc.gc.ca/dhp-mps/alt_formats/pdf/brgtherap/applic-demande/guides/seb-pbu/seb-pbu-2010-eng.pdf.
8. Biologics Price Competition and Innovation Act of 2009, Pub. L. No. 111–148, § 7001, 124 Stat. 119, 804 (2010). http://www.fda.gov/downloads/drugs/guidancecomplianceregulatoryinformation/ucm216146.pdf
9. FDA guidance for sponsors: Scientific Considerations in Demonstrating Biosimilarity to a Reference Product, April 2015. http://www.fda.gov/downloads/DrugsGuidanceComplianceRegulatoryInformation/Guidances/UCM291128.pdf.
10. FDA guidance for industry: Quality Considerations in Demonstrating Biosimilarity of a Therapeutic Protein Product to a Reference Product, April 2015. http://www.fda.gov/downloads/drugs/guidancecomplianceregulatoryinformation/guidances/ucm291134.pdf.
11. FDA draft guidance to industry: Clinical Pharmacology Data to Support a Demonstration of Biosimilarity to a Reference Product, May 2014. http://www.fda.gov/downloads/drugs/guidancecomplianceregulatoryinformation/guidances/ucm397017.pdf.
12. KFDA evaluation guidance for biosimilars, September 2009. http://www.aff.cz/wp-content/uploads/2011/05/Guidelines-on-the-Evaluation-of-Biosimilar-Products.pdf.
13. MCC guidance on biosimilar medicines: Quality, non-clinical and clinical requirements, August 2014. http://www.mccza.com/documents/d259816c2.30_Biosimilars_Aug14_v3.pdf.
14. FDA guidance for sponsors: Statistical Approaches to Establishing Bioequivalence, January 2001. http://www.fda.gov/downloads/Drugs/.../Guidances/ucm070244.pdf.
15. FDA draft guidance for sponsors: Non-inferiority Clinical Trials, 2010. http://www.fda.gov/downloads/Drugs/.../Guidances/UCM202140.pdf (Accessed March 2010).
16. Li, Y., Liu, Q., Wood, P., Johri, A. 2012. Statistical considerations in biosimilar clinical efficacy trials with asymmetrical margins. *Statistics in Medicine* 32(3):393–405.
17. Phillips, K. F. 1990. Power of the two one-sided tests procedure in bioequivalence. *Journal of Pharmacokinetics and Biopharmaceutics* 18(2):137–144.

18. Schuirmann, D. 1987. A comparison of the two one-sided tests procedure and the power approach for assessing the equivalence of average bioavailability. *Journal of Pharmacokinetics and Biopharmaceutics* 15(6):657–680.
19. FDA Briefing Document Oncologic Drugs Advisory Committee Meeting: BLA 125553 EP2006, a proposed biosimilar to Neupogen (filgrastim) Sandoz Inc., a Novartis Company, January 2015. http://www.fda.gov/downloads/AdvisoryCommittees/CommitteesMeetingMaterials/Drugs/OncologicDrugsAdvisoryCommittee/UCM428780.pdf.
20. Gupta, S.K. 2011. Intention-to-treat concept: A review. *Perspectives in Clinical Research* 2:109–112.
21. Njue, C. 2011. Statistical considerations for confirmatory clinical trials for similar biotherapeutic products. *Biologicals* 39:266–269.
22. Sanchez, M., Chen, X. 2006. Choosing the analysis population in non-inferiority studies: Per protocol or intent-to-treat. *Statistics in Medicine* 26:1169–1181.
23. European Agency for the Evaluation of Medicinal Products. 2000. Committee for Proprietary Medicinal Products. Points to consider on switching between superiority and non-inferiority. CPMP, London.

# 2

# *From Isolation to Integration: A Systems Biology Approach for the Discovery of Therapeutic Targets and Biomarkers*

**Attila Seyhan and Claudio Carini**

**CONTENTS**



**ABSTRACT** With the sequencing of whole genomes and the development of a variety of analysis methods and technologies (omics) to measure many of the cellular components, we now have the opportunity to understand the complete descriptions of complex biological systems at a molecular, cellular, tissue, and possibly organismal levels, and to ultimately develop predictive models of human diseases. Systems biology is a biology-based interdisciplinary field applied to biological research using a variety of genome-scale datasets from different omics technologies that focuses on complex interactions within biological systems, using a holistic approach (as opposed to a reductionist approach). This approach analyzes the biology as an informational science, probing biological systems as individual entities as well as a whole and their dynamic interactions with the environment. Systems biology aims to model and discover emergent properties at the cellular and molecular level functioning as a system, which typically involves metabolic and signaling networks. This approach has a significant power in searching for informative novel therapeutic targets and new diagnostic disease biomarkers since it focuses on the underlying mechanistic and molecular network perturbations of a disease. The information gained from network dynamics through experimentation and computational modeling enables us to assess the state of the networks and thus to identify molecular interactions, and derive new hypotheses to better understand the pathogenesis of the disease or prevent its progression by manipulating the network states. This approach, which includes diagnostics and therapeutics, is becoming widely used in clinical and pharmaceutical research.

However, understanding the factors that contribute to the disease state is rather challenging compared to collecting information on the different components involved. By using the newly emerging omics technologies, we can have a deeper understanding of the mechanisms playing a role in the pathogenesis of a specific disease. Thus, systems biology is generating a paradigm shift in our approaches to modeling and experimental levels.

Here, we discuss systems biology as a holistic approach to obtain, integrate, and analyze complex datasets from multiple experimental sources using interdisciplinary tools and review examples of modeling strategies to build cellular models on the basis of detailed multiparametric datasets.

## 2.1 Introduction

The cross-disciplinary research for the understanding of biological interactions in healthy and disease state with the aim to discover novel therapeutic targets and biomarkers has continued to evolve. Multidisciplinary novel technologies along with a better understanding of the ethiopathogenesis of the disease and the development of efficacious therapies have definitively contributed to the development of new diagnostic tools. The sequencing of the human genome has stimulated the development of new technologies. In recent years, the advent of technologies have changed the way we interpret this conundrum of information by exploiting the advancements of the human genome, transcriptome, and proteome, which ultimately will move targets from the stage of discovery to clinical development. Clearly, those efforts lead to the development of useful new methodologies and unprecedented scale-up of data coming from different but yet interconnected disciplines.

However, it is critical to use these technologies since they produce the results needed for deeply understanding, rather than merely describing, the biological systems. This is where systems biology comes into playing a significant role. Systems biology can be viewed as a discipline (a metalanguage) of concepts and models for interdisciplinary usage, which is still evolving. It is a paradigm that aims to incorporate and interconnect many different parameters coming from different disciplines and experimental settings. A systems biology approach aims to describe and understand the complex biological systems at cellular and molecular level and ultimately to develop predictive models of human disease. Contrary to a hypothesis-driven approach that aims to prove or disprove its postulations, systems biology is a hypothesis-free approach that can potentially lead to an unbiased and novel testable hypothesis as an end result. It does this so without assumptions which predict how a biological system should react to a stimulus or altered environment or disease state within a cellular context, across a tissue and time or impact on distant organs.

Gene, functional genome, protein, and metabolite measurements at large-scale "omic technologies" have significantly improved hypothesis generation and testing in human disease models. Bioinformatics and computational tools enabled the integration of information on organ and system level responses resulting in better prioritization of targets and improved decision making. A systems biology approach focuses on the roles of cellular pathways and networks, which when perturbed, and thought to be involved in disease pathophysiology rather than single biomolecules, describe a biological function. Systems biology aims to collectively characterize and quantify large sets of global-scale analytes and biomolecules that can be linked to structure, function, and dynamics of a single organism or multiple organisms. For example, functional genomics which can be described as a subset of genomics aims to identify the gene functions in a given organism. It combines different omics techniques such as transcriptomics and proteomics with mutant collections. In functional genomics, libraries of small molecules, peptides, or oligonucleotides such as small interfering RNAs (siRNAs) can be screened to identify agents that perturb function of a gene or its product (RNA, protein), "perturbagens" that modulate a multitude of functions, including transcriptomic, proteomic, and cellular phenotypic signatures. These molecular agents can be used to deconvolute pathways and networks. For example, in cell-based image analysis named "cytomics" details changes in cellular phenotype that can be quantitatively measured using high-content phenotypic screens. Additionally, changes in a cell's entire transcriptome or proteome can be profiled in detail using transcriptomic or proteomic approaches.

However, integration and analysis of this multiparametric data into systems biology research is challenging. Therefore, concurrent computational developments in data analysis packages and statistical methods are taking place to help understand these complex data and represent them as patterns and relationships within the datasets. These patterns or signatures can point to pathways that are relevant to specific biological processes that may be perturbed in a given disease state making possible the ultimate goal of understanding the biology of a cell at the systems level.

## 2.2 Omics Technologies

A systems biology view of biological systems requires multiple technologies termed "omics" that can generate large multidimensional datasets from many different platform technologies making this approach to drug, drug target, and biomarker discovery increasingly feasible. The power of omics technologies lies in their ability to probe complex biological functions and generate biologically relevant data at unprecedented scales. To accomplish this, various technology platforms are used to study the contribution of genes, RNAs, proteins, metabolites, etc., to disease susceptibility and effects of therapeutic interventions or environmental factors and stimuli (such as pathogens, diet, exercise, and exposure to stresses). Therefore, omics is the study of various collections of biomolecules, biological processes, physiologic functions, and structures as systems, and it aims to query the dynamic interactions between the numerous components of a biological system and represent these interactions as networks, pathways, and interactive relations as genes, transcripts, proteins, metabolites, and cells.[1] A variety of omics technologies such as human genetics (targeted); epigenomics; genomics (genome wide); using a variety of sequencing approaches of the entire genome or exome, transcriptomics (targeted or global transcriptome analysis of RNA species)[2]; proteomics (targeted or global),[3,4] and metabolomics[5,6] and functional genomic screens using RNA interference (RNAi) libraries[7]; and data mining and bioinformatics that capture different dimensions of biological processes and physiological functions and structures as systems are currently being used. These technologies have enabled us to study the function of biological processes in an organism that are controlled at a much higher level of complexity.[8] Additionally, these tools have allowed us to take a holistic approach to understand the underlying factors that may be contributing to disease pathogenesis by systematically characterizing biological processes at various molecular, biological, and temporal levels. Subsequently, efforts have been made to integrate large datasets generated from the omics-based efforts to build pathways and molecular networks to model biological processes associated with disease. Building the interactive networks that underly biological function between normal versus disease, or baseline versus disease state, or control versus treated requires a systems approach by collecting multidimensional data using a variety of omics technologies including transcriptional, translational, and posttranslational responses to genetic, environmental, or pharmacological perturbations. This in turn allowed researchers to gain multidimensional analytical insights to the underlining of the disease state at the molecular level and during various disease states. As a result of this, innovative strategies have emerged to improve the process of novel drug target and more effective and safer (precise) drug development, either by understanding the mechanism of action and side effects involving unanticipated "off-target" interactions of a drug or by identifying novel therapeutic use for an established drug.

Recently, omics technologies have been incorporated into chemical library screening campaigns, genome-wide loss or gain of function genomic screens, and transcriptomic and proteomic profiling leading to the development of a new era of systems biology approach. This facilitated the discovery and development of novel or combination drug targets, novel drugs, and disease- and treatment-specific biomarkers for clinical research by connecting together multiple data types and technologies across DNA, RNA, protein, and metabolite domains. Of course, the need to manage and analyze the large data that reflect the complexity of cellular pathways and interconnecting networks has led to the development of computational biology and bioinformatics, which are now an essential part of omics strategies.

Researchers studying cancer have exploited omics technologies successfully. Application of omics in cancer has enabled the development of multidimensional analytical approaches that led to better understanding of underlying biological changes during various stages of cancer.[9] This led to the discovery of novel drug targets[9,10] and biomarkers,[11,12] which may be translated into practice for novel drug or neoadjuvant drug development, risk stratification, early detection, diagnosis, treatment selection, prognosis, and monitoring for recurrence. Consequently, the omics-based approaches have improved our understanding about cancer and other complex human diseases[1,13–15] and uncovered many disease-specific molecular signatures. Collectively, the omics strategy has been employed effectively to screen a variety of disease-associated biological samples at the molecular and their interaction network levels in searching for novel drug targets and molecular biomarkers, elucidating the biology of target and drug mechanism of action, and identifying potential adverse effects in unexpected interaction. In addition, specialized approaches are being developed to integrate omics information and apply this information to translational research and new therapies, as well as toward the development of personalized medicine.

## 2.3 Systems Science

Systems science is an interdisciplinary field that studies the nature of a wide variety of simple or complex systems in various scientific disciplines, such as biology, sociology, and economics.[16] The objective of systems science is to develop interdisciplinary foundations that are applicable in a variety of areas, such as biology, medicine, physics, chemistry, psychology, cognitive science, sociology, economics, and engineering.[17] The areas commonly emphasized in systems science include (1) holistic view; (2) interaction between a system and its constituents and rooted environment; and (3) complex, often subtle dynamic interactions between systems. These interactions or behaviors are sometimes stable (and therefore reinforcing), whereas at various "boundary situations," they can become unstable (and therefore destructive).

## 2.4 Systems Biology

Systems biology deals with various technology platforms to address many questions that might have arisen from a biological system. Systems biology has gained significant interest in recent years partly due to the realization that traditional approaches focusing only on a few analytes at a specific time point cannot describe the state of pathological processes across a whole cellular, tissue, or organismal level system. Systems biology is an approach that enables the analysis of biological systems at the cellular, tissue, or organ level that perceives biology as an information science. It studies biological systems as a whole and their dynamic interactions with the environment. Systems biology focuses on the fact that biological systems are a network of dynamic information captured in biological networks composed of molecular components (e.g., DNA, RNA, protein, metabolites) and cell types. From this analysis, molecular signatures and patterns emerging from disease-modified networks can be identified. These signatures can then be employed to identify a variety of pathological conditions and be used to segment individuals into subgroups based on variations in genetic and molecular network models of key biological processes perturbed in disease state or during disease progression. Molecular signatures or patterns that are linked to specific pathological processes can then be employed as a panel of "composite" biomarkers consisting of many different types of biomolecules (e.g., DNA, messenger RNA [mRNA], microRNA [miRNA], proteins, and metabolites).

Systems biology relies on a variety of experimental datasets and computational tools including the use of bioinformatics tools and databases in conjunction with clinical and experimental data, and information from the literature to describe a system by tracing observations of complex phenotypes back to information encoded in the genome or its products (e.g., RNA, protein, and metabolites). The addition of clinical laboratory and experimental preclinical measurements means that systems biology need not be entirely reductionist. Furthermore, a systems biology approach also uses complex mathematical tools to model and simulate the system or determine possible associations.

Systems biology is considered as a multitude of information sciences (Figure 2.1), including (1) global biological information and (2) interacting information from the environment which all contribute to the development, physiological responses, and the onset and progression of pathological changes.[18–20] A variety of sources feed into this information sciences, including (1) the measurement of various types of global biological information (e.g., genome, transcriptome, proteome, metabolome; (2) integration of each disparate dataset coming from different omic technology; (3) understanding the interactions between these platforms and environment and subsequent

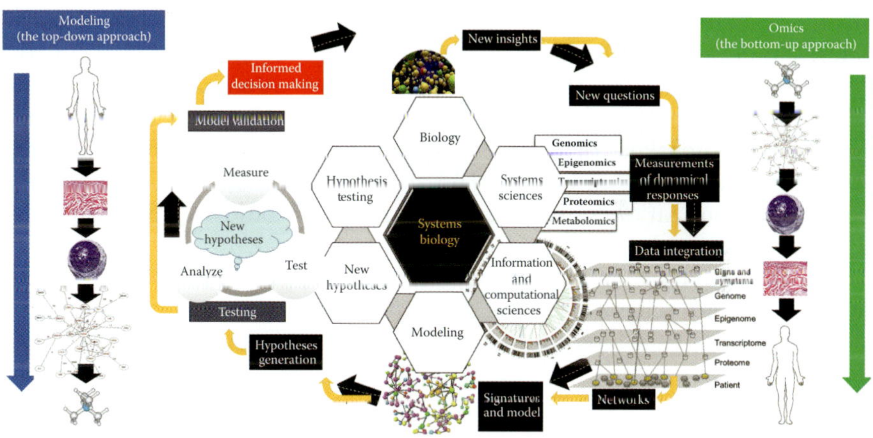


**FIGURE 2.1**
Approaches to systems biology for the discovery of novel therapeutic targets and biomarkers. Omics (the bottom-up) uses a global approach for the identification and global measurement of molecular components. Modeling (the top-down approach) uses integrative (across scales) models of organismal level physiology (e.g., human) and disease. More specifically, such modeling focuses on relatively specific questions at particular scales (e.g., at the mechanics pathway and organ levels). Systems biology attempts to bridge omics and modeling generate profiling data from global profiling experiments designed to incorporate biological complexity at multiple dimensions such as pathways, cell types, and multiple different environments. To achieve this, systems biology uses a variety of often global-scale technologies (omics) that focuses on complex interactions within biological systems, using a holistic approach (as opposed to reductionism) to biological and biomedical research. The goal is to model and discover emergent properties at the cellular, tissue, and organismal level functioning as a system, which typically involve metabolic and signaling networks. Such a complex systems approach addresses the need for data on cell responses to physiological and environmental stimuli and drugs. The ultimate goal of this approach is to better understand the complex mechanisms underlying the specific biological processes (e.g., developmental disease) to be able to properly manipulate them as novel therapeutic targets and biomarkers.

biological responses to the stimuli; (4) understanding the dynamical changes of all biological systems such as networks and signaling pathways as they respond to the stimuli; (5) modeling the biological system through the integration of global and dynamic data; (6) generating hypotheses and testing them experimentally; and (7) enhancing the models via a series of iterative prediction and comparison testing. Once the models closely match the data from biological system responses, these models can then be employed to predict the responses to molecular network perturbations for identifying possible underlying causes for disease, for predicting disease development and progression, and for designing better treatment strategies to improve better patient outcomes.

Systems biology approach is often applied to studying healthy and disease states and their corresponding functions, prediction of disease development and progression as well as response to treatments. The overall goal of these applications is to establish an action strategy informed from diverse sets of information describing biological events and responses to environmental perturbants or stimuli or effects of interventions on different biological scales. Subsequently, the information gained from these efforts help to make informative and useful decisions such as the identification of biomarkers or to assess drug effects or identify novel mechanisms as potential drug targets. The approach may be dynamic and may require customization for each task as each result could suggest a different approach required.

Due to the nature of diverse range of data types and analysis methods, systems biology relies on diverse scientific expertise including clinical and preclinical scientists, bioinformaticians, and biostatisticians.

## 2.5 Systems Biology for Understanding the Molecular Pathways and Regulatory Networks Underlying the Specific Biological Processes

Systems biology aims to understand physiology and pathophysiology from the level of molecular pathways, regulatory networks, specific cell types, tissues, organs, and organismal level. Systems biology is an integrated system as it collects, integrates, and analyzes complex datasets from multiple experimental sources using interdisciplinary tools and a variety of technology platforms. The sources of molecular information may include genomics, epigenomics, transcriptomics, proteomics, metabolomics, lipidomics, and more recently biomics (systems analysis of the biome). Systems biology focuses on the integrated roles of cellular pathways and networks rather than single biomolecules as targets as done earlier. The systems biology approach often involves the development of mechanistic models. Mechanistic models involve dynamic reconstruction of cellular networks using parameters coming from chemical kinetics and control theory.[21,22] Because of the involvement of large data, variables, and constraints in cellular networks, numerical and computational techniques are often used (e.g., flux balance analysis—a mathematical method for simulating metabolism in genome-scale reconstructions of metabolic networks).

A systems biology approach utilizes datasets generated from a variety of omics technologies that can generate and analyze large multidimensional datasets. The changes in transcriptional, protein, metabolomic networks are evaluated against collections of small molecules, peptides, or RNA-based perturbants such as siRNAs to probe the function of genes and to identify agents that modulate the cellular phenotypic signatures. Such agents that perturb the function of their targets (individual biomolecules or pathways) can be used to analyze pathways of genes and proteins or metabolite networks. The power of this approach is its ability to generate signatures of complex biological information in pathophysiological state as compared to physiological state or during disease onset before and after therapeutic interventions. These patterns can then identify new pathways and targets that are relevant to drug discovery. This provides an opportunity for future systems biology approaches to disease treatment based on the ability to identify and assess the state of the perturbed networks as well as the dynamic evolution of such networks under a variety of environmental conditions, genetic background, and perturbations. Information about the dynamics of the networks and their interactions temporally and spatially will enable us to define the state of the pathological process of a disease at the biological network level, predict the progression of the pathology based on network and pathway perturbations and interactions, and derive more targeted interventions to restore the perturbed networks to the normal state.[20] An improved understanding of the systems behavior reflected in changes in cellular signaling pathways and networks, such as identification of key nodes or regulatory hubs as well as cross talk between pathways[23] and networks may help to predict drug target or biomarker effects and their translation to cellular, organ, and organismal level physiology. Information gained about the precise states of the biological networks and the way in which these networks change over time at the molecular level by the assessment of a panel of informative biomarkers will enable us to develop new strategies to specifically manipulate a mechanistic network to prevent or delay the predicted evolution of disease. Thus, the future of systems biology will enable us to discover and develop circulating (e.g., blood) biomarkers that correlate with, and are causally related to, key pathologies. These biomarkers will provide information about the underlying molecular alterations within pathologies specifically associated with state of key networks and regulatory pathways. This advance in deciphering the molecular complexity will enable a more comprehensive understanding of disease and its progression at molecular levels. An improved understanding of network dynamics and the effects of a variety of potential perturbations will lead to a diagnostic-therapeutic systems biology (or medicine) approach based through identifying and manipulating the state of perturbed biological networks. However, the genetic differences among individuals will affect the networks and modify their function and responses to perturbations, further complicating the association between network state and specific disease.

In addition to finding new targets and cellular pathways and networks, sophisticated counter-screening approaches are also used to discover and validate novel targets and pathways.[24] G-protein-coupled receptors (GPCRs) are widely accepted therapeutic targets with great success as medicines. However, it may be more efficient and effective if GPCR modulators are assessed in terms of signaling pathway selectivity, species selectivity, and selectivity against closely related family members at the stage of screening.

Systems biology of cancer is a good example in this regard as it often begins with a focused objective, such as tumorigenesis and treatment of cancer. It begins by collecting the specific data, such as patient samples; high-throughput genome data in patient tumor samples and tools to validate these findings in cancer cell lines; *in vivo* rodent models of tumorigenesis and xenograft; and large-scale perturbation methods, including gene based (RNAi-based functional genome screenings, overexpression of wild-type and mutant genes); chemical approaches using small-molecule libraries; and computational modeling of the lead targets (e.g., mutations).[25,26] Consequently, the ultimate goal of systems biology of cancer is to better diagnose and characterize cancer, and better predict the outcome of a suggested treatment, which is the basis for personalized medicine.

## 2.6 Systems Biology Approach for the Discovery of Therapeutic Drug Targets

Systems biology has emerged as a new field, which takes a holistic approach to biological science by integrating information obtained from various omics technologies and building networks and pathways to model biological processes for target identification and disease association. There are two main approaches for target discovery: (1) a system approach and (2) a molecular approach.[27] The systems approach is a strategy that selects targets through the study of diseases in whole organisms using information derived from clinical trials and a variety of preclinical omics-based studies, whereas the molecular approach, the mainstream of current target discovery strategy,[28,29] aims to identify "druggable" targets where activities can be modulated through interactions with candidate pharmaceuticals or biopharmaceuticals.

Traditionally, global genomics, transcriptomics, and proteomic strategies have been used for hypothesis generation, rather than hypothesis testing, by identifying sets of genes, RNAs, proteins, or their respective networks or pathways perturbed in a specific disease. Global omics technologies can now be used to identify molecular targets associated with a specific disease, providing researchers information on the mechanism of action of new drugs. Because of this, mechanism-based and genome-based technologies, other molecular tools and sensors, and animal models including the use of gene knockout (deletion), suppression, knock-in (replace endogenous gene with new gene with mutation), or ectopic overexpression of a gene of interest while comparing the influence of lead molecules with and without genetic disruption have been used. Information on potential targets is elucidated from increased sensitivity with decreased gene dosage for a certain drug concentration[10] or by enhanced resistance when a target is overproduced[30] or its expression is inhibited.[12] Consequently, by examining the overlap of gene/protein interaction networks with the data obtained from chemical genetic sensitivity screens, candidate pathways that are perturbed by drugs can be identified.[31–35] To be a validated target, first the candidate target must be confirmed in preclinical studies *in vitro* and *in vivo* (animal models) to confirm the effect of target on mechanism and its link to human disease. In preclinical validation, the target expression or modulation must be shown as disease tissue and cell type. Expression level must correlate with disease severity and the modulation of level of activity of target in cell culture and in animal models must be relevant to disease pathophysiology. Finally, modulation of level of target activity level in humans must be associated with disease pathophysiology. Clinically validated target is a molecular target of a known therapeutic agent.

To have pharmaceutical utility, a target must be "druggable," i.e., a target must be accessible to candidate drug molecules (e.g., small molecules or biologics) and bind them in such a way that a desirable biological effect is inflicted. Druggable genome comprises only a fraction of the entire genome, hence many key proteins remain "undrugged" either because they are unknown or they cannot be targeted by current therapeutics. This in fact provides an opportunity to develop novel therapies that can target genes and their products that are currently outside of reach with current therapies and reveal novel disease-specific targets or molecular pathways as well as biomarkers to monitor drug efficacy and patient response to treatments. Presently, the majority of "druggable" targets are GPCRs and protein kinases. Because the biological mechanisms of human diseases are rather complex, the most crucial task in target discovery is not only to identify, prioritize, and select reliable "druggable" targets but also to understand the cellular interactions underlying disease phenotypes, to provide predictive models, and to construct biological networks for human diseases.[27] Because of this, a systems biology approach that enables the use of new omics technologies coupled with high-throughput, genome-scale, and multidimensional and multivariate comprehensive functional analyses could enable the discovery and development of novel drug targets more effectively. However, these are in the end tools and platform technologies bringing us new candidates as targets. A target and changes in its expression or modulation must be critical for disease or pathway associated with the disease and safe (i.e., its activity can be modulated by a therapeutic agent to inhibit or reverse disease onset or progress). Furthermore, modulation of a therapeutic target by a candidate drug should alter the levels of biological pathways, crucial "nodes" on a regulatory network, and ideally selected disease biomarkers. Access to such "surrogate biomarkers" can contribute significantly to a successful drug development research; therefore, development of biomarkers for diseases is also an important part of the target development and validation process.

In addition, the increase of biomedical data and information requires better use of data mining and analysis strategies. This requires extensive gathering and filtering of a multitude of available heterogeneous data and information.[29] For instance, MEDLINE/PubMed currently contains more than 18 million literature abstracts, and more than 60,000 new abstracts are added monthly and the number of chemical, genomic, proteomic, and metabolic data are rapidly growing and have been estimated to double every 2 years. The growth of available data and information is providing opportunities for discovery and development of novel drug targets and biomarkers in support of the drug development research.[29] The bioinformatics of data and text mining of literature, microarray, and proteomic data filter valuable targets by combining biological ideas with computer tools or statistical methods. These curated data sets have been growing rapidly to support the discovery and development of novel targets.[28] With the recent development of high-throughput proteomics and chemical genomics, another two data mining approaches, proteomic data mining and chemogenomic data mining, have surfaced. Due to these new scientific discoveries, there is a need to develop efficient data mining methods.

## 2.7 Systems Biology Approach for the Discovery of Biomarkers

Biomarkers, defined as any analyte or biomolecule, which can be objectively measured, experimentally validated, and clinically relevant to disease,[36] can be used to predict molecular and phenotypical changes before they occur, assess the efficacy and safety of drugs, and stratify patients. Biomarkers are useful molecular markers for disease detection and monitoring and may be treated as intermediate phenotypes of disease. They indicate the physiological status at a given time and vary during the disease development. Genetic mutations, epigenetic modifications, alterations in gene transcription and translation, and their protein products or metabolites can all serve as molecular biomarkers for disease.[37] Biomarkers have the utility to assess molecular and physiological changes associated with disease initiation; progression and onset before, during, and after the therapeutic intervention is essential for the early diagnosis and prediction of complex diseases and could be used to improve drug development.[38–40] Biomarkers can be used to predict molecular and phenotypical changes before they occur to assess the efficacy and safety of drugs and to stratify patients. Additionally, biomarkers can be used for early diagnosis of disease without apparent pathophysiological changes (identify silent phenotypes), identify those with suspected disease and assist in monitoring of disease progression, and identify those modified by treatment or remission of disease. Consequently, biomarkers have gained recognition by pharmaceutical industry and clinical researchers as such that if translated into clinical practice, they can be used for diagnosis, treatment risk stratification, early detection, treatment selection, prognostication, and the monitoring for recurrence.

Systems biology approaches facilitate the discovery of informative biomarkers by extracting a number of key information such as (1) pathways and gene to protein networks are perturbed in disease states; (2) cellular, tissue, and organ-specific components of these networks can be used to infer the state of specific networks; (3) panels of multiple circulating markers including organ-specific and process-specific markers in the blood and other suitable bodily fluids (e.g., plasma, serum, urine) provide information about the state of the affected cell types and tissues; and (4) the selected analytes that are released into the circulation provide key information for the evaluation of the state of perturbed networks.

A variety of omics-based genome-scale technology has been used extensively for the discovery and development of biomarkers for cancer[11] and other diseases. A systems biology approach for the discovery and development of informative biomarkers often begins by collecting key information from (1) networks that are perturbed from their normal states during disease; (2) linking these networks to their tissue or organ-specific components to infer the state of specific networks in the targeted organs; (3) generate a panel of multiple blood markers (composite biomarkers) including organ-specific and process-specific markers in the blood that produce useful information on the perturbed mechanisms in the affected tissues, organs, and cell types; and (4) the identified candidate analytes (proteins, DNA fragments, RNAs, miRNAs, metabolites, lipids, cell types) that are released into the blood provide assessment of the state of perturbed networks.

## 2.8 Multiomics Data Integration and Analysis

The interdisciplinary science of modern systems biology continues to evolve, thereby continuing to bring more multidisciplinary novel multiomics technologies and scientific understanding of the disease development to the biomedical, clinical, and basic science research laboratories. In recent years, the field has experienced the advent of technologies that change the way we approach target biology (the human genome project), build compound collections (combinatorial, automated, and contract synthesis), conduct screening (high-throughput and high-content screens), and ultimately advance compounds from discovery to development. In the following years, we will see more technology-driven advances as the regulation raises the bar for a safer and more efficacious and targeted or personalized medicines with an accelerated development period. The rationale behind the omics approach is that a complete understanding of the responses of a system requires knowledge of all of its component parts. Therefore, the omics technologies focus on the building blocks of complex systems such as genes, RNAs, proteins, metabolites, and lipids with an aim to target identification and validation for generating hypotheses and for experimental analysis in traditional hypothesis-based methods. Omics approach has been used to probe the functions of genes, proteins or phosphorylation states of proteins and whether their expression levels are modified in disease state, subsequently generating a testable hypothesis that the altered state of these components are involved in disease initiation or development. Hence, integration of multiomics measurements within the context of functional genomics or drug perturbations of complex cell or animal models in the context of clinical data forms the foundation of the systems biology. Omics classification of disease states have the ability to identify therapeutic targets that are more relevant to disease state and if done at individual patient level, this may potentially lead to personalization of therapies by identifying specific pathways perturbed in particular disease state of an individual.[41] Furthermore, omics technology has been successfully used for the identification of surrogate markers for disease detection, for assessing the efficacy of therapies,[10,39] and for the identification of potential drug-resistant patients.[42] Despite omics approaches facilitating the generation of novel mechanistic hypotheses and clinical information on disease, the system as a whole cannot be predicted from the individual components (i.e., RNA or proteins or metabolites). A systems biology approach requires information of key pathways and organism level responses captured in global gene and protein expression data. Studies in simple organisms involving global functional genome analyses, identification of coregulated components, and protein–protein interaction studies produced new information on pathway functions and signaling networks. This was most successful in well-defined biological processes such as cell proliferation or the response to environmental stimuli or metabolic perturbation.[32,43–45] However, for the obvious reasons (e.g., the added levels of complexity in human disease and computational limitations), applying omics as a sole approach to human disease is challenging for systems level understanding. Despite these shortcomings, omics approach provides a road map to define mechanistic pathways and networks that are involved in disease that can be used in in top-down models of cell-signaling networks.[46]

As illustrated in Figure 2.2, the more of the disparate systems measured, the more complex the analysis. One way to integrate various omics experimental datasets is to analyze each set independently and then integrate those identified as positive analytes or alternatively to integrate the data before analysis. This can be accomplished by (1) combining all experimental datasets into a single master dataset, and (2) first identifying biological relationships between the molecules and forming networks and subsequently analyzing the networks. Emerging analysis tools such as Ondex are designed to analyze multiomics datasets[47]; however, it does not have the multiomics statistical approaches.[47] Another tool termed Mixomics is an R package, which uses correlation between molecules to identify groups of related molecules corresponding to a particular disease or disease state[48] that can be used to analyze two omics sets simultaneously.

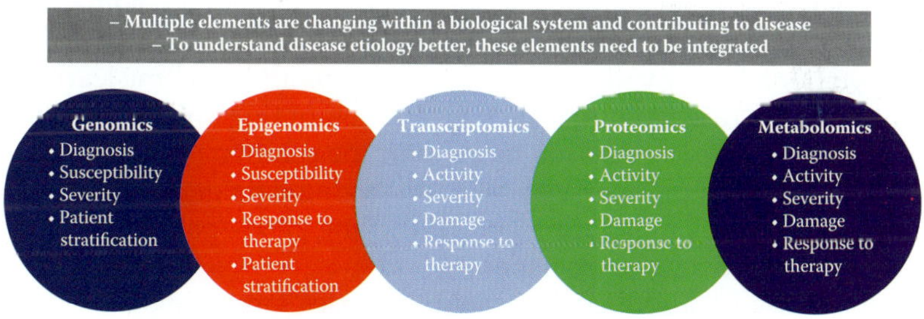


| Platforms | Target profilling | Tools |
|---|---|---|
| Genomics | Gene/genome sequencing, SNP | Next gen sequencing, SNP arrays, etc. |
| Transcriptomics | Differential gene expression | Microarray, qRT-PCR |
| Protemics | Differential protein expression | Mass Spec, ELISA, and other cell-based assay |
| Metabolomics | Differential metabolite expression | NMR, GC-MS, and LC-MS, |

| | | |
|---|---|---|
| Control | Versus | Treated |
| Wild type | Versus | Transgenic, knockout |
| Baseline | Versus | Time course |

**FIGURE 2.2**
Multiomics for the identification of novel drug targets and biomarkers. This is achieved by providing enabling technologies and products that can be incorporated into innovative multiple endpoint platforms, which facilitate more accurate predictive assays for safety and efficacy. Biomarkers offer a means to affect rational drug design early in the development process and accelerate translational drug development from animal to man.

## 2.9 Bioinformatics and Computational Approaches for the Integration of Multiomics Data

The systems biology approach often involves the development of mechanistic models, including the reconstruction of dynamic systems from the quantitative properties of their elementary building blocks.[21,22] Because of the large number of datasets coming from high-throughput molecular profiling studies and variables and constraints in cellular networks, numerical and computational techniques are often used (e.g., flux balance analysis). Also, the systems biology approach generates large and often disparate sets and data types from multiple and different high-throughput omic sources and analysis of these has become a major bottleneck requiring sophisticated computational and statistical methods and skill sets.[49] Some computational approaches and mechanistic models need to be employed for the interpretation of complex datasets. Novel computer-aided algorithms and methodologies for pattern recognition, visualization, and classification of distribution metrics for interpreting large sets of data have been effectively used. This is where the bioinformatics and computational biology play a critical role in linking biological knowledge with clinical practice: they are the interface between the clinical development process of drug target and biomarker discovery and development.

Computational biology uses computational tools and machine learning for data mining, whereas bioinformatics applies computing and mathematics to the analysis of biological datasets to support the solution of biological problems. Bioinformatics plays a key role in analyzing data generated from different omic platforms annotating and classifying genes/pathways for target identification and disease association.

Bioinformatics is described as a field that uses large biological datasets which must be manipulated via computation and tested with robust statistics. Data storage and algorithm development are key challenges in this field and the goal is usually a description of that individual dataset by statistics alone or by also integrating annotations and interpreting the enriched dataset. Bioinformaticians uses computational methods to predict factors (genes and their products) using (1) a combination of mathematical modeling and search techniques, (2) mathematical modeling to match and analyze high-level functions, and (3) computational search and alignment techniques to compare new biomolecules (DNA, RNA, protein, metabolite, etc.) within each functional omics platform. Combination of these and patient datasets are then used to generate hypotheses. Bioinformatics and computational biology enable fine tuning of hypotheses.[50] These fields often require specialized tools and skills for data exploration, clustering, regression, and supervised classification[51,52]; pattern recognition and selection[53]; and development of statistical filtering or modeling strategies and classifiers, including neural networks or support vector machines. The integration of clinical and omic datasets has allowed the exploitation of available biological data such as functional annotations and pathway data.[54–56] Consequently, this has led to the generation of prediction models of disease occurrence or responses to therapeutic intervention.[51,57]

## 2.10 Integration of Different Types of Datasets

Recent advances in global omics approaches have led to the generation of large datasets that are complex and multiparametric. One of the challenges using a variety of disparate multiparametric datasets is the need to integrate large and often complex disparate multiparametric data types into the overall analysis, and interpret and represent integrated data within the context of actual biological and pathobiological processes. Another challenge is to produce a meaningful and biologically relevant interpretation of massive and often disparate datasets that reflect the complexity of mechanistic pathways networks. Systems biology addresses this complexity[58,59] by accommodating the roles of networks and pathways in the physiological and pathophysiological state of biological systems and organisms, allowing us to have a higher level of understanding of the true multidimensionality of biology.

Most efforts up to now have used a single omics platform, which reveals a facet of the multidimensional biological processes and interactive networks, which comprises the biological behavior and responses. Multiomics platforms can concurrently test multiple biological processes at multiple levels of complexity including changes in transcriptome, proteome, phosphoproteome, and protein interactome in response to external factors or genetic stimuli. For example, researchers used both proteomics and transcriptomic technologies to study global protein expression and subcellular localization patterns in fractions of Jurkat T-leukemic cells[60] and identified a total of 5381 unique proteins. However, when combined with transcriptomic data to eliminate the false positives and rescue proteins identified by single peptides, 6271 unique proteins resulted, which is still a large set of candidates that requires further curation and validation. The coupling of omics technologies to systems level analytics and bioinformatics will enable elucidation of biological processes and responses in both normal and diseased states. Additionally, coupling of various omics technologies to phenotypic screening to identify compound-specific targets and molecular pathways with novel biological activity and interactive proteomics to identify candidate drug–target interactions can facilitate drug discovery and identify disease and compound-specific biomarkers for clinical research.

These multiparametric and multidimensional datasets generated by these technologies such as application of phenotypic classifiers using supervised learning approaches and characterization of feature data using statistical methods are analyzed to derive meaningful and biologically relevant knowledge. Accomplishing this requires a standardized analytical processes of normalization, outlier detection, imputation of missing values, and univariate statistical analysis to identify analytes whose levels are significantly altered as a consequence of experimental conduct. Several considerations including signal intensity thresholds, fold change, and ambiguity in molecular identification must all be considered in this statistical analysis. The advantages of unsupervised discovery approaches used in systems biology are that large and often genome-scale datasets can be rapidly analyzed for those significant features representing responses to biological perturbations. The candidate features then are ascribed to biological mechanisms or processes before a "systems biology"-based understanding can be applied.

The number of analytes contributed by different data platforms can vary over several orders of magnitude (>55,000 gene probe pairs on a gene chip versus >1,000 miRNA gene probe pairs or proteomics measurements that can constitute a total of approximately 293,000 nonredundant peptides[61]). A large human proteome catalog covering approximately 84% of human protein coding genes of the human proteome using high-resolution mass spectrometry is available as an interactive web-based resource at http://www.humanproteomemap.org. This will complement available human genome and transcriptome data to accelerate biomedical research in health and disease.[61] It is apparent that the sheer number of data coming from each omic platform underscores the need for further statistical treatments and filtering approaches (e.g., secreted proteome) to balance the effective contributions from each platform, so that the biological significance of a low-density dataset would not be missed.

## 2.11 Data Interpretation and Presentation

Due to the nature of the high level of complexity of the typical systems biology datasets, consisting of many more measurements than subjects, this complexity requires the application of a number of pattern recognition techniques within the data. For example, a dataset may be queried to assess whether different classes of subjects emerge. This is achieved by a supervised learning analysis (i.e., knowing that a case–control relationship already exists or that treated/untreated subjects are present) or by unsupervised means (how many statistically significantly different groups can be identified?) by using a variety of multivariate techniques. These include factor analysis and principal component analysis that can be used to identify patterns in multidimensional datasets.[62,63] For example, in factor analysis, an investigator attempts to understand the patterns of relationships among many dependent variables and to discover independent variables that describe the relationships (the "factors").[63] In the case of principal component analysis, a technique transforms a number of potentially related variables into a small number of unrelated variables and then attempts to describe the variability in a dataset. The first principal component will describe the greatest amount of the variability as possible, the second will describe the next greatest amount of variability, etc., through a potentially infinite series of components that explain all variability in the dataset. Principle component analysis results in a large reduction in the complexity and dimensionality of the data, where classes of subjects can be distilled into, often in two- or three-dimensional representations. The next task is a high-level understanding of biological significance of these discrete classes or clusters of data. The high degree of redundancy in biological systems as well as the scale-free network trafficking of biomolecules preclude absolute assignment of discrete biological process changes. Individual analyte changes rarely point to a fundamental biological process that explains the classes identified by multivariate analysis. Statistical treatment of these changes as part of higher- order biological processes that rely upon ontological assignments of individual analytes helps to the assignment of discrete biological processes. The ontological treatment of analytes is designed to indicate what fundamental biological pathways and processes are in the system. Gene set enrichment analysis (GSEA)[64] was one of the earlier examples in the use of ontological categorization of genes. Genes are attributed to ontological groups, including gene ontology (GO) or Kyoto Encyclopedia of Genes and Genomes (KEGG) and a nonparametric ranking tool based upon the Kolmogorov–Smirnov statistic. Gene networks and pathways with significant contributions from single nucleotide polymorphisms (SNPs), differential gene expression microarrays, proteomic analytes, metabolites and other candidate molecular signatures and pathways (i.e. hits) can be elucidated, and a biological or ontological assessment of disease or treatment impact can be supported through statistical analysis. The existence of well-standardized and annotated gene chips have facilitated the use of this technology, but a similar degree of standardization and annotation has yet to be made for the other platforms. In addition to these ontological tools, other information sources have been successfully mined to include biological context to systems biology data.

More recently, text mining programs are being used to parse text from the scientific literature. Global text mining from multiple sources in scientific literature serve as a means of contextualizing systems biology data to derive hypotheses about pathways.[65] This is done by using subject–verb/object relationships-based search terms, which can then contextualize data from different datasets generated from a variety of omics platforms. Databases such as the Connectivity Map,[34] KEGG,[66] Pathway Interaction Database (PID; pid.nci.nih.gov), Human Protein Interaction Database (http://wilab.inha.ac.kr/hpid/), and the Bimolecular Interaction Network Database (BIND; www.bind.ca) are publicly available resources allowing investigators to identify potential interaction partners within biological networks in physiological or pathophysiological settings. By accompanying these, new tools to graphically illustrate pathways and build models can serve as an illustrative means to generate new hypotheses based on complex systems biology datasets.

Network representation of systems biology data enabled the generation of easily understandable graphical models. A variety of computational tools of biological processes such as the Systems Biology Markup Language (SBML); http://sbml.org), and a more complex Cytoscape (http://cytoscape.org), can utilize a variety of input formats that includes, but is not limited to SBML and can help to develop predictive hypotheses that can be then tested in an experimental setting. Cytoscape is a tool primarily designed for network visualization and analysis; it makes use of a wide variety of plug-ins to extend its functionality that are designed by the scientific community. Subsequent modeling of network behavior provides predictive capability to generate testable hypotheses. The biological processes are frequently described as pathways, where biomolecules interact physically and are frequently transformed.

The physical interaction of biomolecules are being cataloged in a variety of ontology databases such as the ones previously mentioned—PID, Human Protein Interaction Database, and BIND—and are a few examples of assembled knowledge for protein–protein interactions. A similar approach has been used with transcription factors that bind specific nucleic acid sequences (TRANSFAC),[67] which can inform us about pathways that could be regulated through perturbation of one of the many known transcription factors.

## 2.12 Computational Modeling—From Pathways to Disease

Modeling provides a foundation and scaffold for hypothesis generation and disease prediction based on the information of molecular networks and pathways emerged from the omics data analysis and clinical data on disease biology across multiple timescales (from healthy state to disease state and response to therapy) and molecular distances (multiple networks and regulatory pathways at the levels of cell, tissue, or organ).[59] Thus, the advantage of modeling is the use of computational power within a set of predefined principles to simulate a particular environment such as perturbation of a system component(s) and predicting the subsequent outcome.[68] Building a whole-cell model involves new modeling approaches and integration of models specific to each cell type and cellular processes.[69] Although the field is still emerging, progress is being made in developing and testing computational and experimental methods for an integrated modeling of cellular, tissue, and organismal responses to environment and disease, and therapeutic interventions at different scales. A variety of hybrid approaches has been used for building a whole-cell model[69] using top combination of ordinary differential equations (ODEs), and constraints using Boolean methods have been used for integrating individual biological processes and modeled them according to the overall state of the cell.[70,71] Understanding of key regulatory pathways such as identification of key nodes in networks and cross talk between pathways can also help predict drug target effects and their translation to organ and organismal level physiology.

However, several issues need to be addressed before models that aim to integrate complexity at multiple levels can be successfully applied to systems biology. One difficulty is the integration of molecular, cellular, tissue and organ level responses to environment, bioactive stimuli, disease state, and therapeutic interventions. As discussed by Butcher et al.,[59] one approach could be that each level of complexity can be integrated with increasing complexity into an organ level framework in a modular format (e.g., cell–cell communication through cytokine networks, cellular inflammation, and cell-specific molecular signaling).[59]

As for cell and organ level models, simulations of signaling networks often use time-dependent differential equations and model the pathway under specific conditions.[46,72] A cross-talk analysis between pathways brings an additional layer to the model.[23] Computational models have been developed using organ level disease physiology framework such as chronic asthma that incorporated interactions of different cell types and some of the responses to each other and their environment.[73] More complex models of glucose metabolism involving multiple tissue responses to changes in glucose metabolism are a good example in this regard. Cell and organ level models of glucose metabolism and homeostasis based on relationships between glucose and insulin levels have evolved to more complex and integrated models that incorporate multiple tissue responses and their involvement in glucose metabolism has been used.[74,75] Computational modeling enables the determination of the dosing regimen and the number of patients required for the each arm of the clinical trial before the actual trial is conducted, hence saving time and cost and increasing the chances of success of the clinical trial.

## 2.13 Challenges in Validating the Candidate Targets and Biomarkers

Advances in a variety of omics technologies are now utilized to identify molecular targets including biomarkers that can reveal the disease state or the ability to respond to a treatment, thus providing scientists with the molecular insights of the disease pathogenesis. Despite the advances, approximately only 100 biomarkers out of 150,000 so far that appeared in literature have made it to the clinic.[49,76,77] This is because the majority of biomarkers either could not be validated or cannot be linked to a disease.[78,79] Therefore, there is still much to be done. Furthermore, the recent advances in genome-wide omics-based methodologies even add to the complexity of the successful development of useful biomarkers. Therefore, the development of validated biomarkers is in much need to facilitate much improved decision-making process during the preclinical phase of drug development and in more informed execution of personalized medicine in the clinical phase. Biomarker development still requires (1) analytical technologies that deconstruct complex biological systems into their integral molecular constituents, and (2) access to specimens from human subjects and confirmation of these observations from *in vitro* tissue culture models and animal models of human disease. Noninvasive lifestyle independent predictive biomarkers can, therefore, help to predict diseases before the manifestation of disease and enable physicians to stratify individuals at risk of developing disease and identify best treatment options. However, as mentioned above only a few biomarkers have been validated and routinely used in clinical practice. It appears that an insufficient linkage of biomarkers to disease pathogenesis is the main cause for failure of many biomarkers as well as drug targets. Therefore, it is critical to link the target to the disease pathogenesis using datasets enabling us to develop better and more precise therapies by selecting up-front responders, expediting safer and more efficacious clinical studies, and reducing costs. Identifying biomarkers that can be translated from animal models to humans is challenging. While inhibiting an enzyme in an animal model may be effective, this may not be the case in humans. This is either because the pathway has diverged or humans have some compensatory mechanisms or the models are simply the wrong model for the disease. A treatment may change a biomarker but may be irrelevant to a specific disease. Therefore, a true biomarker must be intrinsically linked to the pathogenesis of the disease. Once a biomarker is identified, it is difficult to understand whether it is associated with a specific disease or multiple diseases or if it is a reflection of poor health.

There is a heightened interest from both pharmaceutical companies and medical researchers, as well as regulatory agencies to develop validated biomarkers so that they can be used for decision making. Unfortunately, there is no consensus on the criteria to date identifying which biomarkers should be validated. The risk of using the wrong biomarker or selecting the wrong set of biomarkers may lead to the wrong decision of discontinuing a good drug because the adopted biomarker strategy was inaccurately selected. To overcome this problem, pharmaceutical companies tend to rely on their decision-making process of several biomarkers with a hope that multiple biomarkers can be more effective to segment responders from nonresponders. However, using too many biomarkers is not only complex because of the difficulty of data interpretation but also costly. The better strategy for supporting the decision-making process of biomarkers may require fewer, and combination of, nucleic acid (RNA, DNA), protein, and metabolite or lipid biomarkers with complementary predictive properties.

Another challenge in biomarker development is the identification of robust molecular markers that can be measured in readily accessible samples (e.g., blood) that are specific to diseased organ or tissue. Biomarkers should correlate with disease onset or pathogenic process, differentiate pathologies, be proportional to degree of severity of pathology, and be readily released upon development of pathology. Additionally, biomarkers should be sensitive, specific, rapidly and readily detected, predictive, should have a long half-life, be robust and reproducible with a high degree of cross-species selectivity in a noninvasive fashion in various biologic specimens, and should have clinical utility.[80,81]

## 2.14 Conclusions

Recent advances in various omics technologies in conjunction with sophisticated data analysis and computational and statistical analysis methods have made a systems biology approach to drug, drug target, and biomarker discovery more feasible. A majority of omics studies are often one-dimensional. They often rely on a single technology platform, which results in a single layer of information on what is in reality, a set of complex, multilayer, multidimensional, and interactive and highly dynamic networks of a complex system. Therefore, simultaneously interrogating multiple levels of biological complexity including inherited changes in the genome, inherited or modulated changes in the epigenome, modulations in the cellular transcriptome and protein interactome in response to environmental factors and stimuli or therapeutic interventions coupled with systems level analytics may provide a better understanding of biological processes in both physiological or pathophysiological states in temporal and spatial scales.

One approach to streamline and facilitate downstream data analysis is to have a central database linking with all biological datasets that are obtained from different processes and omics technology platforms.

To model complex processes at organismal level, samples from multiple tissues or organs of the same subject need to be evaluated using multiomics data. Because access to human tissue is challenging and in some instances impossible, comparative systems biology using proper animal models may be an option. Blood is in close contact with every organ in an organism; thus, the blood is important medium to assess multiorgan biological processes in disease state and responses to therapeutic interventions. Blood biomarkers that correlate with and are causally related to disease development and progression can help to identify key network states and their association with disease. For example, using organ-specific protein or RNA (e.g., miRNA) biomarkers for diagnostics is one way to obtain information about the state of that specific organ. The rationale is that pathology arises from dynamically disease-associated networks and that diseased or damaged organs will release their contents including RNAs, proteins, and other biomolecules into the circulation. Circulating miRNA biomarkers due to their high degree of tissue specificity, their roles in regulation of multitude of genes and pathways, and their association with specific pathological development of several different diseases may be a complementary approach for the discovery and development of circulating blood biomarkers. For example, we observed that a panel of pancreatic islet β-cell enriched miRNAs were significantly elevated in individuals with impaired glucose tolerance (IGT, prediabetes), type 2 diabetes as well as individuals with latent autoimmune diabetes of adults (LADA), and type 1 diabetes (unpublished results). We also observed that a number of inflammatory cytokines regulated by these miRNAs were also altered in the circulation of these individuals.

Combining these organ- or tissue-specific miRNAs with proteins can help to develop highly informative panels of "composite" biomarkers to identify and stratify various diseases.

While the field of systems biology analytics is evolving, the statistical treatment of individual platform data remains the core activity. These include but are not limited to integration of disparate datasets and biological contextualization through ontologies to reveal high-order biological processes.

To better model complex organisms, it may be necessary to collect samples from multiple tissues of the same set of individuals ideally longitudinally to better reflect natural course of disease evolution. However, acquiring the relevant tissues from humans is difficult and in some instances impossible. Therefore, samples that are readily available (including blood, serum, plasma, urine) through noninvasive or minimally invasive techniques are desired.

Accurate analyses and validation of disparate and multiparametric large datasets are fundamental for identifying, assessing, and tracking these molecular signatures that reflect disease-modified networks as molecular targets with potential therapeutic value. In summary, these molecular signatures associated with specific pathological processes can be used as biomarkers for disease diagnosis, predicting disease development and monitoring disease progression, assessing response to therapeutic interventions, and developing new treatment strategies for better patient outcome.

## Acknowledgments

We thank Quilin Mars for critical reading of this chapter and editorial support. Publicly available information on PubMed and other Internet sites were used for this literature review. We focused on identifying the articles published on the use of multiple technologies for the discovery and development of clinically relevant biomarkers. The research was restricted to the most recent studies in this field, and all research was limited to human studies published in English.

## References


1. Keusch, G.T. What do -*omics* mean for the science and policy of the nutritional sciences? *Am J Clin Nutr* 83, 520S–522S (2006).
2. Zhu, J., Zhang, B., & Schadt, E.E. A systems biology approach to drug discovery. *Adv Genet* 60, 603–35 (2008).
3. Smith, J.C. & Figeys, D. Proteomics technology in systems biology. *Mol Biosyst* 2, 364–70 (2006).
4. Bernas, T., Gregori, G., Asem, E.K., & Robinson, J.P. Integrating cytomics and proteomics. *Mol Cell Proteomics* 5, 2–13 (2006).
5. Rochfort, S. Metabolomics reviewed: A new "omics" platform technology for systems biology and implications for natural products research. *J Nat Prod* 68, 1813–20 (2005).
6. Weckwerth, W. Metabolomics in systems biology. *Annu Rev Plant Biol* 54, 669–89 (2003)
7. Seyhan, A.A. & Ryan, T.E. RNAi screening for the discovery of novel modulators of human disease. *Curr Pharm Biotechnol* 11, 735–56 (2010).
8. Cho, C.R., Labow, M., Reinhardt, M., van Oostrum, J., & Peitsch, M.C. The application of systems biology to drug discovery. *Curr Opin Chem Biol* 10, 294–302 (2006).
9. Cho, W.C.S. (ed). *An omics perspective on cancer research*. Springer, Dordrecht, The Netherlands (2010).
10. Seyhan, A.A. et al. A genome-wide RNAi screen identifies novel targets of neratinib sensitivity leading to neratinib and paclitaxel combination drug treatments. *Mol Biosyst* 7, 1974–89 (2011).
11. Cho, W.C. Cancer biomarkers. In: Hayat, E.M. (ed) *Methods of Cancer Diagnosis, Therapy and Prognosis*. Springer, Dordrecht, The Netherlands (2010).
12. Seyhan, A.A., Varadarajan, U., Choe, S., Liu, W.a., & Ryan, T.E. A genome-wide RNAi screen identifies novel targets of neratinib resistance leading to identification of potential drug resistant genetic markers. *Mol Biosyst* 8, 1553–70 (2012).
13. Finn, W.G. Diagnostic pathology and laboratory medicine in the age of "omics": A paper from the 2006 William Beaumont Hospital Symposium on Molecular Pathology. *J Mol Diagn* 9, 431–6 (2007).
14. Hamacher, M., Herberg, F., Ueffing, M., & Meyer, H.E. Seven successful years of Omics research: The Human Brain Proteome Project within the National German Research Network (NGFN). *Proteomics* 8, 1116–7 (2008).
15. Nicholson, J.K. —Omics dreams of personalized healthcare. *J Proteome Res* 5, 2067–9 (2006).
16. Strijbos, S. Systems thinking. In: Klein, J.T. & Mitcham, C. (eds) *The Oxford Handbook of Interdisciplinarity*, p. 453. Oxford University Press, Oxford, United Kingdom (2010).
17. Hieronymi, A. Understanding systems science: A visual and integrative approach. *Syst Res Behav Sci* 30, 580–95 (2013).
18. Han, J.D. et al. Developmental systems biology flourishing on new technologies. *J Genet Genomics* 35, 577–84 (2008).
19. Hood, L., Heath, J.R., Phelps, M.E., & Lin, B. Systems biology and new technologies enable predictive and preventative medicine. *Science* 306, 640–3 (2004).
20. Wang, K., Lee, I., Carlson, G., Hood, L., & Galas, D. Systems biology and the discovery of diagnostic biomarkers. *Dis Markers* 28, 199–207 (2010).

21. di Bernardo, D. et al. Chemogenomic profiling on a genome-wide scale using reverse-engineered gene networks. *Nat Biotechnol* 23, 377–83 (2005).
22. Gardner, T.S., di Bernardo, D., Lorenz, D., & Collins, J.J. Inferring genetic networks and identifying compound mode of action via expression profiling. *Science* 301, 102–5 (2003).
23. Bhalla, U.S. & Iyengar, R. Emergent properties of networks of biological signaling pathways. *Science* 283, 381–7 (1999).
24. Swanson, R. & Beasley, J.R. Pathway-specific, species, and sub-type counterscreening for better GPCR hits in high throughput screening. *Curr Pharm Biotechnol* 11, 757–63 (2010).
25. Bianconi, F. et al. Computational model of EGFR and IGF1R pathways in lung cancer: A systems biology approach for translational oncology. *Biotechnol Adv* 30, 142–53 (2012).
26. Materi, W. & Wishart, D.S. Computational systems biology in cancer: Modeling methods and applications. *Gene Regul Syst Bio* 1, 91–110 (2007).
27. Lindsay, M.A. Target discovery. *Nat Rev Drug Discov* 2, 831–8 (2003).
28. Sakharkar, M.K. & Sakharkar, K.R. Targetability of human disease genes. *Curr Drug Discov Technol* 4, 48–58 (2007).
29. Butcher, S.P. Target discovery and validation in the post-genomic era. *Neurochem Res* 28, 367–71 (2003).
30. Brown, E.D. & Wright, G.D. New targets and screening approaches in antimicrobial drug discovery. *Chem Rev* 105, 759–74 (2005).
31. Parsons, A.B. et al. Exploring the mode-of-action of bioactive compounds by chemical-genetic profiling in yeast. *Cell* 126, 611–25 (2006).
32. Hughes, T.R. et al. Functional discovery via a compendium of expression profiles. *Cell* 102, 109–26 (2000).
33. Giaever, G. et al. Chemogenomic profiling: Identifying the functional interactions of small molecules in yeast. *Proc Natl Acad Sci USA* 101, 793–8 (2004).
34. Lamb, J. et al. The Connectivity Map: Using gene-expression signatures to connect small molecules, genes, and disease. *Science* 313, 1929–35 (2006).
35. St Onge, R.P. et al. Systematic pathway analysis using high-resolution fitness profiling of combinatorial gene deletions. *Nat Genet* 39, 199–206 (2007).
36. Wagner, J.A., Williams, S.A., & Webster, C.J. Biomarkers and surrogate end points for fit-for-purpose development and regulatory evaluation of new drugs. *Clin Pharmacol Ther* 81, 104–7 (2007).
37. Wulfkuhle, J.D., Paweletz, C.P., Steeg, P.S., Petricoin, E.F., 3rd, & Liotta, L. Proteomic approaches to the diagnosis, treatment, and monitoring of cancer. *Adv Exp Med Biol* 532, 59–68 (2003).
38. Shendure, J., Mitra, R.D., Varma, C., & Church, G.M. Advanced sequencing technologies: methods and goals. *Nat Rev Genet* 5, 335–44 (2004).
39. Seyhan, A.A. Biomarkers in drug discovery and development. *Eur Pharm Rev,* 19–25 (2010).
40. Guay, C., Roggli, E., Nesca, V., Jacovetti, C., & Regazzi, R. Diabetes mellitus, a microRNA-related disease? *Transl Res* 157, 253–64 (2011).
41. Weston, A.D. & Hood, L. Systems biology, proteomics, and the future of health care: Toward predictive, preventative, and personalized medicine. *J Proteome Res* 3, 179–96 (2004).
42. Seyhan, A.A., Varadarajan, U., Choe, S., Liu, W., & Ryan, T.E. A genome-wide RNAi screen identifies novel targets of neratinib resistance leading to

identification of potential drug resistant genetic markers. *Mol Biosyst* 8, 1553–70 (2012).
43. Covert, M.W., Knight, E.M., Reed, J.L., Herrgard, M.J., & Palsson, B.O. Integrating high-throughput and computational data elucidates bacterial networks. *Nature* 429, 92–6 (2004).
44. Davidson, E.H. et al. A genomic regulatory network for development. *Science* 295, 1669–78 (2002).
45. Ideker, T. et al. Integrated genomic and proteomic analyses of a systematically perturbed metabolic network. *Science* 292, 929–34 (2001).
46. Ideker, T. & Lauffenburger, D. Building with a scaffold: Emerging strategies for high- to low-level cellular modeling. *Trends Biotechnol* 21, 255–62 (2003).
47. Kohler, J. et al. Graph-based analysis and visualization of experimental results with ONDEX. *Bioinformatics* 22, 1383–90 (2006).
48. Le Cao, K.A., Boitard, S., & Besse, P. Sparse PLS discriminant analysis: Biologically relevant feature selection and graphical displays for multiclass problems. *BMC Bioinformatics* 12, 253 (2011).
49. Poste, G. Bring on the biomarkers. *Nature* 469, 156–7 (2011).
50. Azuaje, F., Devaux, Y., & Wagner, D. Computational biology for cardiovascular biomarker discovery. *Brief Bioinform* 10, 367–77 (2009).
51. Camargo, A. & Azuaje, F. Identification of dilated cardiomyopathy signature genes through gene expression and network data integration. *Genomics* 92, 404–13 (2008).
52. Frank, E., Hall, M., Trigg, L., Holmes, G., & Witten, I.H. Data mining in bioinformatics using Weka. *Bioinformatics* 20, 2479–81 (2004).
53. Saeys, Y., Inza, I., & Larranaga, P. A review of feature selection techniques in bioinformatics. *Bioinformatics* 23, 2507–17 (2007).
54. Deschamps, A.M. & Spinale, F.G. Pathways of matrix metalloproteinase induction in heart failure: Bioactive molecules and transcriptional regulation. *Cardiovasc Res* 69, 666–76 (2006).
55. Camargo, A. & Azuaje, F. Linking gene expression and functional network data in human heart failure. *PLoS One* 2, e1347 (2007).
56. Ginsburg, G.S., Seo, D., & Frazier, C. Microarrays coming of age in cardiovascular medicine: standards, predictions, and biology. *J Am Coll Cardiol* 48, 1618–20 (2006).
57. Ideker, T. & Sharan, R. Protein networks in disease. *Genome Res* 18, 644–52 (2008).
58. Butcher, E.C. Can cell systems biology rescue drug discovery? *Nat Rev Drug Discov* 4, 461–7 (2005).
59. Butcher, E.C., Berg, E.L., & Kunkel, E.J. Systems biology in drug discovery. *Nat Biotechnol* 22, 1253–9 (2004).
60. Wu, L. et al. Global survey of human T leukemic cells by integrating proteomics and transcriptomics profiling. *Mol Cell Proteomics* 6, 1343–53 (2007).
61. Kim, M.S. et al. A draft map of the human proteome. *Nature* 509, 575–81 (2014).
62. Rajasethupathy, P., Vayttaden, S.J., & Bhalla, U.S. Systems modeling: A pathway to drug discovery. *Curr Opin Chem Biol* 9, 400–6 (2005).
63. Young, D.W. et al. Integrating high-content screening and ligand-target prediction to identify mechanism of action. *Nat Chem Biol* 4, 59–68 (2008).
64. Subramanian, A. et al. Gene set enrichment analysis: A knowledge-based approach for interpreting genome-wide expression profiles. *Proc Natl Acad Sci USA* 102, 15545–50 (2005).

65. Jensen, L.J., Saric, J., & Bork, P. Literature mining for the biologist: From information retrieval to biological discovery. *Nat Rev Genet* 7, 119–29 (2006).
66. Kanehisa, M., Goto, S., Furumichi, M., Tanabe, M., & Hirakawa, M. KEGG for representation and analysis of molecular networks involving diseases and drugs. *Nucleic Acids Res* 38, D355–60 (2010).
67. Wingender, E., Dietze, P., Karas, H., & Knuppel, R. TRANSFAC: A database on transcription factors and their DNA binding sites. *Nucleic Acids Res* 24, 238–41 (1996).
68. Robinson, S.W., Fernandes, M., & Husi, H. Current advances in systems and integrative biology. *Comput Struct Biotechnol J* 11, 35–46 (2014).
69. Covert, M.W., Xiao, N., Chen, T.J., & Karr, J.R. Integrating metabolic, transcriptional regulatory and signal transduction models in *Escherichia coli*. *Bioinformatics* 24, 2044–50 (2008).
70. Karr, J.R. et al. A whole-cell computational model predicts phenotype from genotype. *Cell* 150, 389–401 (2012).
71. Macklin, D.N., Ruggero, N.A., & Covert, M.W. The future of whole-cell modeling. *Curr Opin Biotechnol* 28, 111–5 (2014).
72. Eungdamrong, N.J. & Iyengar, R. Modeling cell signaling networks. *Biol Cell* 96, 355–62 (2004).
73. Burrowes, K.S. et al. Multi-scale computational models of the airways to unravel the pathophysiological mechanisms in asthma and chronic obstructive pulmonary disease (AirPROM). *Interface Focus* 3, 20120057 (2013).
74. Kumar, A. et al. Multi-tissue computational modeling analyzes pathophysiology of type 2 diabetes in MKR mice. *PLoS One* 9, e102319 (2014).
75. Kansal, A.R. Modeling approaches to type 2 diabetes. *Diabetes Technol Ther* 6, 39–47 (2004).
76. Wang, Q. et al. miR-17-92 cluster accelerates adipocyte differentiation by negatively regulating tumor-suppressor Rb2/p130. *Proc Natl Acad Sci USA* 105, 2889–94 (2008).
77. Heneghan, H.M., Miller, N., McAnena, O.J., O'Brien, T., & Kerin, M.J. Differential miRNA expression in omental adipose tissue and in the circulation of obese patients identifies novel metabolic biomarkers. *J Clin Endocrinol Metab* 96, E846–50 (2011).
78. Rifai, N., Gillette, M.A., & Carr, S.A. Protein biomarker discovery and validation: The long and uncertain path to clinical utility. *Nat Biotechnol* 24, 971–83 (2006).
79. Wang, J.F. et al. Serum miR-146a and miR-223 as potential new biomarkers for sepsis. *Biochem Biophys Res Commun* 394, 184–8 (2010).
80. Illei, G.G., Tackey, E., Lapteva, L., & Lipsky, P.E. Biomarkers in systemic lupus erythematosus. I. General overview of biomarkers and their applicability. *Arthritis Rheum* 50, 1709–20 (2004).
81. Etheridge, A., Lee, I., Hood, L., Galas, D., & Wang, K. Extracellular microRNA: A new source of biomarkers. *Mutat Res* 717, 85–90 (2011).

# 3

# *Immunogenicity of Biological Products: Current Perspectives and Future Implications*

**Candida Fratazzi, Attila Seyhan, and Claudio Carini**

**CONTENTS**



**ABSTRACT** This chapter reflects on the limitations for the interpretation of the relative immunogenicity of biologics. Currently, there is a considerable interest in the development and clinical use of biologics and biosimilars to treat a wide range of diseases. However, there is a growing concern regarding the development of adverse effects (AEs) like immunogenicity in the form of antidrug antibodies (ADA) production and neutralizing antibodies (Nabs). Immunogenicity to biologics and biosimilars represents a significant impediment in the continuing therapy of patients. Several attempts aiming to reduce the incidence of immunogenicity have been made to identify factors that contribute toward the onset of immunogenic response to biologics/biosimilars. An in-depth understanding of the cellular and molecular mechanism sustaining the immunogenic response will likely ameliorate the safety profile of biologics/biosimilars. This chapter addresses the mechanistic basis of ADA generation to biologics/biosimilars, the importance of patient populations in generating an immunogenic response, the impact of ADA and Nab on the safety profile of a drug, and the importance of pursuing the appropriate assays to measure immunogenicity in patients treated with biologics/biosimilars and the potential differences between innovators and biosimilars. Of course, the ultimate goal will be the identification of specific factors that influence the immunogenic response and consequently, the management of immunogenicity to biologics and biosimilars.

## 3.1 Introduction

The immune response to biologics is still a very elusive process governed by a large number of factors. Here, we will cover the different factors involved in the development of the immune response toward biologics and strategies to reduce immunogenicity. We will also address the implications of the complex immune response to the development of biosimilars.

Biologics comprise a rapid growing class of therapeutic molecules including monoclonal antibodies, cytokines, and growth factors that play a crucial role in modulating specific biological functions. Monoclonal antibodies are typically designed to target specific disease pathways [1,2]. Biosimilars are original versions of the (innovator) biologic molecule with demonstrated similarity in structure, function, efficacy, and safety profiles to the reference product. Biologic drugs, including biosimilars, have the potential to elicit an immunogenic response (immunogenicity), which may have an impact on the product safety and/or efficacy. However, in some cases, immunogenicity has been shown to have a significant effect on safety with induction of infusion site reactions, hypersensitivity reactions, and cytokine storm reactions. Immunogenicity is characterized by the presence of ADA detected in the circulation of individuals after the administration of a biopharmaceutical. The formation of ADA [3–6] can cross-react with endogenous counterpart foreign tertiary structures, thus having an impact on the efficacy of the biological product by generating Nabs and affecting the clearance as well [7–9]. For all these reasons, the immunogenicity is measured during drug development, and very often surveillance of immunogenicity goes on long after the study has ended. One of the most feasible factors responsible for an immune response to biologics is the level of nonself of the biological products. Many examples have been reported in the literature, the oldest being insulin, which has been in use since 1920. Several factors may be responsible for the induction of immunogenicity such as structural changes of the protein and presence of aggregates. Indeed, partial unfolding of monomeric proteins may elicit an immune response, especially if the unfolding results in exposure of hidden antigen sites. However, it is still unclear whether this mechanism does play any role in the development of immunogenicity. Unfolded molecules tend to aggregate rapidly forming a nonnative aggregate, which can be potentially immunogenic. Several reports in the literature have shown that nonhuman carbohydrate residues may be immunogenic. Another aberration may be represented by nonnative glycosylation patterns, including the exposure of protective antigen site on the protein. Few evidences have proven that altered glycosylation patterns of self-proteins are implicated in the development of autoreactive clones, thus generating an immune response. Aggregates may represent another risk factor for the induction of an immune response to a variety of protein drugs and high level of aggregates generally raises alerts with the regulatory agencies. Far more elusive is the effect of the product-related factors. Those factors are not part of the active ingredients found in the final product such as degradation products, process-related impurities, and additives. The combinations of those factors together with the compound coadministration generate a significant activation of the immune system that also attacks the therapeutic drug, which enhances the other weak immunogenic response. It is impossible to narrow down the danger signals that will induce immunogenicity toward a specific compound. Aside from the different factors introduced by the drug, the characteristics of the patient to be treated play another important role in the induction of immune response toward biologics. Many factors like genetic and epigenetic footprint of the patient may play a crucial role in eliciting various strengths of the immune response. Furthermore, the pathogenic milieu of a specific disease may reduce or exacerbate the activity of the immune system, and hence reduce or increase the potential for an immune response to the biologics. Dose and dose regimens do also play a role in inducing an immune response. It is well accepted that a high dose followed by frequent administration have a higher chance of triggering a robust immune response toward the biologics compared to low doses and less frequent administration. The route of administration also plays an important role in the elicitation of the immune response. The strength of the immune response to an antigen can be ordered by the route of administration namely subcutaneous, intramuscular, and intravenous. The relationship between the route of administration and the induction of the immune response has been well documented. Several attempts have been made to reduce immunogenicity of specific products such as optimizing the structure, modifying the biomacromolecule, and improving the formulation and clinical measures (proper handling of the product will avoid unexpected adverse events). In summary, the cause of unwanted immunogenicity and antigenicity of the biologics are still not well understood (Figure 3.1).

However, given that the number of new biologics and biosimilars continue to grow there is considerable value in standardizing methods for evaluating and monitoring immunogenicity to unravel the factors that contribute to the elicitation of immunogenicity. Considerable attention has been given to the structure of the product itself, the mode of administration, comorbidities, the underlying disease, and patient's genetic milieu [10–13]. Thus, it is critical that immunogenicity is evaluated throughout the various phases of clinical development and during postmarketing surveillance. The evaluation of the ADA formation is a common practice for monitoring immunogenicity in patients treated with biological products [14–16].

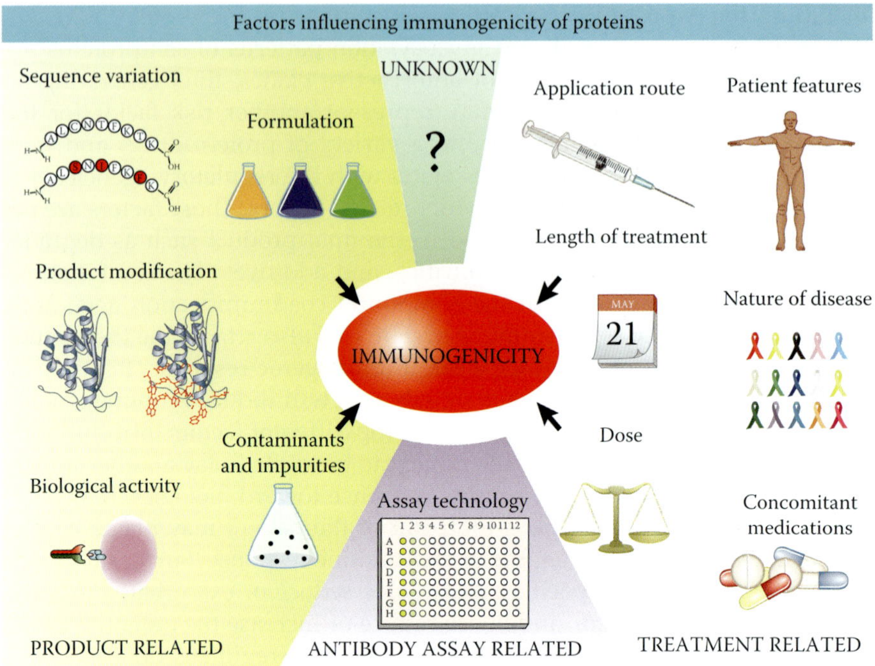


**FIGURE 3.1**
The immunogenic potential of therapeutic proteins can be reduced by the design of the production system and downstream processing. However, some of the factors involved are still unknown. Redrawn from Sugiyama, N., http://www.epivax.com/wp-content/uploads/2013/05/Dr.-Sugiyama_Pfizer_EpiVax-Immunogenicity-Seminar_May2013.pdf

A considerable attention has also been given to the detectable levels of ADA and Nabs to assess the immunogenicity of a given biological product. However, new data on the immunogenicity of a biological product are now generated by measuring pharmacogenomics markers that have not previously been used to evaluate the level of immunogenicity toward a specific biological product. Altogether, this new information will provide a better understanding of the clinical implications of immunogenicity.

## 3.2 Importance of Patient Population on Generating Immune Response

Different patient populations with different genetic and epigenetic background will give rise to different immune response and consequently to different immunogenicity toward a specific biological product.

Thus, a meaningful interpretation of the immunogenicity data should take in the account the history of the patient, including the treatment history as well as the knowledge of the disease that is intended to be treated. The evaluation of the immunogenic response toward a specific biological product can be assessed either in healthy volunteers who currently are not receiving any therapy except the study drug or in patients affected by a specific disease for which the therapeutic use of a biological product is indicated. Different disease status as well as the use of concomitant medications (e.g., immunosuppressive drugs) may give rise to different immunogenic response among those patients. It is a common practice to control the potential immunogenic response in patients treated with biologics by treating them on a background of immunosuppressive drugs. This is the case, for instance, of rheumatoid arthritis (RA), where the biological drug is administered on a background of methotrexate (MTX). There are several reports in the literature about the importance of immunosuppressive drugs like MTX prior to biologics administration and their effect in tempering immunogenicity.

The history of prior exposure as well as frequency, duration, consistency of the treatment, and the biologic dose administered should be taken into account during the immunogenicity risk assessment evaluation. Clearly the treatment regimens may be highly variable as for instance is the case with Factor VIII. For all the other biological products, the treatment regime is more consistent with period of interruption, the so-called drug holidays during chronic dosage schedule. This is done in an attempt to control adverse events. This strategic measure tends to reduce and control the risk of immunogenicity. Another important aspect that should be considered is that in the case of biological products the drug tends to stay onboard for a considerable length of time. Monoclonal antibodies have often a long half-life, thus in some occasions drugs stay onboard up to 2 years after the last dose. Thus, the number of days of drug staying onboard can be much greater than number of treatment days. In that case, immunogenicity is affected by cumulative doses and exposure days. Those two parameters need to be accurately determined for each biological product used. Naturally, while the determination of the doses and treatment days is relatively straightforward, that is not the case with exposure days related to the biological product concentrations. Clinical assessment is typically conducted at interim time points along the duration of the study. Thus, time to endpoint is an additional variable that should be taken in consideration when evaluating the impact of immunogenicity on the outcome.

## 3.3 Development of Immunogenic Response against a Drug

The immune response toward a biological product has generally been assessed by measuring ADA response. However, it is important to underline that the immune response against a biological product comprises the innate and adaptive immune responses. As a result of those two components, the administered biological product may coadminister impurities, or the specific nature of the disease pathogenesis may elicit proinflammatory or anti-inflammatory cytokines, chemokines, and other signals that impact the efficiency of antigen presentation and drug-specific lymphocytic responses (T and B lymphocytes) that determines whether the level of B cell activation is sufficient to elicit high-titer, high-affinity ADA response that could have an impact on the efficacy and safety (e.g., hypersensitivity reactions or immune complexes [ICs] formation) of the drug administered. The T lymphocyte activation also plays a role in mediating adverse events such as infusion reactions and ICs formation. In conclusion, both compartments, namely T and B, should be taken in the account when measuring the immunogenicity profile of a specific biological product.

The immunogenicity profile of a specific drug and the clinical consequences are very much based on the characteristics of ADA, which are heterogeneous, containing a mixture of different isotypes, specificities, and affinities [5,17]. The typical pattern of an immune response is primarily based on a low affinity and transient immunoglobulin (Ig) M response, which is difficult to detect during normal ADA monitoring. The story is different when ICs are formed that occasionally may activate complement [18]. Switching to other class or subclass of isotypes occurs along with random somatic mutation of the Ig variable region, complementarity determining regions (CDRs), genes when CD4+T helper cells get activated. As a result of it, a phenomenon known as "affinity maturation" leads to the production of ADA with higher affinity for the biological product. Isotype composition of ADA determines a potential for clinical effects such as complement activation, antibody-dependent cellular cytotoxicity (ADCC), mast cell sensitization, and interactions with the specialized neonatal Fc receptor, which controls cross-epithelial and placental transport as well as the serum half-life of ADA [19]. ADAs that bind epitope(s) close to the target-binding site are likely to block or "neutralize" the target biological activity. ADAs that bind to the target can easily compromise the pharmacokinetic (PK) of the drug by increasing or decreasing the clearance of the drug [9,20]. If the immune response continues, further expansion of the B cell compartment does occur that results in a phenomenon called "epitope spreading" in which ADA are becoming more diverse in their specificity to bind different structures on the biological product. There are reported cases in which ADA responses so-called transient immune response may decrease and even disappear over time, even in the presence of continuous administration of the biological product due to the development of a partial immune tolerance [20,21].

## 3.4 Antidrug Antibody Assays

Given the nature of ADA heterogeneity, it becomes obvious that the use of reliable analytical methods is critical to appropriately evaluate the ADA response and determine the potential impact on the clinical outcome.

Different ADA assay formats are available, each with pros and cons like limitations in sensitivity and specificity of the assay. Although most biological products are immunogenic under certain conditions, often immunogenicity is observed in some subjects over the course of treatment, and only a small number of patients will typically have a detectable and measurable ADA levels. Using current technology and reagents, it is possible to develop highly sensitive ADA screening assays capable of detecting the most prevalent classes of ADA (IgM, IgG, and IgA); however, due to the low IgE level in circulation, specific assays needs to be adopted. Specific clinical studies with biological products need to establish a cut point that allows sufficient sensitivity/specificity in order to assure the detection of true positive samples. The confirmatory assay usually consists of a competitive inhibition assay, in which samples are tested spiked and unspiked with an excess of the biological product. The excessive amount of the biological product binds the specific ADA, preventing it from binding to the assay capture reagent, causing a signal inhibition in the assay relative to the signal generated by the unspiked sample. Qualitative ADA results (positive/negative) may be supplemented with measurements of the relative magnitude of ADA responses (e.g., titers) to provide more useful information for the interpretation of ADA data. In conclusion, the ADA levels are not "clinically relevant" in the sense that identifying a sample as positive for ADA is not an indicator that the level of ADA present in the sample is sufficient to cause a clinically meaningful effect (e.g., alter PK, efficacy, or cause adverse effect [AE]). However, sensitive assays capable of detecting all ADA generated definitively help to establish the clinical effects of the measured ADA when initially studying the immunogenicity profile of a specific biological product. Sensitive ADA assays are also needed to correlate ADA development with underlying causes of immunogenicity and identify markers of immune response, e.g., markers of early events in triggering an immune response to the drug or indications of incomplete activation of the immune system that could lead to immune tolerance by the biological product.

Other assays may be developed to further characterize ADA positive samples and provide additional data to a more extensive understanding and better interpretation of the clinical relevance of the ADA response to a specific biological product. For example, an assay that specifically measures ADA that neutralize the biological effect of a product may be useful in determining the impact of ADA on pharmacodynamics (PD) effect or efficacy, whereas an assay that measures drug-specific IgE may help to identify the underlying cause of hypersensitivity reactions. A variety of different assay formats may be used for screening. Because of the abovementioned limitations, ADA data should be usually interpreted in combination with PK, PD, and efficacy data to define the immunogenicity profile of the specific biological product studied. Prior to use, ADA assays should be analytically validated to assure reliable performance over time and establish which changes in ADA measurements are likely to be meaningful [22–24]. An underlying conclusion to be drawn from all of those

biosimilar and the innovator. Of course, it may be argued that the biosimilar may be safer than the innovator. Indeed, in the last few decades, the manufactures have improved quite a bit. The production process has been improved so considerably that it is difficult to make a product that will be as bad as the innovator with respect to the amount of impurities and product degradation. However, since the production host and site and facilities will be different from the innovator, the biosimilar may have other impurities and degradation products. Thus, the potential for a biosimilar of inducing immunogenicity may be greater than the innovator. In addition, the use of other formulation principles, materials, and procedures during storage and administration may affect the level of degradation products upon the actual administration of the biosimilar.

Many factors, as previously discussed, can influence immunogenicity, such as changes in glycosylation patterns that may expose or hide antigenic components, alter solubility, or influence protein degradation. Importantly, data have demonstrated that presence of aggregates, impurities, or contaminants can induce undesired immune responses. Thus, alterations in manufacturing processes/storage conditions may result in altered immunogenicity of biosimilars compared with reference products. In biosimilars as with the innovators, the effects of ADA include reduction in serum levels, adverse events, and formation of Nabs. The immunogenicity concern has been highlighted by the increase in number of cases of pure red cell aplasia associated with a specific formulation of epoetin alfa [28–30]. This episode raised considerable apprehension in the medical and regulatory community and made the world to look at biosimilars with extreme caution. The immunological form of pure red cell aplasia was determined by the production of Nabs against endogenous epoetin. Most of the cases occurred in patients treated with Eprex, the biosimilar of epoetin alfa, produced outside of the United States. The most plausible cause was a subtle change in the manufacturing process. Precisely, in the formulation of Eprex, the human albumin stabilizer was replaced by polysorbate 80 and glycine. Polysorbate 80 was supposed to be responsible for the generation of increased immunogenicity of Eprex by eliciting the formation of epoetin-containing micelles or by interacting with leachates released by the uncoated rubber stoppers of prefilled syringes [31]. In another study, many patients treated with recombinant interferons demonstrated the presence of Nabs that significantly suppressed their own production [6]. The development of pegylated thrombopoietin megakaryocyte growth and development factor was stopped in clinical trials because of treatment-associated thrombocytopenia in 13 of 325 healthy volunteers [32,33].

The recent EMA guidelines on comparability of biosimilars state that preclinical data may be insufficient to demonstrate immunologic safety of some biosimilars. In these cases, the immunological safety can only be demonstrated in cohorts of patients enrolled in clinical trials and postmarketing surveillance. The current available assays though more specific and sensitive than previous ELISA still present some considerable limitations to assess the detectable level of immunogenicity. Thus, there is a need to validate and standardize those assays. Due to limited clinical database at the time of approval of a biosimilar, vigorous pharmacovigilance is required.

Immunogenicity is a unique safety issue with biosimilars. However, lack of validation and standardization of methods for detecting immunogenicity further implies the necessity for robust pharmacovigilance programs. The monitoring data of adverse reactions to drugs should be exhaustive, including the type of adverse event and data about drug such as proprietary name, international nonproprietary name (INN), and dosage given.

## 3.7 One versus Two Screening Assays

The revised guidelines on immunogenicity for biosimilars products recommend that two assays should be performed with both the reference and biosimilar molecules in parallel to measure the immune response against the product that was received by each patient. However, even for high complex and relatively immunogenic molecules like infliximab, duplicative testing in parallel assays (one using the innovator and the other the biosimilar version) have not shown appreciable differences. The use of two distinct assays requires a high burden for reagent quality control. The use of separate assays might decrease assay precision and specificity when it comes to comparing results. To limit any bioanalytical bias associated with different assays and different reagents, it would be better to use a single assay to test both the innovator and the biosimilar. The screening assay will be using both the unlabeled candidate biosimilar and reference products as competing antigens. This approach should be able to detect ADA that recognize new epitopes on the biosimilars while avoiding the additional level of assay variability associated with use two different assays.

## 3.8 Conclusions

There is no doubt that biologics shall become a relevant part of the future healthcare landscape. With more and more patents expiring, biosimilars will increasingly become available and play a critical role in the therapeutic landscape. Immunogenicity has been and continues to be a major concern when developing a biological product either as an innovator or biosimilar. Especially in biosimilars the limited clinical data currently available pose a considerable challenge to the regulatory agencies and the developers to assess the immunogenicity biosimilarity. It is important that we get a good overview on the immunogenicity clinical data especially when it comes to biosimilars.

## References


1. Dimitrov DS. Therapeutic proteins. *Methods Mol Biol*. 2012;899:1–26.
2. Leader B, Baca QJ, Golan DE. Protein therapeutics: A summary and pharmacological classification. *Nat Rev Drug Discov*. 2008;7(1):21–39.
3. McKoy JM, Stonecash RE, Cournoyer D, Rossert J, Nissenson AR, Raisch DW, et al. Epoetin-associated pure red cell aplasia: Past, present, and future considerations. *Transfusion*. 2008;48(8):1754–62.
4. Buttel IC, Chamberlain P, Chowers Y, Ehmann F, Greinacher A, Jefferis R, et al. Taking immunogenicity assessment of therapeutic proteins to the next level. *Biologicals*. 2011;39(2):100–9.
5. Brinks V, Weinbuch D, Baker M, Dean Y, Stas P, Kostense S, et al. Preclinical models used for immunogenicity prediction of therapeutic proteins. *Pharm Res*. 2013;30(7):1719–28.
6. Li J, Yang C, Xia Y, Bertino A, Glaspy J, Roberts M, et al. Thrombocytopenia caused by the development of antibodies to thrombopoietin. *Blood*. 2001;98(12):3241–8.
7. Wolbink GJ, Vis M, Lems W, Voskuyl AE, de Groot1 E, Nurmohamed MT, et al. Development of antiinfliximab antibodies and relationship to clinical response in patients with rheumatoid arthritis. *Arthritis Rheum*. 2006;54(3):190–7.
8. Bertolotto A, Sala A, Malucchi S, Marnetto F, Caldano M, Di Sapio A, et al. Biological activity of interferon betas in patients with multiple sclerosis is affected by treatment regimen and neutralising antibodies. *J Neurol Neurosurg Psychiatry*. 2004;75(9):1294–8.
9. Chirmule N, Jawa V, Meibohm B. Immunogenicity to therapeutic proteins: Impact on PK/PD and efficacy. *AAPS J*. 2012;14(2):296–302.
10. Rosenberg AS, Worobec AS. A risk-based approach to immunogenciity concerns of therapeutic protein products. Part 1. Considering consequences of the immune response to a protein. *Biopharm Int*. 2004;17:22–6.
11. Rosenberg AS, Worobec AS. A risk-based approach to immunogenicity concerns of therapeutic protein products. Part 2. Considering host-specific and product-specific factors impacting immunogenicity. *Biopharm Int*. 2004;17:35–41.
12. Rosenberg AS, Worobec AS. A risk-based approach to immunogenicity concerns of therapeutic protein products, Part 3: Effects of manufacturing changes in immunogenicity and the utility of animal immunogenicity studies. *Biopharm Int*. 2005;18;452–9.
13. Luetkens T, Schafhausen P, Uhlich F, Stasche T, Akbulak R, Bartels BM, et al. Expression, epigenetic regulation, and humoral immunogenicity of cancer-testis antigens in chronic myeloid leukemia. *Leuk Res*. 2010;34(12):1647–55.
14. Gadzinowski J, Tansey SP, Wysocki J, Kopinska E, Majda-Stanislawska E, Czajka H, et al. Safety and immunogenicity of a 13-valent pneumococcal conjugate vaccine manufactured with and without polysorbate 80 given to healthy infants at 2, 3, 4, and 12 months of age. *Pediatr Infect Dis J*. 2015;34(2):180–5.
15. Mazor R, Eberle JA, Hu X, Vassall AN, Onda M, Beers R, et al. Recombinant immunotoxin for cancer treatment with low immunogenicity by identification and silencing of human T-cell epitopes. *Proc Natl Acad Sci USA*. 2014;111(23):8571–6.

16. Xu ZH, Lee H, Vu T, Hu C, Yan H, Baker D, et al. Population pharmacokinetics of golimumab in patients with ankylosing spondylitis: Impact of body weight and immunogenicity. *Int J Clin Pharmacol Ther.* 2010;48(9):596–607.
17. Duan F, Duitama J, Al Seesi S, Ayres CM, Corcelli SA, Pawashe AP, et al. Genomic and bioinformatic profiling of mutational neoepitopes reveals new rules to predict anticancer immunogenicity. *J Exp Med.* 2014;211(11):2231–48.
18. van der Kolk LE, Grillo-Lopez AJ, Baars JW, Hack CE, van Oers MH. Complement activation plays a key role in the side-effects of rituximab treatment. *Br J Haematol.* 2001;115(4):807–11.
19. Ward ES, Ghetie V. The effector functions of immunoglobulins: Implications for therapy. *Ther Immunol.* 1995;2(2):77–94.
20. Chen X, Hickling T, Kraynov E, Kuang B, Parng C, Vicini P. A mathematical model of the effect of immunogenicity on therapeutic protein pharmacokinetics. *AAPS J.* 2013;15(4):1141–54.
21. Wight J, Paisley S. The epidemiology of inhibitors in haemophilia A: A systematic review. *Haemophilia* 2003;9(4):418–35.
22. West TW, Cree BA. Natalizumab dosage suspension: Are we helping or hurting? *Ann Neurol.* 2010;68(3):395–9.
23. Stas P, Lasters I. [Immunogenicity of therapeutic antibodies]. *Med Sci (Paris).* 2009;25(12):1070–7.
24. Stas P, Lasters I. Strategies for preclinical immunogenicity assessment of protein therapeutics. *IDrugs.* 2009;12(3):169–73.
25. EMA. Guideline on Immunogenicity Assessment of Biotechnology-Derived Therapeutic Proteins. Doc Ref. EMEA/CHMP/BMWP/14327/2006.2008.
26. EMA. Guideline on Immunogenicity Assessment of Monoclonal Antibodies Intended for *In Vivo* Clinical Use. Doc Ref. EMA/CHMP/BMWP/86289/2010. 2012.
27. FDA. FDA Guidance for Industry: Assay Development for Immunogenicity Testing of Therapeutic Proteins (Draft Guidance). 2009.
28. Mellstedt H, Crommelin DJA, Aravind SK, et al. Interpretation of the new EMEA guidelines in similar biological medicinal products. *Eur J Hosp Pharm Pract.* 2007;13:68–74.
29. Haselbeck A. Epoetins: Differences and their relevance to immunogenicity. *Curr Med Res Opin.* 2003;19:430–2.
30. Locatelli F, Del Vecchio L, Pozzoni P. Pure red-cell aplasia "epidemic"—Mystery completely revealed? *Perit Dial Int.* 2007;27(Suppl 2):303–7.
31. Oberg K, Alm G. The incidence and clinical significance of antibodies to interferon-α in patients with solid tumors. *Biotherapy.* 1997;10:1–5.
32. Nowicki M. Basic facts about biosimilars. *Kidney Blood Press Res.* 2007;30:267–72.
33. Mellstedt H, Niederwieser D, Ludwig H. The challenge of biosimilars. *Ann Oncol.* 2008;19:411–9.

# 4

# *Interchangeability between Biosimilar and Innovator Drug Products*

**Bo Jin, Sandeep M. Menon, Kerry B. Barker, and Steven Ye Hua**

**CONTENTS**

**ABSTRACT** Biosimilarity does not automatically imply interchangeability. For a biosimilar to be considered interchangeable with a reference product, it has to be shown by sponsors and be approved by health regulatory authorities that the biosimilar produces the same clinical result as the reference product in any given patient, and repeatedly switching or alternating between biosimilar and reference product presents no greater safety or efficacy risk than continued use of the reference product. While these requirements for interchangeability have been made clear by the Biologics Price Competition and Innovation Act (BPCIA) of 2009, there remains to be many challenging and unsolved problems for sponsors on how to demonstrate interchangeability in a scientific, clinically meaningful, and practically feasible way. This chapter presents scientific considerations and new methodologies to evaluate interchangeability between biosimilar and innovator products. Specifically, clinical trial study designs and statistical analyses on interchangeability, as well as interchangeability among several biosimilars and their reference products and its impact on drug pharmacovigilance, are discussed.

## 4.1 Introduction

A biosimilar may be shown to be highly similar to a reference (its branded, original innovator) drug product based on data derived from analytical, animal, and clinical studies. Minor differences are allowed in clinically inactive components if no clinically meaningful differences exist between the proposed biosimilar and the reference product with regard to safety, purity, and potency (presumably pharmacokinetics [PK], pharmacodynamics [PD], clinical safety, and efficacy). Once the biosimilar is shown to be highly similar to reference products, it may be further determined to be interchangeable with the reference product [1].

It follows from the Biologics Price Competition and Innovation Act of 2009 (BPCIA) [2], passed by the U.S. Congress, that a biological product is considered to be interchangeable with the reference originator's product if

1. The biological product is biosimilar to the reference product.
2. It can be expected to produce the same clinical result in any given patient.
3. For a biological product that is administered more than once to an individual, the risk in terms of safety or diminished efficacy of alternating or switching between the use of the biological product and the reference product is no greater than the risk of using the reference product without such alternation or switch.

The first requirement is the foundation of interchangeability (an interchangeable biological product must be shown biosimilar first to a reference product), and the second and the third requirements are specific to interchangeability. In other words, biosimilarity does not automatically imply interchangeability. For a biosimilar to be considered interchangeable with a reference product, it has to be shown by sponsors and be approved by health regulatory authorities that the biosimilar drug product produces the same clinical result as the reference product in any given patient and repeatedly switching or alternating between the biosimilar and the reference product presents no greater safety or efficacy risk than continued use of the reference product.

While the definition by the U.S. Congress on interchangeability seems to have given some directions, the regulatory requirements on interchangeability, however, are still emerging or at least not completely clear from many health and regulatory authorities. In fact, there remains many challenging and unsolved problems for sponsors on how to demonstrate in a scientific, clinically meaningful, and practically feasible way that a biosimilar is interchangeable with the reference product. On the other hand, even if interchangeability has not been established, a prescribing physician may switch medications between biosimilars and reference products, and a pharmacist may substitute a certain prescribed product with another equivalent product without prescribing physicians' knowledge. Such a substitution is considered to be an automatic substitution. In fact, it varies by country as for the current practice of substitution and switching between biosimilars and reference products. In the United States, the Food and Drug Administration (FDA) does not have a clear threshold on interchangeability, and automatic substitution between biosimilar and reference products is determined at state level [3]. Health Canada does not support automatic substitution but allows provinces to determine interchangeability [4]. Pharmaceuticals and Medical Devices Agency (PMDA) in Japan highly discourages interchangeability and automatic substitution [5]. European Medicines Agency (EMA)'s evaluation and approval for a biosimilar does not include recommendations on whether a biosimilar could be used interchangeably with its reference medicine, and the legal decision on interchangeability is left to its member states and in fact, no country has explicitly authorized interchangeability for biologicals including biosimilars [6].

Although the regulatory requirements on the threshold of interchangeability have yet to be established, it is clear that interchangeability needs to be shown through comparability clinical studies by sponsors. In the following sections, we will discuss some clinical and statistical aspects of comparability clinical studies on interchangeability of biosimilars. Section 4.2 introduces the definitions of the two aspects of interchangeability: switching and alternating. Section 4.3 discusses study designs on interchangeability. Statistical methods on testing interchangeability are presented in Section 4.4. Interchangeability among several biosimilars and their reference products, and the interchangeability impact on drug pharmacovigilance are discussed in Section 4.5. Section 4.6 provides some concluding remarks.

## 4.2 Switching and Alternating

As seen in the definition of interchangeability, when a biological product is administered more than once to an individual, interchangeability includes the concept of switching and alternating between a reference biological product and its biosimilars. The concept of switching is referred to as not only the switch from reference to test (R to T) or test to reference (T to R) (the narrow sense of switching) but also reference to reference (R to R) and test to test (T to T) (different R's and T's in the broader sense of switching). As a result, in order to assess switching, R to T, T to R, R to R, and T to T need to be assessed based on certain criteria under a valid study design. The concept of alternating is referred to as either the switch from reference to test and then switch back to reference, i.e., R to T to R or vice versa, i.e., T to R to T. Therefore, the differences between "the switch from R to T" or "the switch from T to R" and "the switch from T to R" or "the switch from R to T" need to be assessed in order to address the concept of alternating. We focus on the interchangeability in the narrow sense in this chapter, and discuss the design and analysis on the interchangeability for biosimilars. We will give a brief discussion on the interchangeability in the broader sense in Section 4.5.1.

## 4.3 Study Designs for Interchangeability

Several study designs to investigate interchangeability (switching and alternating) are discussed by Chow [7]. We describe a few designs in the following context, but readers may refer to the original discussions for more design options and the corresponding details.

1. Balaam Design
2. Two-Stage Design
3. Two-Sequence Dual Design
4. Modified Balaam Design
5. Complete Modified Balaam Design

### 4.3.1 Balaam Design

Balaam design is a design to investigate switching, which is a 4 × 2 (four-sequence two-treatment) crossover design, denoted by (TT, RR, TR, RT). Subjects are randomly assigned to receive one of the four treatment sequences: TT, RR, TR, and RT. A Balaam design is the combination of a parallel design (the first two sequences TT and RR) and a crossover design (the third and the fourth sequences TR and RT). The following comparisons can be assessed by a 4 × 2 Balaam design:

1. Comparisons by sequence.
2. Comparisons by period.
3. T versus R based on the sequences of TR and RT—this is equivalent to a typical 2 × 2 crossover design.
4. T versus R given T based on sequences of TT and TR.
5. R versus T given R based on sequences of RR and RT.
6. The comparison between 1 and 3 for assessment of treatment by period interaction.

### 4.3.2 Two-Stage Design

The design has two stages. In the first stage, subjects are randomly assigned to receive either test product (T) or reference product (R). In the second stage, the subjects in the "T" group in the first stage are re-randomized into two groups (T or R), and so are the subjects in the second stage. That is, at the end of the second stage, the design becomes a four-sequence design of (TT, RR, TR, RT). The comparisons in a Balaam design can also be assessed by a two-stage design.

### 4.3.3 Two-Sequence Dual Design

A two-sequence dual design is a 2 × 3 (two-sequence and three-treatment) crossover design, which is useful to investigate alternating. In this design, subjects are randomly assigned to one of the two treatment sequences: TRT and RTR. Comparisons by sequence, comparisons by period and treatment, and T versus R under this design can be assessed.

### 4.3.4 Modified Balaam Design

Modified Balaam design is a design that combines a Balaam design with a two-sequence dual design, in which subjects are randomly assigned to one of the four treatment sequences: TT, RR, TRT, and RTR. Both switching and alternating can be assessed by this design.

### 4.3.5 Complete Modified Balaam Design

A complete modified Balaam design is to make a modified Balaam design with the same number of periods for all the sequences of treatments. That is, subjects are randomly assigned to one of the four treatment sequences: TTT, RRR, TRT, and RTR. Both switching and alternating can be assessed by this design.

We should point out that for most biological products, it is not feasible or ethical to have a sufficiently long washout period between periods in crossover designs. Significant carryover effects may be presented in the study design, which will make it biased for the true treatment difference estimation. On the other hand, the study designs such as Balaam designs for switching and two-sequence dual designs for alternating may be still used in practice, as they represent possible treatment regimens for physicians and patients, and data collected by these designs may still address the interchangeability for biological compounds. By "possible treatment regimens" it means that different sequences in the crossover designs may be considered as different treatments and the crossover designs may then be viewed as parallel designs with sequences as treatments. The treatment comparisons may be of main interest at the end of each period when switching or alternating occurs. Regardless the "carryover" effects in crossover designs, these comparisons may still address the question whether or not switching or alternating biosimilar and the reference products will present different safety or efficacy risk, compared to continuously using reference products.

Study population and study size are also two critical issues for study design. Regulators require biosimilarity be evaluated in most sensitive populations. It seems not to be clear, though, what it means by the "most sensitive" in terms of interchangeability, and whether interchangeability should be evaluated in the most sensitive population. More research and regulations may need to be conducted to define the most sensitive population to study interchangeability.

Sample size should provide sufficient statistical power to evaluate interchangeability, which certainly will be linked to the statistical methods to be employed. We will discuss the statistical power by different statistical methods in Section 4.4.

## 4.4 Statistical Methods

Although Section 4.3 discusses possible options regarding the statistical study designs to investigate interchangeability, which is similar to those for small-molecule drug products, it should be noted that there are fundamental differences between biosimilars for biological products and generic products for small-molecule drug products in terms of characteristics of study designs and statistical analyses. For small-molecule drug products, therapeutic equivalence can be assumed once bioavailability is shown to be equivalent between generic products and reference products, and population bioequivalence (PBE) and individual bioequivalence (IBE) can be assessed to address interchangeability for generic drugs, using various crossover designs, as discussed by Chow [7]. For biological compounds, therapeutic equivalence needs to be assessed by totality of data including clinical efficacy, safety, and immunogenicity, beside the bioavailability data. Bioequivalence in bioavailability is a necessary but not sufficient condition to determine biosimilarity between a biosimilar and its reference products. The study designs to investigate interchangeability for biosimilars usually take on broader objectives than those for generic drugs for small-molecule products. Meanwhile, there are a few problems utilizing crossover designs for biological products. It may not be ethical and clinically feasible for long washout period; there will be carryover effect due to long half-lives for most biologicals; there will always be changes in clinical status of patients over time; and sometimes there will be absence of benefit and/or deterioration of disease state generated by investigational treatment regimens. All these can make it different for data collection and analysis strategy for interchangeability assessment for biological compounds, even when the same forms of study designs are considered as those for generic small-molecule drug products.

1. Population Bioequivalence and Individual Bioequivalence
2. Evaluations by Period
3. Methods to Assess Interchangeability in Parallel Designs
4. Biosimilarity Index and Interchangeability Index
5. Open Statistical Problems for Interchangeability Assessment

### 4.4.1 Population Bioequivalence and Individual Bioequivalence

Assuming that there is a sufficiently long washout period between periods in crossover designs, population bioequivalence (PBE) and individual equivalence (IBE) can be assessed to determine bioavailability similarity on population and individual level. By "sufficiently long," it means that carryover effects from previous periods can diminish with the washout period. As aforementioned, a sufficiently long washout period is feasible only when a product has a short half-life, which is unusual for biologicals; and in fact having a long washout period for patients usually exposes ethical concerns, depending of the nature of disease. Therefore, it is a strong assumption that there is a sufficiently long washout period between periods, which may not hold for most biological products.

#### *4.4.1.1 Population Bioequivalence*

PBE is to take into account of variability of bioavailability, together with average bioavailability, when assessing the bioequivalence between two products. The following criterion, i.e., population bioequivalence criterion, (PBC) is recommended by the FDA guidance [8]:

$$\mathrm{PBC} = \frac{(\eta_T - \eta_R)^2 + \sigma_{TT}^2 - \sigma_{TR}^2}{\max\{\sigma_{T0}^2, \sigma_{TR}^2\}} < \theta_P, \tag{4.1}$$

where $\eta_T$ and $\eta_R$ are the true mean population response (on log scale) for the test product (T) and the reference product (R), respectively; $\sigma_{TT}^2$ and $\sigma_{TR}^2$ are the total variances for the test product and the reference product, respectively; and $\sigma_{T0}^2$ is a constant that can be adjusted to control the probability of pass PBE, and $\theta_P$ is the prespecified PBE limit.

The numerator on the left-hand side of the PBE criteria is the sum of the squared difference of the traditional population average and the difference between total variances in the test and the reference products, which measures the similarity for the marginal population distribution between the test and the reference products. The denominator on the left-hand side of the PBE criteria is a scaled factor depending on the variability of the drug class of the reference drug product.

The FDA guidance suggests that $\theta_P$ be chosen as:

$$\theta_P = \frac{(\ln 1.25)^2 + \varepsilon_P}{\sigma_{T0}^2}, \tag{4.2}$$

where $\varepsilon_P$ is guided by the consideration of the variance term $(\sigma_{TT}^2 - \sigma_{TR}^2)$ that is added to the average bioequivalence criterion (ABE). As suggested by the guidance, it may be appropriate that $\varepsilon_P = 0.02$. For the determination of $\sigma_{T0}^2$, the guidance suggests to use the population difference ratio (PDR), which is defined as:

$$\mathrm{PDR} = \left(\frac{E(\mathrm{T}-\mathrm{R})^2}{E(\mathrm{R}-\mathrm{R}')^2}\right)^{\frac{1}{2}} = \left(\frac{(\eta_T - \eta_R)^2 + \sigma_{TT}^2 + \sigma_{TR}^2}{2\sigma_{TR}^2}\right)^{\frac{1}{2}} = \left(\frac{\mathrm{PBC}}{2} + 1\right)^{\frac{1}{2}}, \tag{4.3}$$

where $E(\mathrm{T}-\mathrm{R})^2$ and $E(\mathrm{R}-\mathrm{R}')^2$ denote the expected squared differences between T and R (administered to the same subject) and that between R and R′ (two administrations of R to the same subject). Assuming that the maximum allowable PDR is 1.25, it follows that $\sigma_{T0}^2 \approx 0.2$ by the substitution of $(\ln 1.25)^2 / \sigma_{T0}^2$ for PBC without the adjustment of the variance term. As mentioned in the FDA guidance, sponsors or applicants who want to use the PBE approach should contact the agency for further information on $\sigma_{T0}^2$, $\varepsilon_P$, and $\theta_P$.

#### *4.4.1.2 Individual Bioequivalence*

In addition to average bioavailability and variability of bioavailability, we may also consider assessment for the variability due to the subject-by-treatment interaction. This type of bioequivalence is called IBE.

The FDA guidance recommends the following individual bioequivalence criterion (IBC) to test IBE:

$$\text{IBC} = \frac{(\eta_T - \eta_R)^2 + \sigma_D^2 + \sigma_{WT}^2 - \sigma_{WR}^2}{\max\{\sigma_{W0}^2, \sigma_{WR}^2\}} < \theta_I, \tag{4.4}$$

where $\eta_T$ and $\eta_R$ are the true mean population response (on log scale) for the test product (T) and the reference product (R), respectively; $\sigma_{WT}^2$, $\sigma_{WR}^2$, and $\sigma_D^2$ are the intrasubject variances of the test product and the reference product, and the variance component due to subject-by-treatment interaction between drug products, respectively; and $\sigma_{W0}^2$ is the scale parameter specified by the regulatory agency or the sponsor. IBE can be claimed if the one-sided 95% upper confidence bound for IBC is less than a prespecified bioequivalence limit denoted as $\theta_I$.

It can be seen that the numerator on the left-hand side of the criterion is the sum of the squared difference of the average bioavailability, the subject-by-treatment interaction variance, and the difference between within-subject variances, which measures the similarity for the marginal population distribution between the test and reference drug products. The denominator on the left side of the criterion is a scaled factor depending upon the variability of the drug class of the reference product.

The FDA guidance suggests that $\theta_I$ be chosen as:

$$\theta_I = \frac{(\ln 1.25)^2 + \varepsilon_I}{\sigma_{W0}^2}, \tag{4.5}$$

where $\varepsilon_I$ is the variance allowance factor, which is guided by the consideration of the subject-by-treatment interaction variance ($\sigma_D^2$) as well as the variance term ($\sigma_{WT}^2 - \sigma_{WR}^2$) that is added to the ABE. As suggested by the guidance, it may be appropriate that $\sigma_D^2 = 0.03$ and $\sigma_{WT}^2 - \sigma_{WR}^2 = 0.02$, thus giving the recommended value of $\varepsilon_I$ as 0.05. For the determination of $\sigma_{W0}^2$, the guidance suggests to use the individual difference ratio (IDR), which is defined as:

$$\text{IDR} = \left(\frac{E(\text{T}-\text{R})^2}{E(\text{R}-\text{R}')^2}\right)^{\frac{1}{2}} = \left(\frac{(\eta_T - \eta_R)^2 + \sigma_D^2 + \sigma_{WT}^2 + \sigma_{WR}^2}{2\sigma_{WR}^2}\right)^{\frac{1}{2}} = \left(\frac{\text{IBC}}{2} + 1\right)^{\frac{1}{2}}, \tag{4.6}$$

where $E(\mathrm{T}-\mathrm{R})^2$ and $E(\mathrm{R}-\mathrm{R}')^2$ denote the expected squared differences between T and R (administered to the same subject), and that between R and R′ (two administrations of R to the same subject). Assuming that the maximum allowable IDR is 1.25, it follows that $\sigma_{\mathrm{W0}}^2 \approx 0.2$ by the substitution of $(\ln 1.25)^2 / \sigma_{\mathrm{W0}}^2$ for PBC without the adjustment of the variance term. As mentioned in the FDA guidance, sponsors or applicants who want to use the IBE approach should contact the agency for further information on $\sigma_{\mathrm{W0}}^2$, $\varepsilon_{\mathrm{I}}$, and $\theta_{\mathrm{I}}$.

#### *4.4.1.3 Statistical Inference for Population Bioequivalence and Individual Bioequivalence*

Both criteria for PBE and IBE are aggregated moment-based criteria, which involve several variance components including the intersubject and intrasubject variances. Since the criteria are nonlinear functions of the direct drug effect, intersubject and intrasubject variability, and the variability due to subject-by-drug interaction (for the IBE criterion), a typical approach is to linearize the criteria and then apply the method of modified large sample (MLS) or extended MLS for obtaining an approximate 95% upper confidence bound of the linearized criteria. PBE and IBE criteria can be rewritten as linear combinations of parameters as following:

$$\mathrm{PBC}_r = (\eta_{\mathrm{T}} - \eta_{\mathrm{R}})^2 + (\sigma_{\mathrm{TT}}^2 - \sigma_{\mathrm{TR}}^2) - \theta_{\mathrm{P}} \max\{\sigma_{\mathrm{T0}}^2, \sigma_{\mathrm{TR}}^2\} < 0 \tag{4.7}$$

and

$$\mathrm{IBC}_r = (\eta_{\mathrm{T}} - \eta_{\mathrm{R}})^2 + \sigma_{\mathrm{D}}^2 + \sigma_{\mathrm{WT}}^2 - \sigma_{\mathrm{WR}}^2 - \theta_{\mathrm{I}} \max\{\sigma_{\mathrm{W0}}^2, \sigma_{\mathrm{WR}}^2\} < 0. \tag{4.8}$$

The FDA guidance suggests that the variances in Equations 4.7 and 4.8 can be estimated by a mixed effects model using a maximum likelihood or restricted maximum likelihood approach proposed by Chinchilli and Esinhart [9]. Also, it is recommended in the guidance to use procedure proposed by Hyslop et al. [10] to construct confidence intervals (CIs) for $\mathrm{PBC}_r$ and $\mathrm{IBC}_r$. The details for this procedure can be found in the guidance.

We should point out that the procedure by Hyslop et al. [10] requires that the study be a crossover design and uniform within sequence. Note that a crossover design is uniform within sequence if treatment $k$, where $k = 1, 2, \ldots, t$, and $t$ is the number of treatments in total, appears the number of times within each sequence. This is to say, this approach cannot be applied to other types of study designs and may not be appropriate when the study design is a crossover but not uniform within sequence. Among others, a design is not uniform when the sample sizes by sequence are not equal or there are some missing data.

When a study design is not a crossover or is not uniform within sequence, bootstrapping may be employed to obtain CIs for PBC and IBC. The FDA guidance encourages sponsors to discuss their approaches to demonstrate PBC and IBC with Center for Drug Evaluation and Research (CDER) review staff prior to submitting their applications.

#### *4.4.1.4 Open Problems for Population Bioequivalence and Individual Bioequivalence*

Both PBE and IBE are aggregate criteria, compared to the traditional ABE. The PBE criterion accounts for the average bioavailability and variability of bioavailability, while the IBE criterion additionally takes into account the variability due to subject-by-treatment interaction. However, it is not clear whether the IBE criterion is a stricter than ABE or the PBE criterion for the assessment of drug interchangeability. In other words, it is not clear whether or not IBE implies PBE and PBE implies ABE.

A logarithmic transformation is needed to be performed for pharmacokinetic data (e.g., area under the concentration–time curve [AUC] and maximum concentration [$C_{max}$]). For ABE, the interpretation on both original and log scale is straightforward since the difference in arithmetic means on the log scale is the ratio of geometric means on the original scale. The interpretation of the aggregate criteria for both PBE and IBE, however, are not clear on the original scale.

The guidance suggests the constant scale can be used for PBE and IBE if the observed estimators of the variance of reference product ($\sigma_{TR}^2$ or $\sigma_{WR}^2$) is smaller than a constant scale ($\sigma_{T0}^2$ or $\sigma_{W0}^2$). Statistically, however, that the observed estimate of $\sigma_{TR}^2$ or $\sigma_{WR}^2$ is smaller than $\sigma_{T0}^2$ or $\sigma_{W0}^2$ does not mean that the true values of $\sigma_{TR}^2$ or $\sigma_{WR}^2$ is smaller than $\sigma_{T0}^2$ or $\sigma_{W0}^2$. A test is needed on whether $\sigma_{T0}^2$ or $\sigma_{W0}^2$ is statistically smaller than $\sigma_{TR}^2$ or $\sigma_{WR}^2$. Consequently, the FDA-recommended approach is in fact a two-stage test procedure. Theoretically speaking, there is a need to control overall type I error rate and the calculation of power and sample size should reflect this fact accordingly.

Power and sample size determinations are also open questions. Unlike ABE, no closed form exists for the power function by the recommended approaches for PBE and IBE, and thus there is no closed form for sample size determination. The sample size may be only determined based on bootstrapping methods by simulation.

PBE and IBE are commonly used to determine drug interchangeability for small-molecule generic products, where the bioavailability in terms of AUC and $C_{max}$ are of main interest. As previously discussed, PBE and IBE evaluation also rely on crossover study designs. For biological products, the clinical assessment on interchangeability is not only on pharmacokinetic evaluations but also on efficacy, immunogenicity, and safety data. On one hand, the crossover designs could be useful to demonstrate interchangeability in terms of pharmacokinetic profiles when a biological product has a short half-life time; on the other hand, the application of crossover designs and the corresponding statistical analysis strategy may not be suitable to demonstrate interchangeability for biosimilar products, given the fact that most biological products have long half-life times. In the following sections, we discuss in detail the strategy to demonstrate interchangeability for biosimilar products in the context of parallel designs.

1. Evaluations by Period
2. Methods to Assess Interchangeability in Parallel Designs
3. Biosimilarity Index and Interchangeability Index
4. Open Statistical Problems for Interchangeability Assessment

### 4.4.2 Evaluations by Period

For most biological products, it is not feasible or not ethical to have a sufficiently long washout period between periods in crossover designs. Significant carryover effects may be presented in the study design, which will make it biased for the true treatment difference estimation. The approaches for PBE and IBEs then may become invalid. On the other hand, regardless of the "carryover" effects in crossover designs, the treatment comparisons at the end of each period when switching or alternating occurs may still address the question whether switching or alternating biosimilar and the reference products will present different safety or efficacy risk, compared to continuously using reference products. As carryover effects are significant, the evaluations may not be conducted in terms of PBE and IBEs. The evaluations will be conducted similarly as those for parallel designs in which only intersubject variability will be used.

### 4.4.3 Methods to Assess Interchangeability in Parallel Designs

In this section, we will describe following the approach proposed by Dong and Tsong [11] and Dong et al. [12], specifically on the equivalence assessment for interchangeability based on TSE approximation method on consistency index, two-sided test, and two one-sided tests methods, respectively, for parallel-arm designs. Readers may refer to the original papers for the technical details under various study designs.

1. TSE Approximation Method on Consistency Index
2. Two-Sided Tolerance Interval Approach
3. Two One-Sided Tests
4. Comparisons between TSE Method, Two-Sided Test, and Two One-Sided Tests
5. An Example—PLANETAS* Open-Label Extension (OLE) Study

* PLANETAS stands for "**P**rogramme eva**L**uating the **A**utoimmune disease i**N**v**E**stigational drug c**T**-p13 in **A**nkylosing **S**pondylitis patients (PLANETAS)".

#### 4.4.3.1 TSE Approximation Method on Consistency Index

Tse et al. [13] proposed an approximate method for testing two-sided probability of the ratio of two log-normally distributed variables. Following their method, Dong and Tsong [11] derived the approximate test of two-sided interchangeability in a similar way for parallel designs. Consider a parallel-arm trial with a test arm (T) and a reference arm (R). Assume that the responses, $X_T$ in test arm and $X_R$ in reference arm, follow a bivariate normal distribution with independent mean $\mu_T$ and $\mu_R$ and variance $\sigma_T{}^2$ and $\sigma_R{}^2$, respectively, and then the response difference $X_d = X_T - X_R$ follows a normal distribution with mean $\mu_d = \mu_T - \mu_R$ and variance $\sigma_T^2 + \sigma_R^2$.

In this way, interchangeability is concluded if at least 100p% proportion of the random sample difference $X_d = X_T - X_R$ is bounded within a prespecified interval (L, U) with at least more than a prospecified probability $p$, where $0 < p < 1$. Denote that the probability of $X_d = X_T - X_R$ is bounded within a prespecified interval (L, U) as $\theta = \Pr(L < X_T - X_R < U)$. The hypothesis can be stated as following:

$$H_0 : \theta = \Pr(L < X_T - X_R < U) \le p \quad \text{versus}$$
$$H_1 : \theta = \Pr(L < X_T - X_R < U) > p. \tag{4.9}$$

The parameter of $\theta$ is a function of $\mu_d$, $\sigma_T{}^2$, and $\sigma_R{}^2$, which can be further expressed as follows:

$$\theta(\mu_d, \sigma_T^2, \sigma_R^2) = \Pr(L < X_T - X_R < U) = \Phi\left(\frac{U - \mu_d}{\sqrt{\sigma_T^2 + \sigma_R^2}}\right) - \Phi\left(\frac{L - \mu_d}{\sqrt{\sigma_T^2 + \sigma_R^2}}\right). \tag{4.10}$$

Let that $\bar{X}_d = \bar{X}_T - \bar{X}_R$ be the sample mean difference for $\mu_d$, $S^2 = S_T^2 + S_R^2$ is the sample variance of the distribution of $\bar{X}_d$. Then the parameter of $\theta$ can be estimated by

$$\hat{\theta}(\bar{X}_d, S_T^2, S_R^2) = \Phi\left(\frac{U - \bar{X}_d}{\sqrt{S_T^2 + S_R^2}}\right) - \Phi\left(\frac{L - \bar{X}_d}{\sqrt{S_T^2 + S_R^2}}\right). \tag{4.11}$$

Assuming sample size is sufficiently large, the approximate test statistics, denoted as $T_W$, can be obtained using Wald test statistic asymptotically following a normal distribution as

$$T_W = \frac{\hat{\theta} - E(\hat{\theta})}{\sqrt{\mathrm{Var}(\hat{\theta})}} \to N(0,1). \tag{4.12}$$

$E(\hat{\theta})$ is the expectation of $\hat{\theta}$ and $E(\hat{\theta}) = \theta + B(\theta)$. $B(\theta)$ and $\mathrm{Var}(\hat{\theta})$ can be expressed as

$$B(\theta)=\frac{1}{2}\frac{\partial^2\theta}{\partial\mu_d^2}\left(\frac{\sigma_T^2}{n_T}+\frac{\sigma_R^2}{n_R}\right)+\frac{1}{2}\frac{\partial^2\theta}{\partial\left(\sigma_T^2\right)^2}\left(\frac{\sigma_T^4}{n_T-1}+\frac{\sigma_R^4}{n_R-1}\right) \tag{4.13}$$

and

$$\mathrm{Var}(\hat{\theta})=\left(\frac{\partial\theta}{\partial\mu_d}\right)^2\left(\frac{\sigma_T^2}{n_T}+\frac{\sigma_R^2}{n_R}\right)+2\left(\frac{\partial\theta}{\partial\sigma_T^2}\right)^2\left(\frac{\sigma_T^4}{n_T-1}+\frac{\sigma_R^4}{n_R-1}\right). \tag{4.14}$$

$\hat{B}(\hat{\theta})$ and $\widehat{\mathrm{Var}}(\hat{\theta})$ can be obtained, respectively, by substituting $\mu_d$, $\sigma_T^2$, and $\sigma_R^2$ with $\bar{X}_d$, $S_T^2$, and $S_R^2$ corresponding in Equations 4.13 and 4.14. The null hypothesis can be rejected at alpha level of $\alpha$, and interchangeability can be concluded if

$$T_W=\frac{\hat{\theta}-\hat{B}(\hat{\theta})-p}{\sqrt{\widehat{\mathrm{Var}}(\hat{\theta})}}>Z_{1-\alpha}. \tag{4.15}$$

#### 4.4.3.2 Two-Sided Tolerance Interval Approach

Tsong and Shen [14] proposed a two-sided tolerance interval to estimate the CI of $\theta$ for interchangeability with equal sample size and equal variance. A two-sided $(p, 1-\alpha)$ tolerance interval for $X_T - X_R$ is an interval that covers at least 100p% of the distribution with a confidence level of $1-\alpha$. For normally distributed response, the tolerance interval is usually in the form of $(\bar{X}_d-kS,\bar{X}_d+kS)$ and defined as

$$P_{\bar{X}_d,S}[P_{X_T-X_R}(\bar{X}_d-kS<X_T-X_R<\bar{X}_d+kS)>p]=1-\alpha. \tag{4.16}$$

In Equation 4.16, $\bar{X}_d=\bar{X}_T-\bar{X}_R$ is the sample mean difference, $S^2$ is the pooled sample variance of the distribution of $\bar{X}_d$, which can be expressed as

$$S^2=\left(1+\frac{1}{R}\right)\frac{(n_T-1)S_T^2+R(n_R-1)S_R^2}{n_T+n_R-2}, \tag{4.17}$$

where $R=\sigma_T^2/\sigma_R^2$ is assumed to be known, and $k$ is unknown and is called the tolerance factor, which can be obtained by solving Equation 4.16.

Dong and Tsong [11] have shown that for parallel designs,

$$\begin{aligned}&P_{X_T-X_R}(\bar{X}_d-kS<X_T-X_R<\bar{X}_d+kS)\\&=\Phi\left(\sqrt{a}W+k\sqrt{\frac{Y^2}{n_T+n_R-2}}\right)-\Phi\left(\sqrt{a}W-k\sqrt{\frac{Y^2}{n_T+n_R-2}}\right),\end{aligned} \tag{4.18}$$

where $\Phi$ is the cumulative density function of a standard normal, and

$$W = \frac{\bar{X}_d - \mu_d}{\sqrt{\frac{\sigma_T^2}{n_T} + \frac{\sigma_R^2}{n_R}}} \sim N(0,1),$$

$$Y^2 = \frac{(n_T + n_R - 2)S^2}{\sigma_T^2 + \sigma_R^2} \sim \chi^2_{n_T + n_R - 2},$$

and

$$a = \frac{\frac{\sigma_T^2}{n_T} + \frac{\sigma_R^2}{n_R}}{\sigma_T^2 + \sigma_R^2} = \frac{R + \frac{n_T}{n_R}}{n_T(R+1)}.$$

A special case is that $n_T = n_R = n$ and then $a = 1/n$. In this case, considering Equation 4.18, $k$ is the solution to the following equation:

$$P_{W,Y^2}\left[\Phi\left(\sqrt{a}W + k\sqrt{\frac{Y^2}{n_T + n_R - 2}}\right) - \Phi\left(\sqrt{a}W - k\sqrt{\frac{Y^2}{n_T + n_R - 2}}\right) > p\right] = 1 - \alpha. \quad (4.19)$$

Applying the similar way described in Krishnamoorthy and Mathew [15], Equation 4.19 can be further expressed as

$$\sqrt{\frac{2}{\pi}}\int_0^\infty P\left(Y^2 > \frac{(n_T + n_R - 2)\chi^2_{1,p}(aW^2)}{k^2}\right)e^{-\frac{W^2}{2}}\,dW = 1 - \alpha. \quad (4.20)$$

After $k$ is obtained, the two treatments T and R are interchangeable if

$$L < \bar{X}_d - kS < \bar{X}_d + kS < U. \quad (4.21)$$

If variance ratio $R$ is unknown, we can use the following to replace $R$ as proposed by Hall [16]:

$$\hat{R} = \frac{S_T^2(n_R - 3)}{S_R^2(n_R - 1)}. \quad (4.22)$$

The power function of the two-sided tolerance interval can be derived as follows:

$$\begin{aligned} \text{POWER}_{TS} &= \Pr(L < \bar{X}_d - kS < \bar{X}_d + kS < U \mid H_1) \\ &= \int_0^b \left(\Phi\left(\frac{U - \mu_d}{\sqrt{a}\sigma_d} - \frac{k}{\sqrt{a}}\sqrt{\frac{Y^2}{n_1 + n_2 - 2}}\right)\right. \\ &\quad \left.-\Phi\left(\frac{L - \mu_d}{\sqrt{a}\sigma_d} + \frac{k}{\sqrt{a}}\sqrt{\frac{Y^2}{n_1 + n_2 - 2}}\right)\right) f(Y^2)\,d(Y^2), \end{aligned} \quad (4.23)$$

where $b = \frac{(n_1 + n_2 - 2)(\mathrm{U} - \mathrm{L})^2}{4k}$, $\Phi(.)$ is the cumulative density function of the standard normal distribution, and $f(Y^2)$ is the probability density function of $\chi^2_{n_1+n_2-2}$.

The detailed derivation can be found in Dong et al. [12].

The method of two one-sided tests can be applied to binary response data too. Assume that the sample response rates, $r_\mathrm{T}$ in test arm and $r_\mathrm{R}$ in reference arm, follow a bivariate normal distribution with independent mean $R_\mathrm{T}$ and $R_\mathrm{R}$ and variance $\sigma_\mathrm{T}{}^2$ and $\sigma_\mathrm{R}{}^2$, respectively, and then the sample response difference $r_\mathrm{d} = r_\mathrm{T} - r_\mathrm{R}$ follows a normal distribution with mean $R_\mathrm{d} = R_\mathrm{T} - R_\mathrm{R}$ and variance $\sigma_\mathrm{T}^2 + \sigma_\mathrm{R}^2 = R_\mathrm{T}(1-R_\mathrm{T}) + R_\mathrm{R}(1-R_\mathrm{R})$. The corresponding two hypotheses can be stated as following:

$$H_{0\mathrm{L}} : P_\mathrm{r}(r_\mathrm{T} - r_\mathrm{R} < \mathrm{L}) \ge P_\mathrm{L} \quad \text{versus} \quad H_{1\mathrm{L}} : P_\mathrm{r}(r_\mathrm{T} - r_\mathrm{R} < \mathrm{L}) < P_\mathrm{L} \tag{4.34}$$

$$H_{0\mathrm{U}} : P_\mathrm{r}(r_\mathrm{T} - r_\mathrm{R} > \mathrm{U}) \ge P_\mathrm{U} \quad \text{versus} \quad H_{1\mathrm{U}} : P_\mathrm{r}(r_\mathrm{T} - r_\mathrm{R} > \mathrm{U}) < P_\mathrm{U} \tag{4.35}$$

Under the normality assumption, these two hypotheses are equivalent to testing the distribution of $R_\mathrm{d} = R_\mathrm{T} - R_\mathrm{R}$ as follows:

$$H_{0\mathrm{L}} : R_\mathrm{d} - Z_{1-P_\mathrm{L}}\sqrt{\sigma_\mathrm{T}^2 + \sigma_\mathrm{R}^2} \le \mathrm{L} \quad \text{versus} \quad H_{1\mathrm{L}} : R_\mathrm{d} - Z_{1-P_\mathrm{L}}\sqrt{\sigma_\mathrm{T}^2 + \sigma_\mathrm{R}^2} > \mathrm{L} \tag{4.36}$$

$$H_{0\mathrm{U}} : R_\mathrm{d} - Z_{P_\mathrm{U}}\sqrt{\sigma_\mathrm{T}^2 + \sigma_\mathrm{R}^2} \ge \mathrm{U} \quad \text{versus} \quad H_{1\mathrm{U}} : R_\mathrm{d} - Z_{P_\mathrm{U}}\sqrt{\sigma_\mathrm{T}^2 + \sigma_\mathrm{R}^2} < \mathrm{U} \tag{4.37}$$

Consider the following test statistic for Equation 4.36:

$$Z = \frac{r_\mathrm{T} - r_\mathrm{R}}{\sqrt{\frac{r_\mathrm{T}(1-r_\mathrm{T})}{n_\mathrm{T}} + \frac{r_\mathrm{R}(1-r_\mathrm{R})}{n_\mathrm{R}}}}. \tag{4.38}$$

The null hypothesis $H_{0\mathrm{L}}$ is rejected at the alpha level of $\alpha_\mathrm{L}$ if

$$Z > z_\mathrm{L} = z_{1-\alpha_\mathrm{L}} + \frac{z_{1-P_\mathrm{L}}\sqrt{r_\mathrm{T}(1-r_\mathrm{T}) + r_\mathrm{R}(1-r_\mathrm{R})} + \mathrm{L}}{\sqrt{\frac{r_\mathrm{T}(1-r_\mathrm{T})}{n_\mathrm{T}} + \frac{r_\mathrm{R}(1-r_\mathrm{R})}{n_\mathrm{R}}}}. \tag{4.39}$$

And the null hypothesis $H_{0\mathrm{U}}$ is rejected at the alpha level of $\alpha_\mathrm{U}$ if

$$Z < z_\mathrm{U} = z_{\alpha_\mathrm{U}} + \frac{z_{P_\mathrm{U}}\sqrt{r_\mathrm{T}(1-r_\mathrm{T}) + r_\mathrm{R}(1-r_\mathrm{R})} + \mathrm{U}}{\sqrt{\frac{r_\mathrm{T}(1-r_\mathrm{T})}{n_\mathrm{T}} + \frac{r_\mathrm{R}(1-r_\mathrm{R})}{n_\mathrm{R}}}}. \tag{4.40}$$

#### 4.4.3.4 Comparisons between TSE Method, Two-Sided Test, and Two One-Sided Tests

In this section, we discuss the differences for the three methods of assessment for the assessment of interchangeability in parallel designs, TSE method, two-sided tolerance interval approach, and two one-sided tests approach.

For the setup of the criteria of interchangeability, the two one-sided tests exert a more specific and stringent requirement for interchangeability than the two-sided test. For the two-sided test, it is tested whether the proportion within (L, U) is larger than a given number $P$. For two one-sided tests, it is tested whether the proportion less than L is less than a specific value $P_L$ and the proportion greater than U is less than a specific value $P_U$ as well. The two one-sided tests may have broader applications and may be more suitable for some specific situations. For example, when conducting interchangeability assessment using therapeutic endpoint for medicines such as inhaler products, one also needs to show the test treatment is superior to the placebo. When designing a trial with only test and reference treatment arms, one may need to use the probability $P_r(X_T - X_R > L) > P^*$ (or equivalently, $P_r(X_T - X_R < L) < P_1$ and $P_1 = 1 - P^*$) to imply the superiority over the placebo as the noninferiority test. In such a case, $P_r(X_T - X_R < L) < P_1$ may need to be confirmed with a 2.5% type I error rate instead of the 5% type I error rate used in the standard equivalence test. In this scenario, two one-sided tests with different type I error rates ($\alpha_L$ and $\alpha_U$) and different margins $P_L$ and $P_U$ may be more suitable than a two-sided test.

Under the normality assumption, the two one-sided hypotheses of interchangeability can be expressed as a linear combination of the mean difference and total variability, and the exact solutions can be provided. It has been shown by Dong et al. [12] that the two one-sided tests are of size-$\alpha$, as the test statistics are of an exact test. The two one-sided tests do not need the assumptions of equal sample sizes and equal variances assumption.

The two-sided test statistics depend on the assumption of variance ratio and has been shown to be conservative by Dong and Tsong [11] in terms of the type I error rate under the boundary of the null hypothesis. This conservativeness could be extremely serious when the margins are not symmetric. The TSE approximation method will need a large sample size to use asymptotic distribution of test statistics, and it does not control the type I error rate well, especially for small and medium sample sizes. In fact, both bias correction and variance of test statistic are obtained by using only the first two orders of the Taylor expansion. The test statistic could be overestimated when the variance is underestimated by Taylor expansion. This can lead to a higher power for the TSE method, when compared to the two-sided tolerance interval approach. However, given the bias, the TSE method is not recommended for small and medium sample sizes.

#### 4.4.3.5 Example—PLANETAS Open-Label Extension (OLE) Study

CT-P13 is an infliximab (INX) biosimilar recently approved by the European Medicine Agency. PLANETAS was a 54-week randomized double-blind parallel group multicenter Phase I study demonstrating pharmacokinetic equivalence of CT-P13 (5 mg/kg infusion every 8 weeks) with INX, in patients with ankylosing spondylitis (AS) [17]. Here we take its extension phase study as an example to apply two one-sided tests to investigate interchangeability. In this OLE study, a total of 174 patients who completed PLANETAS entered into the extension phase: 88 were continuously treated with CT-P13 (maintenance group) and 86 were switched from INX to CT-P13 (switch group) for 1 additional year. Figure 4.1 shows the study scheme.

At Week 54, ASAS20 and ASAS40 response rates seemed to be similar between groups (CT-P13, 70.5%/58.0%; INX, 75.6%/53.5%, respectively). During the extension, ASAS20/ASAS40 rates seemed to be similar in the maintenance group (70.1%/57.5% at Week 78 and 80.7%/63.9% at Week 102) and the switch group (77.1%/51.8% at Week 78 and 76.9%/61.5% at Week 102). These results, as well as 95% CIs and 75% CIs for the response rate differences, are provided in Table 4.1.

As can be seen from Table 4.1, if an equivalence margin of ±15% is considered, the biosimilarity can be established at the alpha level of 0.125 on both sides between the switch group and the maintenance group at all the three time points for both ASAS20 and ASAS40 response rates. However, if the alpha level of 0.025 is considered on both sides, biosimilarity cannot be established with the equivalence margin of ±15%.

We can use the two one-sided tests to check interchangeability in this case. Consider that $U = -L = 15\%$. Let that $\alpha_L = \alpha_U = 0.125$ and $P_L = P_U = 0.50$. Table 4.2 presents the value of $Z$ and the critical values $z_L$ and $z_U$. When $\alpha_L = \alpha_U = 0.125$ and $P_L = P_U = 0.50$, since $z_L < Z < z_U$ for all three time points for both ASAS20 and ASAS40 response rates, interchangeability can be

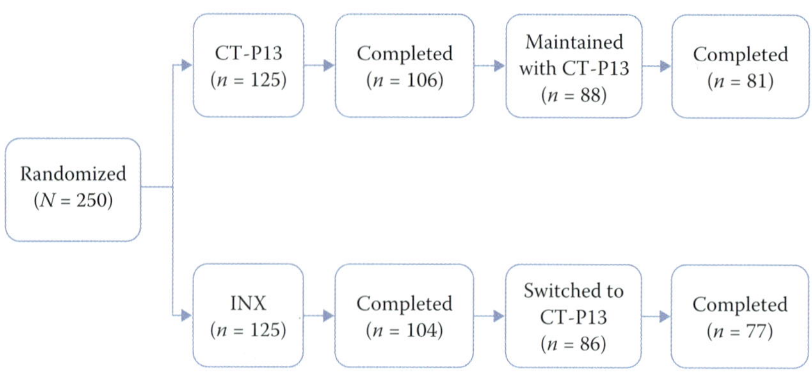


**FIGURE 4.1**
Switching from Remicade® to Remsima®—PLANETAS open-label extension (OLE) study.

**TABLE 4.1**

PLANETAS OLE Study Results

| Efficacy Outcome | Extension Phase Week | CT-P13 Maintenance | Switched from INX to CT-P13 | Response Difference (Switch – Maintenance) (95% CI) (75% CI) |
|---|---|---|---|---|
| ASAS20, *n*/*N* (%) | 54 | 62/88 (70.5) | 65/86 (75.6) | 5.1% (−8.2%, 18.2%) (−2.7%, 12.8%) |
| | 78 | 61/87 (70.1) | 64/83 (77.1) | 7.0% (−6.4%, 20.1%) (−0.8%, 14.7%) |
| | 102 | 67/83 (80.7) | 60/78 (76.9) | −3.8% (−16.7%, 8.9%) (−11.1%, 3.6%) |
| ASAS40, *n*/*N* (%) | 54 | 51/88 (58.0) | 46/86 (53.5) | −4.5% (−19.0%, 10.3%) (−13.1%, 4.2%) |
| | 78 | 50/87 (57.5) | 43/83 (51.8) | −5.7% (−20.4%, 9.3%) (−14.4%, 3.1%) |
| | 102 | 53/83 (63.9) | 48/78 (61.5) | −2.3% (−17.2%, 12.6%) (−11.1%, 6.5%) |

*Notes:* CI, confidence interval; INX, infliximab; OLE, open-label extension.

**TABLE 4.2**

PLANETAS OLE Study Two One-Sided Tests for Interchangeability

| Efficacy Outcome | Extension Phase Week | $Z$ | $\alpha_L = \alpha_U = 0.125$ and $P_L = P_U = 0.50$: $z_L$ | $z_U$ | $\alpha_L = \alpha_U = 0.125$ and $P_L = P_U = 0.20$: $z_L$ | $z_U$ |
|---|---|---|---|---|---|---|
| ASAS20 | 54 | 0.76 | −1.08 | 1.08 | 6.77 | −11.45 |
| | 78 | 1.04 | −1.08 | 1.08 | 6.69 | −11.42 |
| | 102 | −0.59 | −1.18 | 1.18 | 6.36 | −11.88 |
| ASAS40 | 54 | −0.60 | −0.84 | 0.84 | 7.01 | −10.34 |
| | 78 | −0.75 | −0.82 | 0.82 | 6.94 | −10.22 |
| | 102 | −0.31 | −0.82 | 0.82 | 6.73 | −10.22 |

established when $\alpha_L = \alpha_U = 0.125$ and $P_L = P_U = 0.50$. On the other hand, when $\alpha_L = \alpha_U = 0.125$ and $P_L = P_U = 0.20$, interchangeability will not be able to be claimed.

It can be seen that the interchangeability, as its testing considers both mean and variability into test statistics, is more difficult to be claimed than regular equivalence, which considers test statistics on mean only, when the sample margin and the same type I error are considered. On the other hand, the method of two one-sided tests has the flexibility to accommodate different margins of L and U, different tolerance probabilities of $P_L$ and $P_U$, and different type I errors. For example, as can be seen from the case study, interchangeability can be claimed with when $P_L = P_U = 0.50$, whereas interchangeability cannot claimed when $P_L = P_U = 0.20$.

### 4.4.4 Biosimilarity Index and Interchangeability Index

In this session, we describe the development of the biosimilarity index, based on the concept of reproducibility probability proposed by Chow [18] and Chow et al. [19], which leads to the concept of biosimilarity index proposed by Chow [7]. We discuss the use of biosimilarity index and interchangeability index in the assessment of interchangeability.

1. Reproducibility Probability
2. Biosimilarity Index
3. Interchangeability Index

#### *4.4.4.1 Reproducibility Probability*

Suppose that one clinical trial has been conducted and the observed results lead to the rejection of the null hypothesis. That is, the results are statistically significant. It is often of interest to determine whether clinical trials that produced significant clinical results provide substantial evidence to assure that the results will be reproducible in a future clinical trial with the same study protocol. If the two trials are independent, the probability of observing a significant result from the second trial is still of the power function with the same test statistic as for the first trial. However, the information from the first clinical trial should be useful in the evaluation of the probability of observing a significant result in the second trial. This leads to the concept of the reproducibility probability. The reproducibility probability can be defined as an estimated power of the second trial using the data from the first trial. Denote the test statistic as $T$ in the second trial, the true distribution of $T$ under $H_1$ with parameter $\theta$, the critical value of significance as $c$, and the first trial data as $X$. Then, the reproducibility probability is the conditional probability of $|T| > c$ in the future trial given the data $X$, i.e., $P(|T| > c|X)$.

The simple empirical calculation of the reproducibility probability may be replacing the true distribution parameter of $\theta$ by the estimated value $\hat{\theta}$ from the first trial, i.e.,

$$P(|T| > c|X) = P(|T| > c|\theta = \hat{\theta}) \cdot \tag{4.41}$$

In the Bayesian framework, the reproducibility probability can be obtained as

$$P(|T| > c|X) = \int_{\theta} P(|T| > c|\theta)\pi(\theta|X)d\theta, \tag{4.42}$$

where $\pi(\theta|X)$ is the posterior distribution of $\theta$.

Chow [7] discussed the reproducibility probability calculations in terms of Equations 4.41 and 4.42 for different study designs. And readers may refer to the original discussions for details.

#### 4.4.4.2 Biosimilarity Index

Chow [18] and Chow et al. [19] proposed a biosimilarity index based on the concept of the probability of reproducibility as follows:

Step 1: Assess the average biosimilarity between the test product and the reference product based on a given biosimilarity criterion. For the purpose of an illustration, consider a bioequivalence criterion as a biosimilarity criterion. That is, bioequivalence is claimed if the 90% CI of the ratio of means of a given study endpoint falls within the biosimilarity limits of (80%, 125%) or (−0.2231, 0.2231) based on raw (original) data or based on log-transformed data.

Step 2: Once the product passes the test for in Step 1, calculate the reproducibility probability based on the observed data. Thus, the calculated reproducibility probability will take the variability and the sensitivity of heterogeneity in variances into consideration for the assessment of biosimilarity.

Step 3: We then claim biosimilarity if the calculated 95% confidence lower bound of the reproducibility probability is larger than a prespecified number $p_0$, which can be obtained based on an estimate of reproducibility probability for a study comparing a "reference product" to itself (the "reference product"). We will refer to such a study as an R–R study. Alternatively, we can then claim (local) biosimilarity if the 95% confidence lower bound of the biosimilarity index is larger than $p_0$.

The biosimilarity index described earlier has the advantages that (1) it is robust with respect to the selected study endpoint, biosimilarity criteria, and study design; and (2) the probability of reproducibility will reflect the sensitivity of heterogeneity in variance.

Note that the proposed biosimilarity index can be applied to different functional areas (domains) of biological products such as PK, biological activities, biomarkers (e.g., pharmacodynamics), immunogenicity, manufacturing process, efficacy, etc. An overall biosimilarity index or totality biosimilarity index across domains can be similarly obtained as follows:

Step 1: Obtain local biosimilarity index $\hat{p}_i$ (a reproducibility probability) for $i$th domain, where "domain" may stand for a component of totality of data or a period when evaluation by period is conducted.

Step 2: Define the totality biosimilarity index as $\hat{p}_T = \sum_{i=1}^{M} w_i \hat{p}_i$, where $w_i$ is the weight for the $i$th domain, $\sum_{i=1}^{M} w_i = 1$, and $i = 1, 2, \ldots, M$ ($M$ is the total number of domains of evaluations).

Step 3: Claim biosimilarity if the 95% confidence lower bound of $p_T$ is greater than a prespecified value $p_{T0}$.

#### 4.4.4.3 Interchangeability Index

Following the similar idea or biosimilarity index, we may define the interchangeability index in a similar way.

Step 1: Assess interchangeability between the test product and the reference product based on a given interchangeability criterion. For a parallel design, either a two-sided test or two one-sided tests can be considered.

Step 2: Once the product passes the test for in Step 1, calculate the reproducibility probability based on the observed data. The calculated reproducibility probability is the interchangeability index.

Step 3: We then claim interchangeability if the calculated 95% confidence lower bound of the interchangeability is larger than a prespecified number $p_0$.

In the study designs mentioned previously for biological compounds, it is not feasible to have sufficient washout between switching and alternating, and the assessment of interchangeability is in fact by period. And by the end of each period, there are inevitably multiple comparisons between parallel arms. For example, under Balaam's design of (TT, RR, TR, RT) after the switching, there are six comparisons among the four treatment sequences. Correspondingly, six interchangeability indices can be obtained. Similar to overall or total biosimilarity index, the overall interchangeability can be assessed in three ways:

1. Method 1: Total Interchangeability Index.

   Step 1: Obtain local interchangeability index $\hat{p}_i$ for $i$th domain, where "domain" may stand for a component of totality of data, e.g., a comparison between treatment sequence after switching or alternating.

   Step 2: Define the totality interchangeability index as $\hat{p}_T = \sum_{i=1}^{M} w_i \hat{p}_i$, where $w_i$ is the weight for the $i$th domain, $\sum_{i=1}^{M} w_i = 1$, and $i = 1, 2, \ldots, M$ ($M$ is the total number of domains of evaluations).

   Step 3: Claim interchangeability if the 95% confidence lower bound of $p_T$ is greater than a prespecified value $p_{T0}$.

2. Method 2: Minimum Interchangeability Index.

Similar to the switching index for crossover designs, for parallel designs we may use the minimum of all local interchangeability indices to define interchangeability. Let $\hat{p}_{\min} = \min(\hat{p}_i)$, where $i = 1, 2, \ldots, M$. Claim interchangeability if the 95% confidence lower bound of $p_{\min}$ is greater than a prespecified value $p_0$.

The following method provides a possible way to construct the 95% confidence lower bound of $p_{\min}$. Assume that $\hat{p}_1, \hat{p}_2, \ldots, \hat{p}_M$ be a sample from a continuous distribution with probability density function $f(p)$ and cumulative density function $F(p)$. Following David and Nagaraja [20], the probability function of $p_{\min}$, denoted as $f_{p_{\min}}(p)$, can be expressed as

$$f_{p_{\min}}(p) = M(1 - F(p))^{M-1} f(p). \tag{4.43}$$

The expected value and the variance of $p_{\min}$ are given by

$$E(p_{\min}) = M \int_p p(1 - F(p))^{M-1} f(p)dp,$$

and

$$\mathrm{Var}(p_{\min}) = E(p_{\min}^2) - (E(p_{\min}))^2$$

$$= M \int_p p^2 (1 - F(p))^{M-1} f(p)dp - M^2 \left( \int_p p(1 - F(p))^{M-1} f(p)\, dp \right)^2.$$

With a given distribution function $f(p)$ and $F(p)$, the expected value and the variance of order statistics could be derived. However, the population distribution may be unknown or difficult to determine. Distribution-free nonparametric bounds for the moments of order statistics may then be considered. Let $\hat{p}_1, \hat{p}_2, \ldots, \hat{p}_M$ be from a population with expectation $E(p)$ and variance $\mathrm{Var}(p)$. As shown by Arnold and Groeneveld [21],

$$E(p)-\sqrt{(M-1)\mathrm{Var}(p)} \le E(p_{\min}) \le E(p). \tag{4.44}$$

Papadatos [22] showed that

$$\mathrm{Var}(p_{\min}) \le M \times \mathrm{Var}(p). \tag{4.45}$$

The sample mean $\hat{E}(\hat{p})$ and variance $\widehat{\mathrm{Var}}(\hat{p})$ can be used to estimate $E(p)$ and variance $\mathrm{Var}(p)$, respectively. Considering Equations 4.37 and 4.38, an estimate of the lower bound of 95% CI for $p_{\min}$ can be expressed as:

$$\hat{E}(\hat{p})-\left(\sqrt{M-1}+z_{0.975}\sqrt{M}\right)\sqrt{\widehat{\mathrm{Var}}(\hat{p})}. \tag{4.46}$$

3. Method 3: Interchangeability Index Range.

Similar to the switching index for crossover designs, for parallel designs we may use the range of all local interchangeability indices to define interchangeability. Let $\hat{R} = \hat{p}_{\max} - \hat{p}_{\min} = \max(\hat{p}_i) - \min(\hat{p}_i)$, where $i$ = 1, 2,..., $M$. Claim interchangeability if the 95% confidence upper bound of $R$ is less than a prespecified value $R_0$. Following David and Nagaraja [20], the joint probability density function of $p_{\max}$ and $p_{\min}$, denoted as $f_{p_{\max}, p_{\min}}(p_{\max}, p_{\min})$, can be expressed as follows:

$$f_{p_{\max}, p_{\min}}(p_{\max}, p_{\min}) = M(M-1)\left(F(p_{\max})-F(p_{\min})\right)^{M-2} f(p_{\max}) f(p_{\min}). \tag{4.47}$$

The expected value of $R$ can be given by

$$E(R) = M(M-1)\int\int (p_{\max}-p_{\min})\left(F(p_{\max})-F(p_{\min})\right)^{M-2} f(p_{\max}) f(p_{\min})\,\mathrm{d}p_{\min}\mathrm{d}p_{\max}.$$

And the variance of $R$ can be given by

$$\mathrm{Var}(R) = E(R^2) - (E(R))^2,$$

where

$$E(R^2) = M(M-1)\int\int (p_{\max} - p_{\min})^2 \left(F(p_{\max}) - F(p_{\min})\right)^{M-2}$$
$$f(p_{\max}) f(p_{\min}) \mathrm{d}p_{\min} \mathrm{d}p_{\max}.$$

As shown by in Arnold and Groeneveld [21], the upper bound for $E(R)$ is given by

$$E(R) \le \sqrt{2M\mathrm{Var}(p)}. \tag{4.48}$$

And using Cauchy–Schwarz inequality (Casella and Berger [23]), the upper bound for $\mathrm{Var}(R)$ is given by

$$\mathrm{Var}(R) \le 4M\mathrm{Var}(p). \tag{4.49}$$

Substituting $\mathrm{Var}(p)$ with sample variance $\widehat{\mathrm{Var}}(\hat{p})$ and considering Equations 4.48 and 4.49 together, an estimate of the upper bound of 95% CI for $R$ can be expressed as:

$$(\sqrt{2} + 2z_{0.975})\sqrt{M\widehat{\mathrm{Var}}(\hat{p})}. \tag{4.50}$$

### 4.4.5 Open Statistical Problems for Interchangeability Assessment

Although the testing procedures proposed by Dong and Tsong [11] and Dong et al. [12] for parallel designs considered both average mean and variability into interchangeability assessment, there remains a few open questions. One of the challenging situations is that there will always be changes in clinical status of patients over time, and patients may discontinue from the studies for various reasons such as loss of follow-up and deterioration of disease state. The available data may be decreasing over time, and the observed sample size may become smaller in later periods. On the other hand, interchangeability statistical tests, as considering both mean and variability into test statistics, in fact require greater sample size to establish interchangeability if the sample margin and the same type I error are considered as the traditional equivalence tests. The contradiction between the shrinking sample size along time and greater sample size requirement for statistical evaluations on interchangeability imposes an issue on planning and statistical evaluations of interchangeability after the establishment of biosimilarity: Should a study which contains both the period of biosimilarity evaluation and that of switching and/or alternating evaluations be powered in terms of interchangeability, instead of biosimilarity? It seems to be controversial by doing this too, as interchangeability should be evaluated only after the establishment of biosimilarity. Adding formal statistical evaluations on interchangeability into study planning will need a comprehensive evaluation on the trade-offs on cost, benefit, and risk for the development of a biosimilar.

As discussed in Section 4.4.3.4, the method of two one-sided tests may be more flexible than other methods when evaluating interchangeability. However, there remains a number of issues to prespecify the setup of the tests. Without prior knowledge of switching and alternating, it is a difficult task to prespecify the two type I errors, the margins of L and U, and the tolerance probabilities of $P_L$ and $P_U$. Considering that the sample size gets smaller over time and to accommodate practical feasibility of clinical trials, the margins of L and U could be different from those for biosimilarity evaluations, and so are the tolerance probabilities of $P_L$ and $P_U$ and two type I errors as well. Nevertheless, more research will be needed to provide guidance on selecting type I errors, the margins of L and U, and the tolerance probabilities of $P_L$ and $P_U$ for the approach of two one-sided tests.

There remains a number of questions on total biosimilarity index and interchangeability index too. For total biosimilary index or total interchangeability, it is not clear how to determine the weights for each evaluation component. And it is also uncertain how to prespecify criterion $p_{T0}$ without employing two reference treatment arms in a parallel design for the sake of saving cost in practice.

The statistical inference on the total biosimilarity index or interchangeability index may not be straightforward. Depending on the test method and power function, the reproducibility probability may not have a closed form. Consequently, it seems to be a challenging problem to construct CIs of total biosimilarity index or interchangeability index.

The methods described in Section 4.4.4.3 on minimum interchangeability index and interchangeability range may not be feasible due to the conservative approximations of the lower or upper bounds of the constructed 95% CIs, which may lead to a lower power of the tests for interchangeability.

## 4.5 Other Issues on Interchangeability

### 4.5.1 Interchangeability among Several Biosimilars and Their Reference Products

In Sections 4.3 and 4.4, we introduced the study design and analysis methods on the evaluation of a biosimilar and a reference product, and discussed the statistical challenging issues in the study design and analysis. In reality, different biosimilars to the same (or different) reference biologicals may be developed by different sponsors, and comparability studies are performed between a biosimilar by a sponsor and its corresponding reference product, but studies between one biosimilar and another are usually not done.

Two separate biosimilars may have been compared to the same reference but not between themselves. In two separate studies, both biosimilars may have been demonstrated to be biosimilar and even to be interchangeable with the same reference product. However, due to the complexity of different biological compounds such as structural changes, differences in stability and variations of manufacturing quality control, interchangeability between the two biosimilars cannot be assumed or established without additional clinical studies. The evaluation on the interchangeability among several biosimilars and their reference products is an even more challenging task than that on just one biosimilar and its reference product. Little knowledge, few regulations, and no clinical data are available to date to address this issue.

### 4.5.2 Interchangeability and Pharmacovigilance

One reason that some regulators do not endorse interchangeability is that allowing interchangeability may complicate effective pharmacovigilance for biological compounds. In reality, physicians may not be informed in an appropriate or timely fashion when switching or alternating between biosimilars and reference products. Consequently, it may subvert the ability to attribute adverse events to the appropriate agent. Besides, some adverse reactions, including immunogenic reactions, may develop only after several months of treatment. By the time of reporting of the adverse reactions, there will be two or more biological agents (biosimilars or reference products) that have been administered to patients, which then will also make it a difficult task to attribute the adverse events to the appropriate agent. More research and regulations on biological compound pharmacovigilance should be conducted when taking interchangeability into account.

## 4.6 Concluding Remarks

The assessment for interchangeability for a biosimilar is a comprehensive evaluation based on clinical data. This means the interchangeability assessment is based on all the clinical data, including bioavailability, efficacy, safety, and immunogenicity data. This also means that all the prior knowledge on a biosimilar needs to be considered when developing clinical programs to determine interchangeability.

Some useful statistical methods to test interchangeability are discussed in this chapter. The approach of two one-sided tests has the flexibility to accommodate different upper and lower equivalence margins, different type I errors for the two one-sided tests, and different tolerance probability margins. Questions remain, though, of how to prespecify these parameters in design and planning of clinical trials, and how to balance cost, risks, and benefits to investigate interchangeability.

Prior knowledge is probably important to quantitatively decide prespecified margins and/or criteria to evaluate interchangeability. However, the scope of prior knowledge may be broad, which should include, and may not be limited to, the following aspects: known safety issues with reference products, known efficacy by period with reference products, safety signals during biosimilar development, immunogenicity risks for both biosimilar and reference products, and safety and efficacy in different indications, especially when indication extrapolation has occurred. Prior knowledge and current studies data to address interchangeability will constitute the totality of evidence and then be able to provide a robust evaluation of risk and benefit assessments on switching and alternating between biosimilars and reference products.

Interchangeability among several biosimilars and their reference products may not be feasible given the current knowledge of interchangeability. Interchangeability may also complicate drug pharmacovigilance. More research and regulations on these issues should be conducted in future.

## References

1. Chow SC, Endrenyi L, Lachenbruch PA, Mentré F, "Scientific factors and current issues in biosimilar studies," *J Biopharm Stat*. 2014; 24: 1138–53.
2. Biologics Price Competition and Innovation Act of 2009, Pub. L. No. 111–148, § 7001, 124 Stat. 119, 804 (2010). http://www.fda.gov/downloads/drugs/guidancecomplianceregulatoryinformation/ucm216146.pdf.
3. Sherman RE, Biosimilar Biological Products, Biosimilar Guidance Webinar, 15 February 2012. http://www.fda.gov/downloads/Drugs/DevelopmentApprovalProcess/HowDrugsareDevelopedandApproved/ApprovalApplications/TherapeuticBiologicApplications/Biosimilars/ucm292463.pdf.
4. Health Canada Guidance for Sponsors: Information and Submission Requirements for Subsequent Entry Biologics (SEBs), 05 March 2010. http://www.hc-sc.gc.ca/dhp-mps/alt_formats/pdf/brgtherap/applic-demande/guides/seb-pbu/seb-pbu-2010-eng.pdf.
5. MHLW Guideline for Ensuring Quality, Safety and Efficacy of Biosimilar Products, 4 March 2009. http://www.pmda.go.jp/files/000153851.pdf.
6. EMA, Questions and answers on biosimilar medicines (similar biological medicinal products), 27 September 2012. http://www.ema.europa.eu/docs/en_GB/document_library/Medicine_QA/2009/12/WC500020062.pdf.
7. Chow SC, *Biosimilars: Design and Analysis of Follow-on Biologics*, Chapman & Hall/CRC Biostatistics Series, Chapman & Hall/CRC, Boca Raton, FL, 2013.
8. FDA, Guidance for Industry: Statistical Approaches to Establishing Bioequivalence, January 2001.
9. Chinchilli VM and Esinhart JD, "Design and analysis of intra-subject variability in cross-over experiments," *Stat Med*. 1996; 15: 1619–34.
10. Hyslop T, Hsuan F, Holder KJ, "A small-sample confidence interval approach to assess individual bioequivalence," *Stat Med*. 2000; 19: 288–97.

11. Dong X, Tsong Y, "Equivalence assessment for interchangeability based on two-sided tests," *J Biopharm Stat.* 2014; 24: 1312–31.
12. Dong X, Tsong Y, Shen M, "Equivalence tests for interchangeability based on two one-sided probabilities," *J Biopharm Stat.* 2014; 24: 1332–48.
13. Tse S-K, Chang J-Y, Su W-L, Chow S-C, Hsiung C, Lu Q, "Statistical quality control process for traditional Chinese medicine," *J Biopharm Stat.* 2006; 16: 861–74.
14. Tsong Y, Shen M, "An alternative approach to assess exchangeability of a test treatment and the standard treatment with normally distributed response," *J Biopharm Stat.* 2007; 17: 329–38.
15. Krishnamoorthy K, Mathew T, *Statistical Tolerance Regions: Theory, Applications, and Computation*, John Wiley & Sons, Hoboken, NJ, 2009.
16. Hall IJ, "Approximated one-sided tolerance interval for the difference or sum of two independent normal variables," *J Qual Tech.* 1984; 16: 15–9.
17. Park W, et al., "Efficacy and safety of switching from reference infliximab to CT-P13 compared with maintenance of CT-P13 in ankylosing spondylitis: 102-week data from the PLANETAS extension study," *Ann Rheum Dis.* 2016, doi:10.1136/annrheumdis-2015-208783.
18. Chow SC, On scientific factors of biosimilarity and interchangeability. Presented at FDA Public Hearing on Approval Pathway for Biosimilar and Interchangeable Biological Products, Silver Spring, MD, November 2–3, 2010.
19. Chow SC, Endrenyi L, Lachenbruch, PA, Yang LY, Chi E, "Scientific factors for assessing biosimilarity and drug interchangeability of follow-on biologics," *Biosimilars*, 2011; 1: 13–26.
20. David H, Nagaraja H, *Order Statistics*, John Wiley & Sons, New York, NY, 2003.
21. Arnold B, Groeneveld R, "Bound on expectations of linear systematic statistics based on dependent samples," *Ann Stat.* 1979; 7: 220–3.
22. Papadatos N, "Maximum variance of order statistics," *Ann Inst Stat Math.* 1995; 47: 185–93.
23. Casella G, Berger R, *Statistical Inference*, 2nd edn. Duxbury, Pacific Grove, CA, 2002.

# 5

# *Bridging a New Biological Product with Its Reference Product*

**Jianjun (David) Li and Jin Xu**

**CONTENTS**



**ABSTRACT** Unlike most small-molecule drugs, biological products are known to have a large variability although this variability does not impact its purity, potency, and safety in any clinically meaningful ways. This unique fact creates challenges in assessing similarity of a follow-on biologic and its reference product. A biosimilar follow-on biologic should be "highly similar" to its reference product. But how similar is highly similar? How do we measure the similarity? These are hard questions and there has been no consensus on how to address these questions. This chapter discusses different metrics to measure the similarity and puts forward two scientific principles, which can be used to establish the threshold for similarity in each metric. The first principle is that a biosimilar criterion should be determined in a way that it allows the reference product to claim similarity to itself with a high probability. And the second is that all commercial lots of the reference product should meet a preset lot consistency criterion with a high probability. Following the proposed metrics and established thresholds, the corresponding statistical approaches are proposed for evaluating the similarity. Simulations are provided to compare different statistical approaches given at the end of this chapter.

## 5.1 Introduction

The biological products are distinctly different from small-molecule drugs. Unlike small-molecule drugs, a biological product is seldom a product with molecules of identical structure. Instead, it is usually composed of a mixture of molecules with slightly different structures, like all snowflakes are similar but not identical to each other. This inherent heterogeneity of a biological product comes mainly from its complex molecular structure and its complicated manufacture process.

Compared with small-molecule drugs, biological products are much larger in molecular weights and have more complex structures. Take two examples that we are familiar with, a small-molecule drug Zocor for lowering cholesterol level and a large biological product Humira for treating autoimmune diseases (Zocor Structure; Humira Structure). Humira's average molecular weight is 144,190, which is 300 times larger than Zocor, which is 418. Humira's structure is also more complex, involves more layered structures, which are folded in place by weak forces among various components that are sensitive to changes in temperature, pH, and light intensity in the environment and small variations in the manufacture process.

Another significant difference between small-molecule drugs and biological products is the complexity of their manufacturing processes. A small-molecule drug is often produced by a relatively simpler process that can be controlled more precisely and produce the same molecule consistently, but a biological product is either made by or derived from living organisms such as cell lines, yeast, bacteria, animals, or plants that are more sensitive to small variations in their environment. The level of complexity is also reflected in the number of in-process tests used to ensure the quality of the product. According to an European Commission (EC) consensus information paper in 2013 (EC, 2013), there are typically 250 tests for a biological product manufacture process but only about 50 for a small-molecule drug. Consequently, a biological product often has a larger variability among its manufactured lots.

As a result, the licensure pathway for follow-on biologics is different from that for generic versions of small-molecule drugs. There is an established standard for assessing the equivalence between the generic version and brand name product. It typically involves demonstration that the generic product has the same physiochemical properties as the brand name product and its average bioavailability is equivalent to that of the brand name product, typically within 80%–125% of the brand name product's bioavailability. However, it is much more challenging to establish similarity between a follow-on biologic and its original reference product because of the complexity of the manufacturing process and inherent molecule heterogeneity in both the follow-on biologic and the reference product. This challenge is well recognized by regulatory agencies. The European Medicines Agency (EMA) in its 2014 guideline on biosimilar products explicitly stated that the standard generic approach applicable to most chemically derived medicinal products is in principle not sufficient to demonstrate similarity of biological/biotechnology-derived product (EMA, 2014). In 1985, the Food and Drug Administration (FDA) required a full new drug application for biologicals even when the ingredient in the product is thought to be identical in molecule structure to a product that had been previously approved by the FDA (FDA, 1985). In addition to demonstrating similar bioavailability between the follow-on biologic and its reference product by bioassays and pharmacokinetic studies, applicants must also provide "product-specific full safety and efficacy" of the biological product independently. Only after many years' improvements in manufacture process and quality control of the product, the requirement is reduced and now an abbreviated application procedure is available as the Biologic Price Competition and Innovation (BPCI) Act signed into law in March 2010 (BPCI, 2009). The abbreviated procedure is for the sponsor to demonstrate that the follow-on biological is "highly similar" to the reference product but not to demonstrate the safety and effectiveness of the follow-on biologic independently. Essentially, the abbreviated pathway allows the follow-on biologic to piggyback on the safety and effectiveness established by the reference product. In the short period that followed the BPCI Act, great attention has been focused on how to define and demonstrate the high similarity between a follow-on and its reference product. In 2012, the FDA recommended a stepwise approach to establish similarity in terms of structure, function, animal toxicity, human pharmacokinetics and pharmacodynamics, clinical immunogenicity, and clinical safety and effectiveness, and advised the sponsors of the follow-on to meet with the FDA to discuss their development plans and to establish milestone reviews during the development (FDA, 2012a). In the EU, the EMA recommends a similar stepwise approach (EMA, 2014).

To assess similarity between a follow-on biologic and its reference product in light of "totality of the evidence," the FDA suggests to present comparison of the products in a fingerprint-like analysis to characterize the follow-on biologic covering a large number of attributes (FDA, 2012b). A multitiered approach can also be employed where a large number of attributes are subject to varying degrees of statistical evaluation; the hypothesis testing is conducted for the endpoints with the most importance, point estimate and 95% confidence interval calculated for those of median importance, and summary statistics provided for endpoints with less importance. Another approach is to use a biosimilar index (Hsieh et al., 2013), in which the reproducibility of similarity tests regarding individual attributes of the product is weighted by individual attributes' clinical importance and combined to form a global index to measure the overall biosimilarity.

Getting down to an individual attribute or endpoint level, how to assess similarity given the high variability remains a challenge. There is no universally accepted rule to follow for establishing the similarity criterion, including the metric used to measure similarity and threshold to claim

$\mu_{(3)} - \mu_{(1)} < \ln(1.5) = 0.4055$ as the preset consistency criterion in the following. Like the choice of biosimilar level and lot consistency level, the consistency criterion stated in Principle 2 should also be determined based on the specific biologic product and the nature of the disease the biologic is intended to treat.

One approach to evaluate the similarity between a biological product and its reference product is to use the Euclidean distance between the two product means. The similarity is assessed using an equivalence test whose hypotheses are given by $H_0 : \mu_T - \mu_R \leq -\delta$ or $\mu_T - \mu_R \geq \delta$ versus $H_1 : -\delta < \mu_T - \mu_R < \delta$, where $\delta$ is a prespecified similarity threshold, and $\mu_T$ and $\mu_R$ are the population means of the follow-on biologic and the reference product, respectively.

Traditionally, $\delta = \ln(1.25) = 0.2231$ has been used for small-molecule drugs. However, given the larger variability of biologics, 0.2231 may not be appropriate. Intuitively, the choice of biosimilar threshold $\delta$ should be based on the tolerable variation limit of the reference product. If the reference product has a large variability, which has been demonstrated to have no meaningful impact on the product purity, potency, and safety, then $\delta$ for assessing biosimilarity of the follow-on product may accordingly be set relatively large.

Assume that the reference product has an overall across-lot mean $\mu_{R0}$ and a variance $\sigma_{R0}^2$, that is, $\mu_R$ has a normal distribution $N(\mu_{R0}, \sigma_{R0}^2)$. Consider any two lots of the reference product. By Principle 1, these two lots should be able to be declared "biosimilar" to each other with 95% probability. That is, $\delta$ should be chosen such that $\Pr(-\delta < \mu_{R2} - \mu_{R1} < \delta) = 95\%$, where $\mu_{R1}$ and $\mu_{R2}$ are the means of the two lots. A straightforward calculation gives the relationship

$$\delta = 1.960\sqrt{2}\sigma_{R0} = 2.772\sigma_{R0}. \tag{5.1}$$

Per Principle 2, if $\mu_{(3)} \leq \mu_{(2)} \leq \mu_{(1)}$ are ordered means from three lots, we expect

$$\Pr(\mu_{(3)} - \mu_{(1)} < 0.4055) = 95\%. \tag{5.2}$$

As it is intended, Equation 5.2 helps to quantify the variability of the reference product lots. Per Appendix 5.1,

$$\Pr(\mu_{(3)} - \mu_{(1)} < 0.4055) = 6E\left[\Phi\left(\frac{0.4055}{\sigma_{R0}} + \pi_1\right)\left\{1 - \Phi(\pi_1)\right\} - \Phi(\pi_1)\Phi(\pi_1)\right], \tag{5.3}$$

where $\pi_1$ denotes the standard normal variable and $\Phi(\cdot)$ the cumulative distribution function of the standard normal variable. Then we get $\sigma_{R0} = 0.1210$. Now substitute $\sigma_{R0} = 0.1210$ to Equation 5.1 and we have

$$\delta = 2.772\sigma_{R0} = 2.772 \times 0.1210 = 0.3354. \tag{5.4}$$

Thus, we established a framework for deriving a biosimilar threshold for the given Euclidean distance. The biosimilar threshold $\delta$ depends on three factors for a given metric: (1) desired reference biosimilar level, (2) required reference lot consistency level, and (3) lot consistency criterion. If a large difference among various lots of the reference product does not impact its efficacy and safety, then the lot consistency criterion can be less stringent, the lot consistency level can be lower, and/or the biosimilar level can be higher, consequently $\delta$ can be larger.

### 5.2.2 Impact of Selecting Reference Product

Using the traditional Euclidean distance, the similarity can be assessed by testing hypotheses

$$H_0 : |\mu_T - \mu_R| \geq 0.3354 \quad \text{versus} \quad H_1 : |\mu_T - \mu_R| < 0.3354. \tag{5.5}$$

Note that one needs to choose one lot of the reference product for testing the hypotheses. Different selection of the reference lot, or equivalently, different selection of $\mu_R$, will impact the probability of rejecting the null hypothesis and consequently the probability of claiming biosimilar. For example, a follow-on biologic with $\mu_T = 0$ is biosimilar to the reference product with $\mu_{R0} = 0$. However, as indicated in Figure 5.1, the probability of claiming biosimilarity can range from <3% to 100% depending on which reference lot, i.e., $\mu_R$, has been chosen. The probabilities are 84% and 31% when $\mu_R = \sigma_{R0} = 0.1210$ and $\mu_R = 2\sigma_{R0} = 0.2420$, respectively.

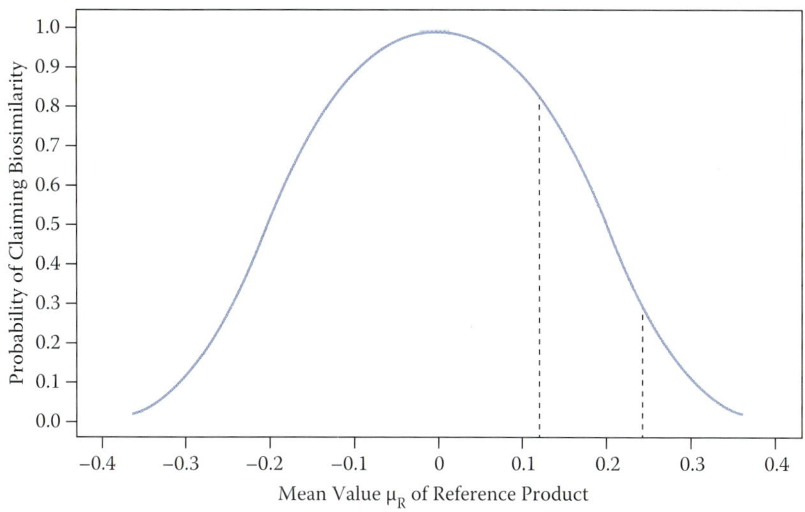


**FIGURE 5.1**
Probability of claiming biosimilarity when $\mu_T = 0$ and $\mu_R$ is sampled from $N(0, 01210^2)$.

### 5.2.3 Alternative Metrics and Thresholds

Given the impact of selecting a different reference lot, stated in Section 5.2.2, one's natural thinking is to use more than one lot from the reference product, in which case an alternative approach to assess similarity is to test

$$H_0: \left|\mu_T - \frac{\mu_{R1}+\mu_{R2}}{2}\right| \geq \delta^* \quad \text{versus} \quad H_1: \left|\mu_T - \frac{\mu_{R1}+\mu_{R2}}{2}\right| < \delta^*, \tag{5.6}$$

where $\mu_{R1}$ and $\mu_{R2}$ are means of two separate lots from the reference product. So $\mu_{R1}$ and $\mu_{R2}$ are independent and have the identical normal distribution $N(\mu_{R0}, \sigma_{R0}^2)$.

Following the framework stated in Section 5.2.1, $\delta^*$ should be chosen such that a hypothetical third lot $\mu_{R3}$ from the same reference product can be claimed "biosimilar" to the two selected reference lots with 95% probability, which means $\Pr\left(\left|\mu_{R3} - \frac{\mu_{R1}+\mu_{R2}}{2}\right| < \delta^*\right) = 95\%$. Simple calculation results in $\delta^* = 1.960 \cdot \sqrt{3/2}\sigma_{R0} = 2.401\sigma_{R0}$. Using $\sigma_{R0} = 0.1210$ from Section 5.2.1, we have $\delta^* = 0.2905$. So Equation 5.6 becomes

$$H_0: \left|\mu_T - \frac{\mu_{R1}+\mu_{R2}}{2}\right| \geq 0.2905 \quad \text{versus} \quad H_1: \left|\mu_T - \frac{\mu_{R1}+\mu_{R2}}{2}\right| < 0.2905. \tag{5.7}$$

The second alternative is based on a modification to the relative distance metric that Kang and Chow (2013) have proposed. The relative distance is defined as the absolute ratio of two differences, the difference between the follow-on biologic and the reference product, and the difference between the two reference lots, i.e., $\left|\frac{\mu_T - \frac{\mu_{R1}+\mu_{R2}}{2}}{\mu_{R2}-\mu_{R1}}\right|$. The rationale behind the relative distance is the recognition of potential large difference between reference lots even after the reference product has established consistency. Therefore, any difference between the follow-on biologic and reference product should be evaluated in the context of the difference between two reference lots. A larger difference between lots of reference product should allow a larger difference between the follow-on biologic and the reference product. However, we realized that the denominator in the relative distance is quite likely close to 0 as the two lots are chosen from the same reference product. In this case, the relative distance is very sensitive to the minor changes of $\mu_{R1}$ or $\mu_{R2}$. So we use a modified version of relative distance and propose to assess similarity by testing

$$H_0: \frac{\left|\mu_T - \dfrac{\mu_{R1}+\mu_{R2}}{2}\right|}{\max\left(\left|\mu_{R2}-\mu_{R1}\right|,\ \sqrt{2}\sigma_{R0}\right)} \ge \delta^{**} \quad \text{versus} \quad H_1: \frac{\left|\mu_T - \dfrac{\mu_{R1}+\mu_{R2}}{2}\right|}{\max\left(\left|\mu_{R2}-\mu_{R1}\right|,\ \sqrt{2}\sigma_{R0}\right)} < \delta^{**},$$

where $\mu_{R1}$ and $\mu_{R2}$ again are the means of the two lots from the reference product and are independently distributed as $N(\mu_{R0}, \sigma_{R0}^2)$. Note that $\mu_{R1}-\mu_{R2}$ has a standard deviation (SD) of $\sqrt{2}\sigma_{R0}$. So if $|\mu_{R1}-\mu_{R2}|$ is smaller than its SD $\sqrt{2}\sigma_{R0}$, $\sqrt{2}\sigma_{R0}$ is used in the denominator.

Assuming that a hypothetical third lot $\mu_{R3}$ from the same reference product will be "biosimilar" to the two selected reference lots with 95% probability, then $\Pr\left(\frac{\left|\mu_{R3} - \frac{\mu_{R1}+\mu_{R2}}{2}\right|}{\max\left(\left|\mu_{R2}-\mu_{R1}\right|,\ \sqrt{2}\sigma_{R0}\right)} < \delta^{**}\right) = 95\%$. It can be calculated $\delta^{**} = 1.598$. Thus, the similarity can be assessed by testing

$$H_0: \frac{\left|\mu_T - \dfrac{\mu_{R1}+\mu_{R2}}{2}\right|}{\max\left(\left|\mu_{R2}-\mu_{R1}\right|, 0.1711\right)} \ge 1.598 \quad \text{versus} \quad H_1: \frac{\left|\mu_T - \dfrac{\mu_{R1}+\mu_{R2}}{2}\right|}{\max\left(\left|\mu_{R2}-\mu_{R1}\right|, 0.1711\right)} < 1.598. \tag{5.8}$$

If the two selected lots are so different that their difference is more than 1 SD of the difference, then $\max\left(\left|\mu_{R2}-\mu_{R1}\right|, 0.1711\right) = \left|\mu_{R2}-\mu_{R1}\right|$ and Equation 5.8 becomes

$$H_0: \frac{\left|\mu_T - \dfrac{\mu_{R1}+\mu_{R2}}{2}\right|}{\left|\mu_{R2}-\mu_{R1}\right|} \ge 1.598 \quad \text{versus} \quad H_1: \frac{\left|\mu_T - \dfrac{\mu_{R1}+\mu_{R2}}{2}\right|}{\left|\mu_{R2}-\mu_{R1}\right|} < 1.598. \tag{5.9}$$

Then the similarity is assessed using the relative distance metric $\left|\frac{\mu_T - \frac{\mu_{R1}+\mu_{R2}}{2}}{\mu_{R2}-\mu_{R1}}\right|$ proposed by Kang and Chow (2013). On the other hand, if the two lots are close to each other such that their difference is within 1 SD, Equation 5.8 becomes

$$H_0: \left|\mu_T - \frac{\mu_{R1}+\mu_{R2}}{2}\right| \ge 0.2734 \quad \text{versus} \quad H_1: \left|\mu_T - \frac{\mu_{R1}+\mu_{R2}}{2}\right| < 0.2734 \tag{5.10}$$

and the similarity is assessed using the Euclidean distance metric $\left|\mu_T - \frac{\mu_{R1}+\mu_{R2}}{2}\right|$.

## 5.3 Statistical Approach to Assess Biosimilar

Section 5.2 described three different metrics and corresponding thresholds to assess biosimilarity. For testing the hypotheses in Equation 5.5, the clinical study is a two-arm parallel group design, with one arm using a lot selected from a reference product and the other using follow-on biologic. Assume that there are $n$ subjects in each arm.

Let $Y_{Ti}$, $i=1,\cdots,n$ and $Y_{Ri}$, $i=1,\cdots,n$ denote the response variables from the follow-on biologic and the reference product, respectively, and further assume that they independently follow the normal distributions with the means $\mu_T$ and $\mu_R$, respectively, and the common known variance $\sigma$. The null hypothesis in Equation 5.5 can then be rejected and biosimilarity claimed if

$$\frac{\sqrt{n}\left(\bar{Y}_T - \bar{Y}_R - 0.3354\right)}{\sqrt{2}\sigma} < -z_\alpha \quad \text{and} \quad \frac{\sqrt{n}\left(\bar{Y}_T - \bar{Y}_R + 0.3354\right)}{\sqrt{2}\sigma} > z_\alpha, \tag{5.11}$$

where $z_\alpha$ is the upper $\alpha$ quantile of the standard normal distribution, and $z_\alpha = 1.645$ if $\alpha = 0.05$. We refer to this testing method as Method 1 in the following sections.

For testing hypotheses in Equations 5.7 and 5.8, a three-arm study will be conducted, which includes one arm for the follow-on biologic and two reference arms, each using a different lot of the reference product. Assume that there are $n$ subjects enrolled in the follow-on biologic arm and $n/2$ subjects enrolled in each reference arm for a total of $2n$ subjects, the same total number of subjects as the two-arm study has. Using a similar notation to that used for the two-arm study, denote $Y_{Ti}$, $i=1,\cdots,n$ and $Y_{R1i}$, $Y_{R2i}$ $i=1,\cdots,n/2$ the response variables from the follow-on biologic and the reference product in the second and third arms. Similarly, assume that they independently follow the normal distributions with the means $\mu_T$, $\mu_{R1}$, and $\mu_{R2}$, respectively, and the common known variance $\sigma$. The null hypothesis in Equation 5.7 can be rejected at the significance level $\alpha$ and the biosimilarity claimed if

$$\frac{\sqrt{n}\left(\bar{Y}_T - \left(\bar{Y}_{R1} + \bar{Y}_{R2}\right)/2 - 0.2905\right)}{\sqrt{2}\sigma} < -z_\alpha \quad \text{and} \quad \frac{\sqrt{n}\left(\bar{Y}_T - \left(\bar{Y}_{R1} + \bar{Y}_{R2}\right)/2 + 0.2905\right)}{\sqrt{2}\sigma} > z_\alpha. \tag{5.12}$$

We refer to this testing method as Method 2 in the following sections.

For testing the hypotheses in Equation 5.8, we need to first determine whether $|\mu_{R2} - \mu_{R1}| > 0.1711$ because the hypotheses for testing biosimilarity are different depending whether it is true or not. When $\mu_{R2} - \mu_{R1} > 0.1711$, Equation 5.8 becomes

$$H_0 : \mu_T - \frac{\mu_{R1} + \mu_{R2}}{2} - 1.598\left(\mu_{R2} - \mu_{R1}\right) \geq 0$$

or

$$\mu_T - \frac{\mu_{R1}+\mu_{R2}}{2} + 1.598(\mu_{R2}-\mu_{R1}) \le 0$$

versus

$$H_1: -1.598(\mu_{R2}-\mu_{R1}) < \mu_T - \frac{\mu_{R1}+\mu_{R2}}{2} < 1.598(\mu_{R2}-\mu_{R1}). \qquad (5.13)$$

When $\mu_{R2}-\mu_{R1} < -0.1711$ or equivalently $\mu_{R1}-\mu_{R2} > 0.1711$, Equation 5.8 becomes

$$H_0: \mu_T - \frac{\mu_{R1}+\mu_{R2}}{2} - 1.598(\mu_{R1}-\mu_{R2}) \ge 0$$

or

$$\mu_T - \frac{\mu_{R1}+\mu_{R2}}{2} + 1.598(\mu_{R1}-\mu_{R2}) \le 0$$

versus

$$H_1: -1.598(\mu_{R1}-\mu_{R2}) < \mu_T - \frac{\mu_{R1}+\mu_{R2}}{2} < 1.598(\mu_{R1}-\mu_{R2}). \qquad (5.14)$$

When $|\mu_{R2}-\mu_{R1}| \le 0.1711$, Equation 5.8 becomes

$$H_0: \left|\mu_T - \frac{\mu_{R1}+\mu_{R2}}{2}\right| \ge 0.2734 \quad \text{versus} \quad H_1: \left|\mu_T - \frac{\mu_{R1}+\mu_{R2}}{2}\right| < 0.2734. \qquad (5.15)$$

Statistically, we will reject the hypothesis $\mu_{R2}-\mu_{R1} \le 0.1711$ and conclude $\mu_{R2}-\mu_{R1} > 0.1711$ at the significance level $\alpha$ if $\frac{\sqrt{n}\left(\bar{Y}_{R2}-\bar{Y}_{R1}-0.1711\right)}{2\sigma} > z_\alpha$. On the other hand, we will reject the hypothesis $\mu_{R1}-\mu_{R2} \le 0.1711$ and conclude $\mu_{R1}-\mu_{R2} > 0.1711$ at the significance level $\alpha$ if $\frac{\sqrt{n}\left(\bar{Y}_{R1}-\bar{Y}_{R2}-0.1711\right)}{2\sigma} > z_\alpha$. So together we will claim biosimilarity if

$$\frac{\sqrt{n}\left(\bar{Y}_{R2}-\bar{Y}_{R1}-0.1711\right)}{2\sigma} > z_\alpha \text{ and } \frac{\sqrt{n}\left(\bar{Y}_T-\left(\bar{Y}_{R1}+\bar{Y}_{R2}\right)/2-1.598\left(\bar{Y}_{R2}-\bar{Y}_{R1}\right)\right)}{\sigma\sqrt{1+(1/2+1.598)^2\cdot 2+(1/2-1.598)^2\cdot 2}} < -z_\alpha \text{ and}$$

$$\frac{\sqrt{n}\left(\bar{Y}_T-\left(\bar{Y}_{R1}+\bar{Y}_{R2}\right)/2+1.598\left(\bar{Y}_{R2}-\bar{Y}_{R1}\right)\right)}{\sigma\sqrt{1+(1/2+1.598)^2\cdot 2+(1/2-1.598)^2\cdot 2}} > z_\alpha$$

or

$$\frac{\sqrt{n}\left(\bar{Y}_{R1}-\bar{Y}_{R2}-0.1711\right)}{2\sigma}>z_{\alpha} \text{ and } \frac{\sqrt{n}\left(\bar{Y}_{T}-\left(\bar{Y}_{R1}+\bar{Y}_{R2}\right)/2-1.598\left(\bar{Y}_{R1}-\bar{Y}_{R2}\right)\right)}{\sigma\sqrt{1+(1/2+1.598)^2\cdot 2+(1/2-1.598)^2\cdot 2}}<-z_{\alpha} \text{ and }$$

$$\frac{\sqrt{n}\left(\bar{Y}_{T}-\left(\bar{Y}_{R1}+\bar{Y}_{R2}\right)/2+1.598\left(\bar{Y}_{R1}-\bar{Y}_{R2}\right)\right)}{\sigma\sqrt{1+(1/2+1.598)^2\cdot 2+(1/2-1.598)^2\cdot 2}}>z_{\alpha}$$

or

$$\frac{\sqrt{n}\left(\bar{Y}_{R2}-\bar{Y}_{R1}-0.1711\right)}{2\sigma}\le z_{\alpha} \text{ and } \frac{\sqrt{n}\left(\bar{Y}_{R1}-\bar{Y}_{R2}-0.1711\right)}{2\sigma}\le z_{\alpha} \text{ and }$$

$$\frac{\sqrt{n}\left(\bar{Y}_{T}-\left(\bar{Y}_{R1}+\bar{Y}_{R2}\right)/2-0.2734\right)}{\sqrt{2}\sigma}<-z_{\alpha} \text{ and } \frac{\sqrt{n}\left(\bar{Y}_{T}-\left(\bar{Y}_{R1}+\bar{Y}_{R2}\right)/2+0.2734\right)}{\sqrt{2}\sigma}>z_{\alpha}. \quad (5.16)$$

We refer to this testing method as Method 3 in the following sections. By construction, Method 1 and Method 2 control the type I error rate at the targeted level. We have done simulations and confirmed that Method 3 controls type I error rate at the targeted level as well.

## 5.4 Simulations to Compare the Three Testing Methods

We compare the probability of claiming biosimilarity by the three testing methods via simulations. The simulation setup is as follows:

1. Choose $\mu_T$ equal to some number, e.g., $\mu_T = 0$.
2. Draw $\mu_{R1}$ and $\mu_{R2}$ independently from a normal distribution $N(0, 0.1210^2)$. For Method 1, $\mu_R = \mu_{R1}$.
3. Draw independent samples $Y_{Ti}$, $i = 1, \cdots, 300$ from $N(\mu_T, 0.5^2)$ and $Y_{R1i}$, $Y_{R2i}$ $i = 1, \cdots, 150$ from $N(\mu_{R1}, 0.5^2)$ and $N(\mu_{R2}, 0.5^2)$, respectively, for each given triplets $(\mu_T, \mu_{R1}, \mu_{R2})$. For Method 1, additional $Y_{Ri}$=$Y_{R1i}$, $i = 1, \cdots, 150$ are drawn from $N(\mu_{R1}, 0.5^2)$.
4. For each set of samples simulated in Step 3, the decision at $\alpha = 0.05$ by each method per Equation 5.11 or 5.12 or 5.16 is recorded as rejection = 1 and 0 otherwise.
5. Repeat Step 3 and Step 4 10,000 times and calculate the probability of claiming biosimilarity by each method as the proportion of rejections out of 10,000 times.

To compare the three methods, $\mu_T$ is chosen as 0, 0.1, 0.2, 0.5, 0.6, and 0.7. For $\mu_{R1}$ and $\mu_{R2}$, 200 random draws are made and four of them are deleted as they do not meet condition $|\mu_{R1} - \mu_{R2}| < \log(1.5)$, the consistence criterion. The mean of the probability of claiming biosimilarity over these 196 scenarios by each method is reported in Table 5.1. Other statistics reported in Table 5.1

TABLE 5.1
Probability of Claiming Biosimilarity for Different $\mu_T$ Over Randomly Drawn Pair ($\mu_{R1} = \mu_R, \mu_{R2}$)

| $\mu_T$ | Method | Mean | SD | Min | P5 | Q1 | Median | Q3 | P95 | Max |
|---|---|---|---|---|---|---|---|---|---|---|
| 0.0 | Method 1 | 0.9734 | 0.1134 | 0.0302 | 0.8856 | 0.9991 | 1.0000 | 1.0000 | 1.0000 | 1.0000 |
| | Method 2 | 0.9886 | 0.0678 | 0.1306 | 0.9505 | 0.9988 | 0.9999 | 1.0000 | 1.0000 | 1.0000 |
| | Method 3 | 0.9862 | 0.0492 | 0.5648 | 0.9171 | 0.9973 | 0.9998 | 1.0000 | 1.0000 | 1.0000 |
| 0.1 | Method 1 | 0.9179 | 0.2158 | 0.0009 | 0.3483 | 0.9973 | 1.0000 | 1.0000 | 1.0000 | 1.0000 |
| | Method 2 | 0.9179 | 0.1858 | 0.0228 | 0.4350 | 0.9463 | 0.9991 | 1.0000 | 1.0000 | 1.0000 |
| | Method 3 | 0.9048 | 0.2043 | 0.0456 | 0.2908 | 0.9263 | 0.9983 | 1.0000 | 1.0000 | 1.0000 |
| 0.2 | Method 1 | 0.7666 | 0.3673 | 0.0000 | 0.0015 | 0.6770 | 0.9888 | 1.0000 | 1.0000 | 1.0000 |
| | Method 2 | 0.6277 | 0.3869 | 0.0000 | 0.0051 | 0.2094 | 0.8000 | 0.9867 | 0.9999 | 1.0000 |
| | Method 3 | 0.6162 | 0.3738 | 0.0000 | 0.0038 | 0.2704 | 0.7524 | 0.9692 | 0.9998 | 1.0000 |
| 0.5 | Method 1 | 0.0313 | 0.1255 | 0.0000 | 0.0000 | 0.0000 | 0.0000 | 0.0004 | 0.2138 | 0.9969 |
| | Method 2 | 0.0023 | 0.0302 | 0.0000 | 0.0000 | 0.0000 | 0.0000 | 0.0000 | 0.0004 | 0.4228 |
| | Method 3 | 0.0187 | 0.0942 | 0.0000 | 0.0000 | 0.0000 | 0.0000 | 0.0003 | 0.0749 | 0.7645 |
| 0.6 | Method 1 | 0.0038 | 0.0438 | 0.0000 | 0.0000 | 0.0000 | 0.0000 | 0.0000 | 0.0004 | 0.6076 |
| | Method 2 | 0.0000 | 0.0003 | 0.0000 | 0.0000 | 0.0000 | 0.0000 | 0.0000 | 0.0000 | 0.0037 |
| | Method 3 | 0.0064 | 0.0423 | 0.0000 | 0.0000 | 0.0000 | 0.0000 | 0.0000 | 0.0075 | 0.4204 |
| 0.7 | Method 1 | 0.0001 | 0.0011 | 0.0000 | 0.0000 | 0.0000 | 0.0000 | 0.0000 | 0.0000 | 0.0159 |
| | Method 2 | 0.0000 | 0.0000 | 0.0000 | 0.0000 | 0.0000 | 0.0000 | 0.0000 | 0.0000 | 0.0000 |
| | Method 3 | 0.0014 | 0.0109 | 0.0000 | 0.0000 | 0.0000 | 0.0000 | 0.0000 | 0.0002 | 0.1192 |

*Notes:* Max, maximum value; Min, minimum value; P5, fifth percentile; P95, 95th percentile; Q1, first quartile or 25th percentile; Q3, third quartile or 75th percentile; SD, standard deviation.

**TABLE 5.2**

Probability of Claiming Biosimilar for a Given Set of $\mu_T, \mu_{R1} (= \mu_R), \mu_{R2}$

| | | | $\mu_{R2}$ | | | | | | | | |
|---|---|---|---|---|---|---|---|---|---|---|---|
| $\mu_T$ | $\mu_{R1}$ | **Method** | **−0.3630** | **−0.2420** | **−0.1210** | **−0.0605** | **0** | **0.0605** | **0.1210** | **0.2420** | **0.3630** |
| 0 | 0.3630 | Method 1 | 0.01 | 0.01 | 0.01 | 0.01 | 0.01 | 0.01 | 0.01 | 0.01 | 0.01 |
| | | Method 2 | 1.00 | 1.00 | 0.99 | 0.96 | 0.85 | 0.61 | 0.33 | 0.03 | 0.00 |
| | | Method 3 | 1.00 | 1.00 | 1.00 | 1.00 | 0.99 | 0.85 | 0.44 | 0.01 | 0.00 |
| 0 | 0.2420 | Method 1 | 0.74 | 0.74 | 0.74 | 0.74 | 0.74 | 0.74 | 0.74 | 0.74 | 0.74 |
| | | Method 2 | 1.00 | 1.00 | 1.00 | 1.00 | 0.99 | 0.96 | 0.85 | 0.33 | 0.03 |
| | | Method 3 | 1.00 | 1.00 | 1.00 | 1.00 | 0.99 | 0.92 | 0.74 | 0.20 | 0.01 |
| 0 | 0.1210 | Method 1 | 1.00 | 1.00 | 1.00 | 1.00 | 1.00 | 1.00 | 1.00 | 1.00 | 1.00 |
| | | Method 2 | 0.99 | 1.00 | 1.00 | 1.00 | 1.00 | 1.00 | 0.99 | 0.84 | 0.33 |
| | | Method 3 | 1.00 | 1.00 | 1.00 | 1.00 | 1.00 | 1.00 | 0.98 | 0.73 | 0.44 |
| 0 | 0 | Method 1 | 1.00 | 1.00 | 1.00 | 1.00 | 1.00 | 1.00 | 1.00 | 1.00 | 1.00 |
| | | Method 2 | 0.85 | 0.99 | 1.00 | 1.00 | 1.00 | 1.00 | 1.00 | 0.99 | 0.85 |
| | | Method 3 | 0.99 | 0.99 | 1.00 | 1.00 | 1.00 | 1.00 | 1.00 | 0.99 | 0.99 |
| 0.1 | 0.3630 | Method 1 | 0.55 | 0.55 | 0.55 | 0.55 | 0.55 | 0.55 | 0.55 | 0.55 | 0.55 |
| | | Method 2 | 1.00 | 1.00 | 1.00 | 1.00 | 1.00 | 1.00 | 0.98 | 0.70 | 0.17 |
| | | Method 3 | 1.00 | 1.00 | 1.00 | 1.00 | 1.00 | 1.00 | 0.96 | 0.54 | 0.08 |
| 0.1 | 0.2420 | Method 1 | 1.00 | 1.00 | 1.00 | 1.00 | 1.00 | 1.00 | 1.00 | 1.00 | 1.00 |
| | | Method 2 | 0.93 | 1.00 | 1.00 | 1.00 | 1.00 | 1.00 | 1.00 | 0.98 | 0.70 |
| | | Method 3 | 1.00 | 1.00 | 1.00 | 1.00 | 1.00 | 1.00 | 1.00 | 0.94 | 0.54 |
| 0.1 | 0.1210 | Method 1 | 1.00 | 1.00 | 1.00 | 1.00 | 1.00 | 1.00 | 1.00 | 1.00 | 1.00 |
| | | Method 2 | 0.51 | 0.94 | 1.00 | 1.00 | 1.00 | 1.00 | 1.00 | 1.00 | 0.98 |
| | | Method 3 | 1.00 | 0.99 | 1.00 | 1.00 | 1.00 | 1.00 | 1.00 | 1.00 | 0.96 |
| 0.1 | 0.0000 | Method 1 | 1.00 | 1.00 | 1.00 | 1.00 | 1.00 | 1.00 | 1.00 | 1.00 | 1.00 |
| | | Method 2 | 0.07 | 0.52 | 0.94 | 0.99 | 1.00 | 1.00 | 1.00 | 1.00 | 1.00 |
| | | Method 3 | 0.90 | 0.57 | 0.87 | 0.97 | 1.00 | 1.00 | 1.00 | 1.00 | 1.00 |
| 0.1 | −0.1210 | Method 1 | 0.88 | 0.88 | 0.88 | 0.88 | 0.88 | 0.88 | 0.88 | 0.88 | 0.88 |
| | | Method 2 | 0.00 | 0.07 | 0.52 | 0.78 | 0.94 | 1.00 | 1.00 | 1.00 | 1.00 |
| | | Method 3 | 0.12 | 0.04 | 0.36 | 0.65 | 0.87 | 1.00 | 1.00 | 1.00 | 1.00 |

include the SD, the minimum value (Min), the fifth percentile (P5), the first quartile or 25th percentile (Q1), the median (Median), the third quartile or 75th percentile (Q3), and the maximum value (Max).

To compare the three methods at a specific triplet ($\mu_T, \mu_{R1}, \mu_{R2}$), Step 3 through Step 5 are also repeated for $\mu_T = 0, 0.1, 0.2$, $\mu_{R1} = 0, \pm 0.5 \times 0.1210, \pm 0.1210, \pm 2 \times 0.1210, \pm 3 \times 0.1210$, and $\mu_{R2} = 0, \pm 0.5 \times 0.1210, \pm 0.1210, \pm 2 \times 0.1210, \pm 3 \times 0.1210$. Due to space limitation, some of these results as typical scenarios are reported in Table 5.2.

From Table 5.1, Method 3 performs better in terms of probability of claiming biosimilarity when the follow-on biologic is the closest to the reference product ($\mu_T = \mu_{R0} = 0$) and reference lots are picked randomly. The SD is the smallest among the three methods, which indicates that Method 3 is least sensitive to the selection of reference lots. Also the minimal probability of claiming biosimilarity by Method 3 is 56%, while the other two methods have just 3% and 13%. When $\mu_T = 0.1$, Method 2 seems to perform better as 95% of randomly drawn cases have the probability at least 44%, while the probabilities by the other two methods are 35% and 29%, respectively. When $\mu_T = 0.2$, Method 3 has at least 68% probability of claiming biosimilarity among 75% of cases, while other two methods have probabilities below 30%. When $\mu_T = 0.5$, all three methods have small probabilities to claim biosimilarity, in most cases, if not all. For example, only 5% of cases have a probability of $\geq 22\%$ for Method 1, $\geq 0.04\%$ for Method 2, and $\geq 7.5\%$ for Method 3. These probabilities are even smaller when $\mu_T > 0.5$.

Table 5.2 confirms the findings identified in Table 5.1, and it also provides the probability of claiming biosimilarity when choice of reference lots is controllable, so $\mu_{R1}$ and $\mu_{R2}$ are known or can be approximately estimated.

## 5.5 Summary and Discussions

It is well known that the biological product has large variability, though the variations of the product rarely impact the product's purity, potency, and safety meaningfully. Availability of follow-on biologics has the potential to make a significant contribution to public health. However, conducting biosimilar studies by sponsors and approving biosimilar biologics by regulatory agencies have been challenging. In particular, the issues of how to measure similarity and determine a threshold for endpoints, especially clinically important ones, have been heavily discussed. This chapter discusses different options to formulate metrics to measure the similarity and puts forward two scientific principles to establish the threshold for each metric. The first principle is that the biosimilar criterion should be determined in a way that it allows the reference product to claim similarity to itself with a high probability, and the second is that all commercial lots of the reference product should meet a preset lot consistency criterion with a high probability.

With proposed metrics and derived thresholds, we compare the performance of corresponding statistical approaches in evaluating the similarity of the follow-on biologic and the reference product under various configurations of the follow-on and its reference product.

While the proposed approach helps to set up the specific threshold to assess biosimilarity, its implementation, especially the determination of the reference biosimilar level, the reference lot consistence level, and the consistency criterion, will need to take into consideration the specific disease area and the reference product profile. Therefore, it is important to work jointly with clinical colleagues within the study team and get input from regulatory agencies in implementing the approach.

## References


BPCI (2009). US Congress. Senate. Biologics Price Competition and Innovation. http://www.fda.gov/downloads/Drugs/GuidanceComplianceRegulatoryInformation/UCM216146.pdf (Accessed 15 December, 2014).

EC (2013). European Commission. Consensus Information Paper 2013. What do you need to know about Biosimilar Medicinal Products. http://ec.europa.eu/enterprise/sectors/healthcare/files/docs/biosimilars_report_en.pdf (Accessed 13 December, 2014).

EMA (2014). Guideline on similar biological medicinal products. http://www.ema.europa.eu/docs/en_GB/document_library/Scientific_guideline/2014/10/WC500176768.pdf (Accessed 15 December, 2014).

FDA (1985). Points to consider in the production and testing of new drugs and biologicals produced by recombinant DNA technology. http://www.fda.gov/downloads/BiologicsBloodVaccines/GuidanceComplianceRegulatoryInformation/OtherRecommendationsforManufacturers/UCM062750.pdf (Accessed 4 December, 2014).

FDA (2007). Guidance for Industry: Clinical data needed to support the licensure of pandemic influenza vaccines. http://www.fda.gov/downloads/BiologicsBloodVaccines/GuidanceComplianceRegulatoryInformation/Guidances/Vaccines/ucm091985.pdf (Accessed 15 December, 2014).

FDA (2012a). Guidance for industry—Scientific considerations in demonstrating biosimilarity to a reference product. http://www.fda.gov/downloads/drugs/guidancecomplianceregulatoryinformation/guidances/ucm291128.pdf (Accessed 15 December, 2014).

FDA (2012b). Guidance for Industry—Quality considerations in demonstrating biosimilarity to a reference protein product. http://www.fda.gov/downloads/drugs/guidancecomplianceregulatoryinformation/guidances/ucm291134.pdf (Accessed 15 December, 2014).

Haidar SH, Davit B, Chen ML, Conner D, Lee LM, Li QH, Lionberger R, Makhlouf F, Patel D, Schuirmann DJ, and Yu LX (2008). Bioequivalence approaches for highly variable drugs and drug products. *Pharm. Res.* 1: 237–41.

Hsieh TC, Chow SC, Yang LY, and Chi E (2013). The evaluation of biosimilarity index based on reproducibility probability for assessing follow-on biologics. *Stat. Med.*, 32: 406–14.

Humira Structure. http://www.drugbank.ca/drugs/DB00051 (Accessed 12 December, 2014).

Kang SH and Chow SC (2013). Statistical assessment of biosimilarity based on relative distance between follow-on biologics. *Stat. Med.*, 32: 382–92.

Zhang N, Yang J, Chow SC, Endrenyi L, and Chi E (2013). Impact of variability on the choice of biosimilarity limits in assessing follow-on biologics. *Stat. Med.*, 32: 424–33.

Zocor Structure. http://www.drugbank.ca/drugs/DB00641 (Accessed 12 December, 2014).

## Appendix 5.1

Note that $\mu_1$, $\mu_2$, and $\mu_3$ are independent and have the same normal distribution $N(\mu_{R0}, \sigma_{R0}^2)$. So $\Pr(\mu_{(3)} - \mu_{(1)} < \eta) = 6\Pr(\mu_3 - \mu_1 < \eta,\ \mu_3 > \mu_2 > \mu_1)$. Denote $\pi_i = (\mu_i - \mu_{R0})/\sigma_{R0},\ i = 1, 2, 3$. Let $I_{[\pi_1 < \pi_2]}$ be the indicator function, taking value 1 if $\pi_1 < \pi_2$ and 0 otherwise. Then

$$
\begin{aligned}
\Pr(\mu_{(3)} - \mu_{(1)} < \eta) &= 6\Pr(\mu_1 < \mu_2 < \mu_3 < \eta + \mu_1) \\
&= 6\Pr\left(\pi_1 < \pi_2 < \pi_3 < \frac{\eta}{\sigma_{R0}} + \pi_1\right) \\
&= 6E\left[\left\{\Phi\left(\frac{\eta}{\sigma_{R0}} + \pi_1\right) - \Phi(\pi_2)\right\} I_{[\pi_1 < \pi_2]}\right] \qquad \text{(conditioning on } \pi_1, \pi_2\text{)} \\
&= 6E\left[\Phi\left(\frac{\eta}{\sigma_{R0}} + \pi_1\right) I_{[\pi_1 < \pi_2]}\right] - 6E\left[\Phi(\pi_2) I_{[\pi_1 < \pi_2]}\right] \\
&= 6E\left[\Phi\left(\frac{\eta}{\sigma_{R0}} + \pi_1\right)\{1 - \Phi(\pi_1)\}\right] - 6E\left[\Phi(\pi_2)\Phi(\pi_2)\right] \\
&= 6E\left[\Phi\left(\frac{\eta}{\sigma_{R0}} + \pi_1\right)\{1 - \Phi(\pi_1)\}\right] - 6E\left[\Phi(\pi_1)\Phi(\pi_1)\right] \\
&= 6E\left[\Phi\left(\frac{\eta}{\sigma_{R0}} + \pi_1\right)\{1 - \Phi(\pi_1)\} - \Phi(\pi_1)\Phi(\pi_1)\right].
\end{aligned}
$$

## 6.2 Noninferiority Test Problem and Methods

Suppose the outcome is a dichotomous efficacy variable. For convenience, we will assume that a higher response rate is desirable (if the opposite is true one can always just multiply by –1 to get the desired direction). Let $T$, $C$, and $P$ be response rates of the test drug, active control drug, and putative placebo in the NI trial, respectively. Let $C_0$ and $P_0$ be the response rates of the active control drug and placebo in historical trials, respectively. Note that active control is the reference product. In NI trials there is no placebo arm, but sponsors and regulatory agencies are still usually interested in estimating what the effect size of the test product over placebo would have been if the placebo had been included in the current NI trial. Since no direct comparison is available, we impute a placebo, called a putative placebo, from historical data to assist in this indirect comparison.

Figure 6.1 shows the relationship among response rates of the test drug ($T$), active control drug ($C$), and putative placebo ($P$) in the NI trial; "0" is included to indicate direction.

Formulation of the hypothesis depends on the primary objectives. According to Blackwelder (1982), the general objective of a NI trial is to show the test treatment is not worse than the active control by a prespecified margin, that is,

$$H_0: C - T \geq \delta \text{ versus } H_1: C - T < \delta. \tag{6.1}$$

$C - T$ stands for "difference" between the active control and the test product, and it could be difference, relative risk, odds ratio, LRR, or LOR (mathematic expression can be modified accordingly). The margin $\delta$ is the largest acceptable difference between the two products that would be considered not clinically meaningful and must be carefully defined in advance. Selection of the margin $\delta$ is extremely challenging, involving both careful clinical and statistical judgments (CHMP, 2006; D'Agostino et al., 2003; FDA, 2010; Hung et al., 2003, 2005; Julious, 2011; Wang and Hung, 2003).

The minimum standard for regulatory agencies' approval of a test treatment is to show "superiority over placebo." However, with missing the placebo arm in active controlled clinical trials, direct demonstration of such superiority is impossible. Furthermore, with reference products having already been marketed for years with positive risk–benefit profiles, "superiority over placebo" is a necessary but not sufficient condition to approve a

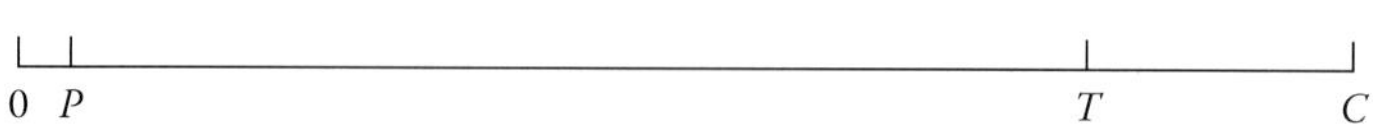


**FIGURE 6.1**
Relationship among response rates of test drug ($T$), active control drug ($C$), and putative placebo ($P$) in noninferiority (NI) trial.

test product. The goal is to choose a margin so that the test product retains some fraction of reference product efficacy (FDA, 1999). If all uncertainties are properly and comprehensively considered, ruling out the margin $\delta$ within an acceptable statistical error from the NI trial can be helpful in also demonstrating superiority over placebo with great confidence.

Given an objective of retaining a portion of the active control treatment efficacy, Equation 6.1 can be rewritten as Equation 6.2:

$$H_0 : C - T \geq (1-\lambda)(C-P) \text{ versus } H_1 : C - T < (1-\lambda)(C-P), \tag{6.2}$$

where $\lambda$ is the level of percent effect retention from previous active trial. A key question is what estimate to use for $C - P$? Does one use the point estimate or should one use a more conservative estimate? A regulatory guidance document suggests using a lower bound of a confidence interval and/or taking "discount" of any related uncertainties. Note that such estimate of effect size of reference product can be either point estimate or lower bound of some confidence interval, or taking "discount" of any related uncertainties (Snapinn, 2004). Our discussions below are based on the retention test hypothesis, Equation 6.2.

### 6.2.1 Fixed Margin Method

This method rejects the null hypothesis $H_0$ in Equation 6.2 and concludes that the test treatment is not inferior to the reference treatment if

$$\hat{C} - \hat{T} + z_\alpha \sigma_{TC} < (1-\lambda)\{\tilde{C}_0 - \tilde{P}_0 - z_\alpha \sigma_{PC0}\}, \tag{6.3}$$

where $z_\alpha$ is the (1 α)th percentile of the standard normal distribution. $\tilde{C}_0$ and $\tilde{P}_0$ are estimators of $C$ and $P$ from historical trial s, and $\sigma_{PC0}$ estimates the standard error of ($C - P$). Similarly, $\hat{C}$ and $\hat{T}$ are estimators of $C$ and $T$ from the current NI trial, and $\sigma_{TC}$ estimates the standard error of ($C - T$).

The NI margin $\delta$ is a function (often taking the smaller value) of a statistical margin and a clinical margin and must be predetermined before the NI trial starts. However, when conducting this NI analysis, the margin is treated as a fixed constant. The clinical margin comes from a comprehensive review of literature combined with clinical judgment, whereas a statistical margin often comes from an analysis of one or more historical superiority trials. In this chapter, we will assume that the statistical margin is smaller than the clinical margin, but we should bear in mind that choosing an FM is always combining both the statistical and the clinical information.

If we use $\alpha = 0.025$, the FM method is known as the 95–95 method, where the first 95 means the 95% confidence interval obtained from the historical trial and the second 95 means the 95% confidence interval obtained from the NI trial. The FM method is also known as confidence interval method. This method is conservative due to the fact that the margin is determined by discounting the lower bound of $\tilde{C}_0 - \tilde{P}_0$. For further details of this method, please refer Hung et al. (2003, 2005, 2007), Laster et al. (2006), Tsong et al. (2003), Wang and Hung (2003), Wang et al. (2002), Wiens (2002), and references therein.

### 6.2.2 Synthesis Method

Syn method rejects the null hypothesis $H_0$ in Equation 6.2 if

$$Z_{\text{pv}} = \frac{\hat{C} - \hat{T} - (1-\lambda)\{\tilde{C}_0 - \tilde{P}_0\}}{\sqrt{\sigma_{\hat{T}C}^2 + (1-\lambda)^2 \sigma_{\tilde{P}C0}^2}} < -z_\alpha, \tag{6.4}$$

where $z_\alpha$ is the $(1 - \alpha)$th percentile of the standard normal distribution. This method is also known as preservation test method.

This method synthesizes two sources of data—current NI study (estimates the effect of test treatment over reference treatment $\hat{C} - \hat{T}$) and historical studies (estimates the effect of reference treatment over placebo $\tilde{C}_0 - \tilde{P}_0$). Here, there is no need to prespecify an NI margin. $\tilde{C}_0 - \tilde{P}_0$ is not a fixed constant but an additional random variable similar to the random variable $\hat{C} - \hat{T}$. Because the test statistic is constructed by dividing a relevant combination of the estimate of test treatment effect and the active control effect by the combined standard error, this method purports to control type I error rate under the constancy assumption. Since the variance of the FM method is larger than the variance of the Syn method, the FM method is more conservative and hence the nominal type I error rate is often much less than the desired target type I error rate (even when the constancy assumption holds). The Syn method has been shown to be very sensitive to the constancy assumption. Violation of the constancy assumption will result in the Syn method being liberal. However, since the FM method uses the worst limit of the confidence interval of the active control effect to define the margin, it may be less sensitive to the violations of the constancy condition, the degree of which depends on the level of preservation specified in the defining the margin. For more details of this method, please refer Hasselblad and Kong (2001), Holmgren (1999), Hung et al. (2003), ICH (1998), Rothmann et al. (2003), Snapinn (2004), Wang and Hung (2002, 2003), Wang et al. (2002), and references therein.

### 6.2.3 Modified Covariate-Adjustment Fixed Margin/Synthesis Methods

Nie and Soon (2010) proposed a covariate-adjustment regression model approach to assess the test treatment effect when population difference between the historical trial and the NI trial causes constancy assumption violation. Applying this approach, they were not only able to measure the impact of population difference on the degree of constancy assumption violation but were also able to re-estimate the effect size of the active control when constancy assumption did not hold. For a historical superiority trial, the following logistic model is used to describe association among dichotomous outcome, treatment arm, and covariate:

$$\text{logit}\left(P(Y=1)\right)=\alpha+\beta * Trt+\beta_1 * X+\gamma_1 * X * Trt, \tag{6.5}$$

where $Y$ is the primary efficacy endpoint (outcome); *Trt* is the treatment arm, 1 for placebo and 0 for reference product; $X$ is a binary covariate, coded as 1 or 0; and $X * Trt$ is the interaction term for treatment and covariate. This basic model can easily extend to a more complicated one, such as including two or more covariates, and some of them may be independent from the treatment arm. IPD is needed for this modeling.

Based on the above model, the effect of active control is $\text{logit}(C_0)-\text{logit}(P_0)=-\beta-\gamma_1\bar{X}_{.H}$, where $\bar{X}_{.H}$ is the mean of covariate $X$ for the historical trial population. The NI trial population can also be used to estimate the mean of covariate $X$. Constancy assumption holds if the difference between such effects using two populations is small. To estimate the effect size of the active control, the current NI trial population is preferable if it is available; otherwise, the historical population can be used to estimate this. We modified Nie and Soon's method by always using the covariate mean of the current NI trial population, because it will give us a more accurate estimator of active control efficacy in the NI test. We further apply this active control effect to the FM method and Syn method for covFM method and covSyn method, respectively.

1. covFM method

   Replace the estimator of $\tilde{C}_0-\tilde{P}_0$ and its standard error $\sigma_{PC0}$ in Equation 6.3 using parameters estimated in Equation 6.5 and covariate mean of current NI trial population.

2. CovSyn method

   Replace the estimator of $\tilde{C}_0-\tilde{P}_0$ and its standard error $\sigma_{PC0}$ in Equation 6.4 using parameters estimated in Equation 6.5 and the covariate mean of the current NI trial population.

### 6.2.4 Two-Stage Covariate-Adjustment Fixed Margin/Synthesis Methods

Often one does not know the true effect of a covariate. In Section 6.2.3, describing modified covariate-adjustment methods, the covariate effect was confirmed via model selection using historical data and did not use current NI data. In the proposed two-stage method, the first stage is to confirm that the effect of covariate is sufficiently present in the current study to such an extent that it should be incorporated in the current analysis, and the second stage is to use either the covariate method or unadjusted method based on the results of stage 1.

Stage 1: Test of covariate

For a given NI trial, suppose $RR_1$ and $RR_2$ are response rates of subgroups defined by a binomial covariate. To confirm the effect of covariate in the first stage, we propose the following hypothesis test using threshold 0.15 instead of commonly used 0.05:

$$H_0 : RR_1 = RR_2 \text{ versus } H_a : RR_1 \neq RR_2. \quad (6.6)$$

Stage 2: Test of NI

In stage 2, use the FM method or Syn method if the null hypothesis in stage 1 is not rejected, i.e., the effect of the covariate is not worth putting into the model; use the covFM method or covSyn method if null hypothesis can be rejected. We will denote the above by 2sFM method if the FM method is used in stage 2, and the 2sSyn method if the Syn method is used in stage 2.

### 6.2.5 Paradigms of the Two Noninferiority Methods: Fixed Margin versus Synthesis

All methods used here involve using either the FM approach or the Syn approach. Note that these two approaches operate under different sets of paradigms. The FM method uses conventional clinical trial inference, which is based on a comparison of two randomized groups within a study. However, the Syn method uses across-study inference, which is based on synthesizing analysis from multiple studies.

## 6.3 Simulation

### 6.3.1 Motivating Example

HER2 is human epidermal growth factor receptor 2, a member of the HER family. This family has four distinct receptors, the epidermal growth factor receptor (EGFR), HER2, HER3, and HER4. HER3/HER2 status is considered a potential strong covariate for HER2+ cancer as it has been shown in some studies that HER3+/HER2+ subjects tend to respond better than HER3−/HER2+ patients.

Consider a hypothetical but realistic scenario. Suppose in a historical trial, 50% of enrolled subjects are HER3+/HER2+, and 50% are HER3−/HER2+. In an active controlled trial, the percent of enrolled subjects with HER3+/HER2+ may vary from 10% to 70%. We will consider four scenarios. The response rates of these four scenarios are as follows:

1. Response rates of taking placebo and active control are 0.18 and 0.50 for HER3+/HER2+ patients; response rates of taking placebo and active control are 0.18 and 0.50 for HER3−/HER2+ patients, respectively.
2. Response rates of taking placebo and active control are 0.28 and 0.60 for HER3+/HER2+ patients; response rates of taking placebo and active control are 0.13 and 0.45 for HER3−/HER2+ patients, respectively.
3. Response rates of taking placebo and active control are 0.40 and 0.60 for HER3+/HER2+ patients; response rates of taking placebo and active control are 0.13 and 0.45 for HER3−/HER2+ patients, respectively.
4. Response rates of taking placebo and active control are 0.18 and 0.78 for HER3+/HER2+ patients; response rates of taking placebo and active control are 0.31 and 0.38 for HER3−/HER2+ patients, respectively.

Figure 6.2 describes the relationship among HER3/HER2 status, response rate, and treatment arms. To determine whether HER3/HER2 status is a covariate, and to what extent it interacts with treatment arm, Table 6.1 gives numerical information.

In scenario 1, HER3/HER2 status is not associated with event rate, so it is not a covariate. While in scenarios 2 to 4, HER3/HER2 status is associated with event rate, and thus it is a covariate. Moreover, in scenario 1, HER3/HER2 status does not interact with the treatment arm. In scenarios 2, 3, and 4, the covariate has mild, moderate, and high interaction with the treatment arm, respectively.

If the covariate is associated with the effect size of the reference product, which means the covariate interacts with the treatment arm, then changes in percent of subjects with HER3/HER2 status will result in the constancy assumption being violated. Otherwise, the change in percent of subjects with HER3/HER2 status will not result in constancy assumption violation.

### 6.3.2 Simulation Details

Simulations were performed in order to evaluate and compare the operating characteristics of the six methods described in Sections 6.2.1 through 6.2.4. The six methods are as follows:

1. FM method
2. Syn method
3. covFM method
4. covSyn method
5. 2sFM method
6. 2sSyn method

In addition, we will examine three different measures of association for each of the six methods. These three measures are difference, LRR, and LOR. The log

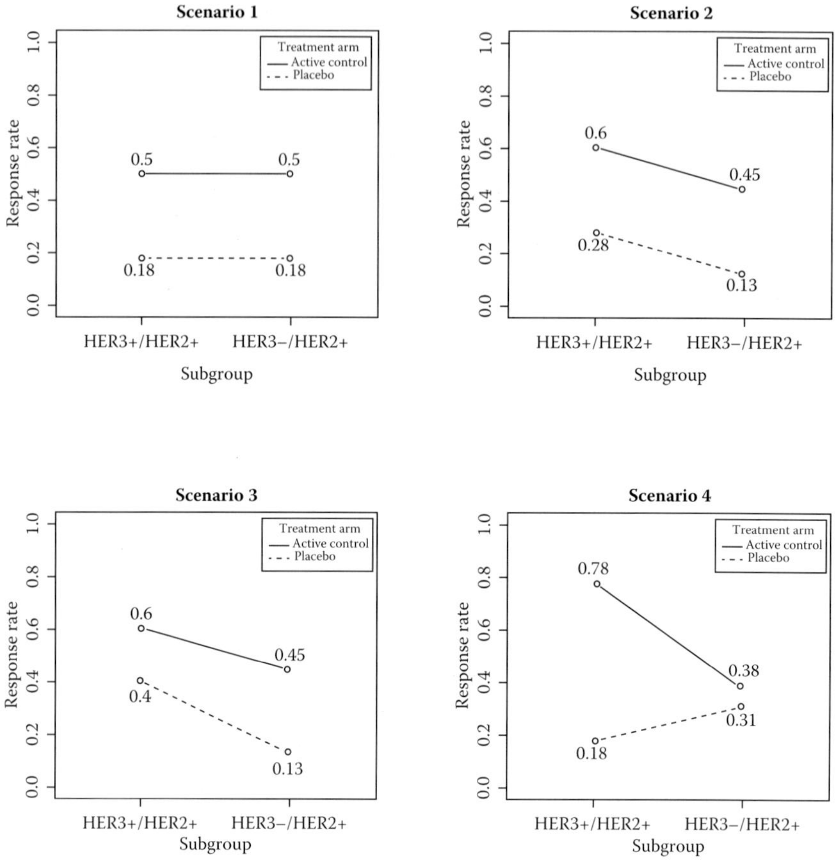


**FIGURE 6.2**
Relationships among response rate, human epidermal growth factor receptor (HER)3/HER2 status, and treatment arm.

scale of relative risk and odds ratio were used because of the following reasons: (1) log(A/B) = log(A) − log(B) = −log(B/A)—in this case, one can interpret the difference between A and B as the inverse of the difference between B and A; (2) log scale data can be approximated with Gaussian distribution theorem.

For each method and measure of association combination, 10,000 simulations were run to:

1. Compare empirical type I error using target alpha level of 2.5%.
2. Compare power using target power level of 80% at the approximate the same empirical alpha level.
3. Perform extensive sensitivity analyses to assess the performance of each method in lieu of violation of the constancy assumption. In particular, to compare the degree of departure of the constancy

**TABLE 6.1**

Numerical Information on Association between HER3/HER2 Status and Outcome (Column 4), Association between HER3/HER2 Status and Treatment Arm (Column 7)

| Scenario | Response Rate (1:1 Randomization) HER3+/HER2+ | HER3−/HER2+ | Fold Change of Response Rate (HER3+/HER2+ versus HER3−/HER2+) | Active Control versus Placebo Odds Ratio HER3+/HER2+ | HER3−/HER2+ | Fold Change of Odds Ratio (HER3+/HER2+ versus HER3−/HER2+) |
|---|---|---|---|---|---|---|
| 1 | 0.34 | 0.34 | 1 | 4.556 | 4.556 | 1 |
| 2 | 0.44 | 0.29 | 1.51 | 3.857 | 5.476 | 0.704 |
| 3 | 0.50 | 0.29 | 1.724 | 2.25 | 5.476 | 0.411 |
| 4 | 0.48 | 0.345 | 1.39 | 16.152 | 1.364 | 11.842 |

*Note:* HER, human epidermal growth factor receptor.

assumption needed to double or triple the empirical type I error rate. Hence, this evaluation will evaluate the robustness of each method to deviations from the assumption used in the analysis.

Since the null hypothesis is composite, we will measure empirical type I error rate when equality in null hypothesis of NI testing holds. Power is to be compared when the constancy assumption holds, i.e., 50% HER3+/HER2+ in both the historical trial and current NI trial. If the constancy assumption is seriously violated, the FM and Syn methods will appear to have good power. However, that is misleading since the type I error rate is inflated. To compare power, assign the response rate of the test product 10 possible values, with maximum equal to the response rate of the reference product and minimum equal to the response rate of the test product used in computing type I error rate. When examining the power plots, the type I error rates when the percent of HER3+/HER2+ is 50% can be also found.

Simulation steps:

1. Use underlying true parameters to generate 1000 per arm (two arms) in the historical trial, 300 per arm (three arms) in the NI trial.
2. Apply each of the six methods to reject/accept $H_0$.
3. Repeat Steps 1 and 2 10,000 times to get the proportion of rejection for all six methods and three measures of association.

### 6.3.3 Simulation Results

For each scenario and measure of association combination, results are presented in a panel of four plots as shown in Figure 6.3 (scenario 2 with difference as the measure of association). Row one presents the type I error rate, while row two presents the power. Column one gives results over broad

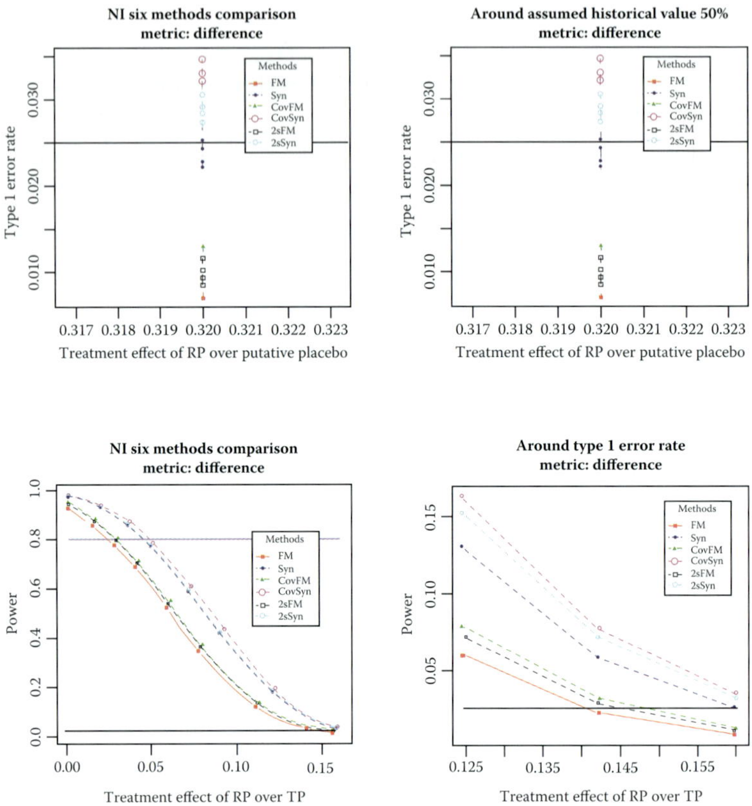


**FIGURE 6.3**
Performance characteristics comparisons—measure of association: difference.

range of all values, while column two zooms in on values of interest. The upper left plot has seven groups of points for each of the six methods (corresponding to percent of HER3+/HER2+ in the NI trial, ranging from 10% to 70% by 10% increments). Note that 50% is the same percent of HER3+/HER2+ in the historical trial, so points around it (40%, 50%, and 60% of HER3+/HER2+ in the NI trial) are zoomed, which are shown on the upper right. The bottom left plot is 10 groups of points for each of the six methods (corresponding to 10 points between ranges of possible test product effect). Note that the 10th group of points is the power when the test product (TP) effect equals that computed in the type I error rate. So they are actually type I error rates when the percentage of HER3+/HER2+ is 50% in the NI trial. A closer look at power around the type I error rate is given in the bottom right plot.

This chapter shows only the results for scenario 2 (mild interaction), since the conclusions drawn from scenario 2 also hold for the other three scenarios. To see simulation results for scenarios 1, 3, and 4, please refer to Xu et al. (2014).

Scenario 2:

Response rates of placebo and active control treatment groups are 0.28 and 0.60 for HER3+/HER2+ patients, respectively; response rates of placebo and active control treatment groups are 0.13 and 0.45 for HER3−/HER2+ patients, respectively.

In this scenario, HER3/HER2 status is a covariate. This covariate does not interact with the treatment arm using metric difference (Figure 6.3), but mildly interacts with the treatment arm using metrics LRR (Figure 6.4) and LOR (Figure 6.5). Thus, change of percent of HER3+/HER2+ in the NI trial will not cause constancy assumption violation for metric difference, but will result in constancy assumption violation for LRR and LOR. Moreover, when using LRR and LOR, increasing the percent of HER3+/HER2+ will decrease the effect of the reference product (RP) over the putative placebo and also decrease the effect of the reference product over the TP. Thus, the 10% point corresponding to the biggest "treatment effect of RP over putative placebo" in type I error plots are shown in Figures 6.4 and 6.5.

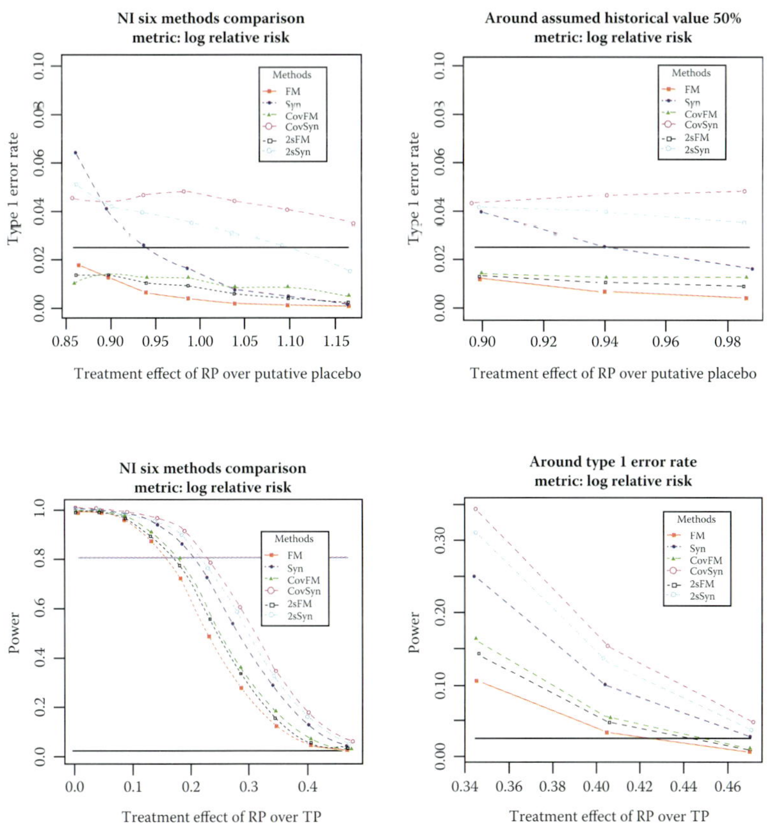


**FIGURE 6.4**
Performance characteristics comparisons—measure of association: log relative risk.

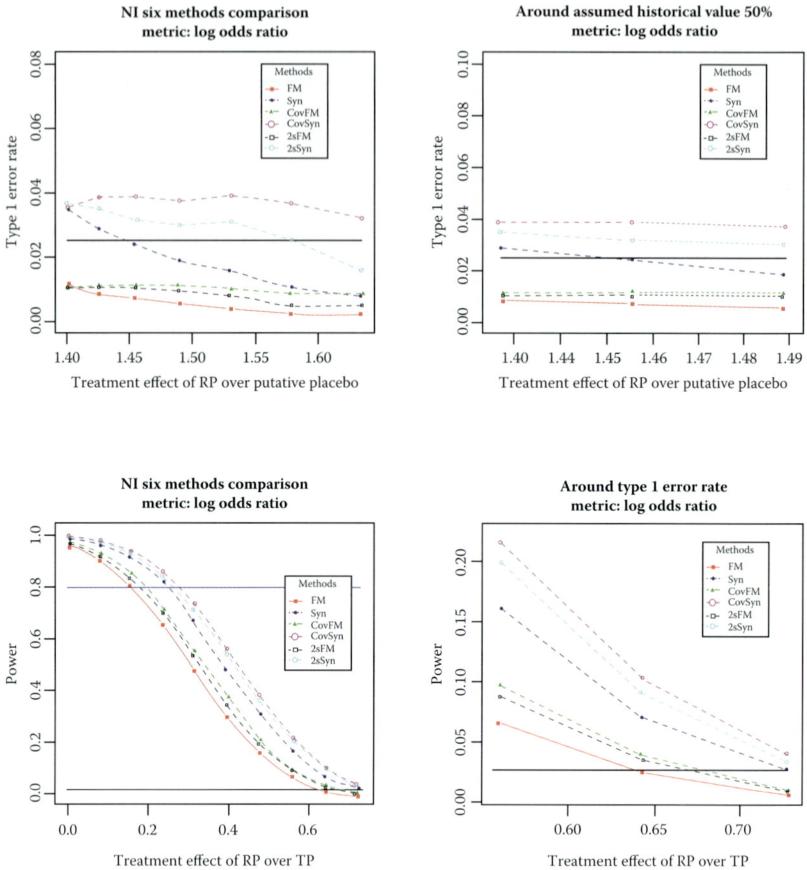


**FIGURE 6.5**
Performance characteristics comparisons—measure of association: log odds ratio.

Type I error rates of FM, CovFM, and s2FM are all under 0.025, while Syn, CovSyn, and 2sSyn have higher type I error rates and can be greater than 0.025 at some points. As can be seen in Figures 6.4 and 6.5, even slight departure from the constancy assumption (50%) causes the type I error rate to inflate. Looking at the upper left plots in Figures 6.3 through 6.5, we see the type I error rates of CovSym and 2sSyn are larger than 0.025 when constancy assumption holds (note this is the case where we adjusted the covariate when it is unnecessary). As can be seen in the upper right plots of Figures 6.4 and 6.5, the Syn method is extremely sensitive to constancy assumption, such that any small departure from constancy assumption and/or any small estimation variation inflates the type I error rate. The FM method is more stable in controlling the type I error rate. CovFM and 2sFM improve the conservativeness of FM, but can still control type I error rate at target value 0.025.

**TABLE 6.2**
Scenario 2—Type I Error Rate

| Metric | Percent of HER3+/HER2+ | *P* | *T* | *C* | FM | Syn | CovFM | CovSyn | 2sFM | 2sSyn |
|---|---|---|---|---|---|---|---|---|---|---|
| Difference | 0.1 | 0.145 | 0.305 | 0.465 | 0.0085 | 0.0279 | 0.0082 | 0.0295 | 0.0085 | 0.0283 |
| | 0.2 | 0.16 | 0.32 | 0.48 | 0.0084 | 0.0251 | 0.0087 | 0.0297 | 0.0084 | 0.0278 |
| | 0.3 | 0.175 | 0.335 | 0.495 | 0.0083 | 0.0241 | 0.0105 | 0.0303 | 0.0095 | 0.0285 |
| | 0.4 | 0.19 | 0.35 | 0.51 | **0.007** | **0.0228** | **0.0106** | **0.033** | **0.0096** | **0.0293** |
| | 0.5 | 0.205 | 0.365 | 0.525 | **0.0086** | **0.0253** | **0.0129** | **0.0347** | **0.0115** | **0.0306** |
| | 0.6 | 0.22 | 0.38 | 0.54 | **0.007** | **0.0222** | **0.0093** | **0.0303** | **0.0083** | **0.0273** |
| | 0.7 | 0.235 | 0.395 | 0.555 | 0.009 | 0.0244 | 0.0114 | 0.0323 | 0.0101 | 0.029 |
| LRR | 0.1 | 0.145 | 0.259663 | 0.465 | 3.00E-04 | 0.0015 | 0.0053 | 0.0357 | 0.0019 | 0.0152 |
| | 0.2 | 0.16 | 0.277128 | 0.48 | 0.001 | 0.0042 | 0.0087 | 0.0407 | 0.0042 | 0.0255 |
| | 0.3 | 0.175 | 0.294321 | 0.495 | 0.0016 | 0.0075 | 0.0083 | 0.044 | 0.0057 | 0.031 |
| | 0.4 | 0.19 | 0.311288 | 0.51 | **0.0035** | **0.0158** | **0.0125** | **0.0478** | **0.0089** | **0.0356** |
| | 0.5 | 0.205 | 0.328062 | 0.525 | **0.0063** | **0.0245** | **0.0124** | **0.0464** | **0.0104** | **0.0394** |
| | 0.6 | 0.22 | 0.344674 | 0.54 | **0.0123** | **0.0397** | **0.0145** | **0.043** | **0.014** | **0.0418** |
| | 0.7 | 0.235 | 0.361144 | 0.555 | 0.0185 | 0.0659 | 0.0107 | 0.0446 | 0.0135 | 0.0519 |
| LOR | 0.1 | 0.145 | 0.277419 | 0.465 | 0.0023 | 0.008 | 0.0083 | 0.0322 | 0.0048 | 0.016 |
| | 0.2 | 0.16 | 0.295434 | 0.48 | 0.0021 | 0.0104 | 0.0087 | 0.0369 | 0.0045 | 0.0258 |
| | 0.3 | 0.175 | 0.313179 | 0.495 | 0.0042 | 0.0159 | 0.0102 | 0.0392 | 0.0078 | 0.0311 |
| | 0.4 | 0.19 | 0.330704 | 0.51 | **0.0055** | **0.0187** | **0.0113** | **0.0376** | **0.0097** | **0.0301** |
| | 0.5 | 0.205 | 0.348049 | 0.525 | **0.0071** | **0.0239** | **0.0119** | **0.0387** | **0.0107** | **0.0316** |
| | 0.6 | 0.22 | 0.365247 | 0.54 | **0.0083** | **0.0289** | **0.0112** | **0.0388** | **0.0103** | **0.0352** |
| | 0.7 | 0.235 | 0.382323 | 0.555 | 0.0112 | 0.0351 | 0.0106 | 0.0356 | 0.0107 | 0.0362 |

*Notes:* Bold rows are percent of HER3+/HER2+ 40%, 50%, and 60%.

C, response rate of active control drug in noninferiority trial; covFM, modified covariate-adjustment fixed margin method; covSyn, modified covariate-adjustment synthesis method; FM, fixed margin method; LOR, log odds ratio; LRR, log relative risk; P, response rate of putative placebo in noninferiority trial; 2sFM, two-stage covariate-adjustment fixed margin method; 2sSyn, two-stage covariate-adjustment synthesis method; Syn, synthesis method; T, response rate of test drug in noninferiority trial.

**TABLE 6.3**

Scenario 2—Power

| Metric | *P* | *T* | *C* | FM | Syn | CovFM | CovSyn | 2sFM | 2sSyn |
|---|---|---|---|---|---|---|---|---|---|
| Difference | 0.205 | 0.507222 | 0.525 | 0.8424 | 0.9244 | 0.8742 | 0.9433 | 0.8628 | 0.9353 |
| LRR | 0.205 | 0.503118 | 0.525 | 0.9898 | 0.9978 | 0.9951 | 0.9989 | 0.9938 | 0.9986 |
| LOR | 0.205 | 0.505339 | 0.525 | 0.9132 | 0.968 | 0.937 | 0.9801 | 0.928 | 0.9751 |

Note the reason why we only see type I error rate inflated in one direction is because the bigger the relative effect of the reference product over the placebo, the bigger is the relative effect of the reference product over the test product. Thus it will make it harder for us to reject the null hypothesis of NI.

The power plots in Figures 6.3 through 6.5 show that CovFM has a higher power than both 2sFM and FM. CovFM has similar operating characteristics across all scenarios, even when there is no interaction effect (Figure 6.3). As expected, 2sFM has a larger power than FM, since 2sFM rejects the null hypothesis in Equation 6.6 when there is a strong observed covariate effect and therefore will use CovFM, which is a model-based regression approach. However, 2sFM has less power than CovFM because of potential type II error associated with testing hypothesis Equation 6.6, i.e., fail to reject the null hypothesis in Equation 6.6 even though the covariate effect is warranted.

Table 6.2 summarizes the type I error rates of the six NI methods, for different percentages of HER3+/HER2+ (10% to 70% by 10% increment) using three different measures of associations (difference, LRR, and LOR).

Table 6.3 summarizes the power of the six NI methods, for the second groups of points in power plots.

## 6.4 Conclusions and Discussion

Both FM and Syn have inflated type I error rates when constancy assumption is seriously violated (scenario 4), and Syn is the more liberal of the two. Syn is also very sensitive to violations of the constancy assumption. Small departures from the constancy assumption and/or small estimation variation could inflate the type I error rate. While not as severe as Syn, both the CovSyn and 2sSyn methods also have inflated type I error rates due to sensitivity of Syn.

FM has empirical type I error rate over the desired value when constancy assumption is seriously violated, although it is not as sensitive as the Syn method. This can be explained mathematically from the formula $\hat{C} - \widehat{T} + z_{0.025}\sigma_{TC} < (1-\eta)\{\tilde{C}_0 - \tilde{P}_0 - z_{0.025}\sigma_{PC0}\}$; if constancy is seriously violated, $\tilde{C}_0 - \tilde{P}_0$ will become smaller and so it is easier to reject the null hypothesis, resulting in inflated type I error rate. When constancy assumption does not hold due to covariate effect, adjusting for this effect will result in significantly less type I error. This is why the CovFM and 2sFM methods perform better than the FM method in controlling the type I error rate. 2sFM may falsely accept the null hypothesis in Equation 6.6. Method CovFM performs consistently well across all scenarios: CovFM method has almost the same power as 2sFM in scenario 1 (no covariate, no interaction) and scenario 4 (covariate and high interaction), while CovFM has a larger power than 2sFM in scenario 2 (mild interaction) and scenario 3 (moderate interaction).

Based on these results, we recommend using the CovFM method, since it controls the type I error rate and has satisfactory power for any of the three measures of association.

The most logical use for this methodology is when a company wants to show NI for a new formulation, for example, a new Sub Q dose for the company's existing IV drug. Thus, the company has IPD. It is the authors' hope that with the emphasis on comparative effectiveness initiatively found in the Patient Protection and Affordable Care Act passed by the U.S. Congress on March 23, 2010, sharing IPD among sponsors/agencies will be possible in the future.

## References


Blackwelder W.C. (1982). "Proving the null hypothesis" in clinical trials. *Controlled Clinical Trials* 3. 345–353.

Broeze K.A., Opmmer B.C., Van Der Veen F., Bossuyt P.M., Bhattachwrya S., Mol B.W. (2010). Individual patient data meta-analysis: A promising approach for evidence synthesis in reproductive medicine. *Human Reproduction Update* 16: 561–567.

Committee for Medicinal Products for Human Use (CHMP) (2006). Guideline on the choice of non-inferiority margin. *Statistics in Medicine* 25: 1628–1638.

D'Agostino R.B., Massaro J.M., Sullivan L. (2003). Non-inferiority trials: Design concepts and issues—the encounters of academic consultants in statistics. *Statistics in Medicine* 22: 169–186.

Fisher L.D. (1999). Advances in clinical trials in the twentieth century. *Annual Review of Public Health* 20: 109–124.

Food and Drug Administration (FDA) (1999). *Summary of CBER Considerations on Selected Aspects of Active Controlled Trial Design and Analysis for the Evaluation of Thrombolytics in Acute MI*. Rockville, MD: U.S. FDA.

Food and Drug Administration (FDA) (2010). *Guidance for Industry: Non-Inferiority Clinical Trials*. Rockville, MD: U.S. FDA.

Hasselblad V., Kong D.F. (2001). Statistical methods for comparison to placebo in active-control trials. *Drug Information Journal* 35: 435–449.

Holmgren E.B. (1999). Establishing equivalence by showing that a specified percentage of the effect of the active control over placebo is maintained. *Journal of Biopharmaceutical Statistics* 9: 651–659.

Hung H.M.J., Wang S.J., O'Neill R. (2005). A regulatory perspective on choice of margin and statistical inference issues in non-inferiority trials. *Biometrical Journal* 47: 28–36.

Hung H.M.J., Wang S.J., O'Neill R. (2007). Issues with statistical risks for testing methods in noninferiority trial without a placebo arm. *Journal of Biopharmaceutical Statistics* 17: 201–213.

Hung H.M.J., Wang S.J., Tsong Y., Lawrence J., O'Neill R. (2003). Some fundamental issues with non-inferiority testing in active controlled clinical trials. *Statistics in Medicine* 22: 213–225.

ICH. (1998). E9 Statistical Principles for Clinical Trials. Rockville, MD: U. S. FDA. Available at http://www.fda.gov/downloads/drugs/guidancecomplianceregulatoryinformation/guidances/ucm073137.pdf.

Julious S.A. (2011). The ABC of non-inferiority margin setting from indirect comparisons. *Pharmaceutical Statistics* 10: 448–453.

Julious S.A., Wang S.J. (2008). Issues with indirect comparisons in clinical trials particularly with respect to non-inferiority trials. *Drug Information Journal* 42: 625–633.

Laster L.L., Johnson M.F., Kotler M.L. (2006). Non-inferiority trials: The 'at least as good as' criterion with dichotomous data. *Statistics in Medicine* 25: 1115–1130.

Metzler C.M. (1974). Bioavilability—A problem in equivalence. *Biometrics* 30: 309–317.

Nie L., Soon G.X. (2010). A covariate-adjustment regression model approach to noninferiority margin definition. *Statistics in Medicine* 29: 1107–1113.

Pocock S.J. (1983). *Clinical Trials: A Practical Approach*. New York, NY: John Wiley.

Rothmann M., Li N., Chen G., Chi G.Y.H., Temple R., Tsou H.T. (2003). Design and analysis of non-inferiority mortality trials in oncology. *Statistics in Medicine* 22: 239–264.

Simmonds M.C., Higgins J.P., Stewart L.A., Tierney J.F., Clarke M.F., Thompson S.G. (2005). Meta-analysis of individual patient data from randomized trials: A review of methods used in practice. *Clinical Trials* 2: 209–217.

Snapinn S.M. (2004). Alternatives for discounting in the analysis of noninferiority trials. *Journal of Biopharmaceutical Statistics* 14: 263–273.

Tsong Y., Wang S.J., Hung H.M.J., Cui L. (2003). Statistical issues on objective, design, and analysis of noninferiority active-controlled clinical trial. *Journal of Biopharmaceutical Statistics* 13: 29–41.

Wang S.J., Hung H.M.J. (2002). Assessing treatment efficacy in noninferiority or equivalence studies. *Controlled Clinical Trials* 23: 2–14.

Wang S.J., Hung H.M.J. (2003). TACT method for non-inferiority testing in active controlled trials. *Statistics in Medicine* 22: 227–238.

Wang S.J., Hung H.M.J., Tsong Y. (2002). Utility and pitfalls of some statistical methods in active controlled clinical trials. *Controlled Clinical Trials* 23: 15–28.

Westlake W.J. (1972). Use of confidence intervals in analysis of comparative bioavailability trials. *Journal of Pharmaceutical Sciences* 61: 1340–1341.

Wiens B.L. (2002). Choosing an equivalence limit for noninferiority or equivalence studies. *Controlled Clinical Trials* 23: 2–14.

Xu S.Y., Barker, K., Menon S., D'Agostino R.B. (2014). Covariate effect on constancy assumption in non-inferiority clinical trials. *Journal of Biopharmaceutical Statistics* 24: 1173–1189.

# 7

# *Novel Method in Inference of Equivalence in Biosimilars*

**Siyan Xu, Steven Ye Hua, Ronald Menton, Kerry B. Barker, Sandeep M. Menon, and Ralph B. D'Agostino**

**CONTENTS**



**ABSTRACT** Equivalence trials aim to demonstrate that new and standard treatments are equivalent within predefined clinically relevant limits. In the presence of unspecified variances, methods such as the likelihood ratio test use sample estimates for those variances; Bayesian models integrate them out in the posterior distribution. These methods limit the knowledge of the extent that equivalence is affected by variability of the parameter of interest. In this chapter, we propose a likelihood approach that retains the unspecified variances in the model and partitions the likelihood function into two components: $F$-statistic function for variances and $t$-statistic function for the ratio of two means. By incorporating unspecified variances, the proposed method can help identify a numeric range of variances where equivalence is more likely to be achieved, which cannot be accomplished by current analysis methods. By partitioning the likelihood function into two components, the proposed method provides more inference information than a method that relies solely on one component. We recommend the proposed likelihood method as a better alternative than current analysis methods for equivalence inference.

## 7.1 Introduction

### 7.1.1 Motivation

In an article (Xu et al., 2014), the authors addressed the inference of bioequivalence for log-normal data with unspecified variances by expressing a likelihood function into the product of two components: $F$-statistic function for variances and $t$-statistic function for the difference of two means. For bioequivalence studies, the U.S. Food and Drug Administration (FDA) (2003) recommends that 90% confidence interval (CI) values for the ratio of the relative means for area under the concentration–time curve (AUC) and maximum concentration of a drug ($C_{max}$) of the new and reference drugs should fall between 0.80 and 1.25. The two pharmacokinetic (PK) parameters, AUC and $C_{max}$, refer to area under the concentration–time curve and the maximum concentration of a drug, respectively. The distribution of the individual PK parameters is often assumed to be log-normal; therefore, bioequivalence is usually assessed on the difference of logarithmically transformed PK parameters. The proposed method in Xu et al. (2014) retains the unspecified variances in the likelihood function and presents them via three parameters: the ratio of two variances ($\gamma^2$), the variance of the reference drug $\sigma_R^2$, and correlation of the two drugs ($\rho$) for crossover studies only. The word "unspecified" means those parameters are included in the model and allowed to vary over a range of values to show the robustness of bioequivalence inference conditional on different values. This method helps identify ranges of variances where bioequivalence is more likely to be achieved, which cannot be accomplished by methods that replace or remove these parameters such as two one-sided tests (TOSTs) or Bayesian analysis. This method applies to both crossover and parallel designs.

When the untransformed variable is normally distributed, Hauschke et al. (1999) gave several examples to justify the need to assess the therapeutic equivalence for two treatments using the ratio of two normal means. Liu and Weng (1994) and Berger and Hsu (1996) showed that analyses based on the original scale are always more powerful than those based on the transformed scale when the distribution is normal. A likelihood ratio test proposed by Sasabuchi (1988a, 1988b) has been suggested by several authors, including Berger and

Hsu (1996), Hauschke et al. (1999), Hua et al. (2013), among others, as appropriate to test the *null hypothesis of nonequivalence* for the ratio of two normal means. Similar to log-normal data, CI inclusion such as the Fieller confidence set (FCS) (Fieller, 1954), operationally equivalent to the likelihood ratio test, is more commonly used to assess equivalence for normal data. However, the extent of inference about equivalence affected by variability (unspecified) of the parameter of interest remains unaddressed in the literature.

### 7.1.2 Outline

In this chapter, we expand the likelihood approach by Díaz-Francés and Sprott (2004) and Xu et al. (2014) and apply it to equivalence for the ratio of two normal means ($\beta$) by expressing the likelihood function in the product of two components: a function of $F$-statistic for variances and a function of the $t$-statistic for $\beta$. In essence, the findings regarding inference of bioequivalence for log-normal data that is affected by the unspecified variances as described before can be applied to the inference of equivalence for the ratio of two normal means. We show that the proposed method is effective in investigating the impact of variances on the inference of equivalence. Since this has already been addressed in Xu et al. (2014), we will discuss it only briefly in this chapter. Our focus in this chapter is to show another benefit of the proposed method. In a general case, when model parameters are independent, the proposed likelihood function method produces results that are the same as the likelihood ratio test and comparable to Bayesian analysis. In the special case when model parameters are dependent, for example, the ratio of two variances is directly proportional to the ratio of two means, the proposed method yields better results in inference about equivalence than either the likelihood ratio test, which relies solely on the $t$-statistic function, or Bayesian analysis that integrates out the variances in the posterior distribution.

The remainder of the chapter is organized as follows: Section 7.2 describes the proposed likelihood method. Section 7.3 presents the Bayesian model for our specific problem. The impact of unspecified variances on equivalence is discussed in Section 7.4. Comparisons of different methods in general and special cases will be shown in Section 7.5, followed by conclusion and discussion in Section 7.6.

## 7.2 Likelihood Method

In this section, we give details on a likelihood function that can be used to characterize equivalence for normal data based on bivariate normal (BVN) distribution. The method can be used in both crossover and parallel designs.

### 7.2.1 Crossover Design

Suppose two variables $x_i$ and $y_i$, where $i = 1,\ldots,n$, follow BVN distribution

$$\begin{pmatrix} x_i \\ y_i \end{pmatrix} \sim \text{BVN}\left(\begin{pmatrix} \beta\mu \\ \mu \end{pmatrix}, \begin{pmatrix} \gamma^2\sigma^2 & \rho\gamma\sigma^2 \\ \rho\gamma\sigma^2 & \sigma^2 \end{pmatrix}\right) \tag{7.1}$$

In the context of equivalence studies, variables $x_i$ and $y_i$ represent individual observations (e.g., an efficacy assessment) for the two treatments (test and reference), respectively. Parameters in model Equation 7.1 are $\beta = E(x_i)/E(y_i), \mu = E(y_i), \rho$, the correlation coefficient between the two drugs, and $\gamma^2$, the ratio of two variances $\left(\gamma^2 = \text{Var}(x_i)/\text{Var}(y_i)\right)$ and $\sigma^2 = \text{Var}(y_i)$. The correlation coefficient $\rho$ is to address crossover designs, where subjects start with one treatment and then the same subjects are switched to the other treatment usually after a washout period, that is, $x_i$ and $y_i$ are observations from the same subject. In parallel designs, $\rho = 0$. Model Equation 7.1 above is a simple model, which assumes there is no sequence or period effect.

#### 7.2.1.1 *Hypothesis and Likelihood Ratio Test*

It follows from Berger and Hsu (1996), Hauschke et al. (1999), and Liu and Weng (1994), and the equivalence hypotheses for the ratio $\beta$ with the prespecified margins $(\theta_1, \theta_2)$ can be stated as,

$$\begin{aligned} &H_{01}: \beta < \theta_1 \text{ or } H_{02}: \beta > \theta_2 \\ &H_A: \theta_1 \leq \beta \leq \theta_2 \end{aligned} \tag{7.2}$$

These authors further indicated that the size-$\alpha$ likelihood ratio test originally proposed by Sasabuchi (1988a, 1988b) is appropriate for the hypotheses in Equation 7.2 and rejects $H_0$ if

$$T_1^c \geq t_{\alpha,\, n-1} \text{ and } T_2^c \leq -t_{\alpha,\, n-1} \tag{7.3}$$

where $T_h^c = \dfrac{\bar{x} - \theta_h \bar{y}}{\hat{\sigma}_{(\bar{x}-\theta_h\bar{y})}} =, h = 1, 2.\ \bar{x} = \dfrac{\sum_{i=1}^{n} x_i}{n}$, $t_{\alpha,\,v}$ is the (1 − $\alpha$) percentile of the central $t$-distribution with $v$ degrees of freedom (df). The letter "c" in superscript means crossover design. For convenience, we chose the margins $\theta_1 = 0.8$, $\theta_2 = 1.25$ to assess equivalence for the ratio of two normal means; however, readers should always consider clinically relevant margins in their research and practice.

#### 7.2.1.2 *Fieller Confidence Set*

A CI for the ratio of two means can be constructed using the generalized Fieller theorem (Fieller, 1954). By solving the quadratic equation

$T_h^{c\ 2} = t_{\alpha,\ n-1}^2$ from Equation 7.3, we obtained the Fieller confidence limits as follows:

$$\theta_{\pm}^{c} = \frac{(\overline{xy} - a_c\rho\gamma) \pm \sqrt{(\overline{xy} - a_c\rho\gamma)^2 - (\bar{x}^2 - a_c\gamma^2)(\bar{y}^2 - a_c)}}{\bar{y}^2 - a_c},\ a_c = \frac{\hat{\sigma}^2}{n} t_{\alpha,n-1}^2 \quad (7.4)$$

After some algebraic manipulation and rearrangement, it can be shown that inequalities in Equation 7.3 are operationally equivalent to

$$\theta_{-}^{c} \geq \theta_1 \text{ and } \theta_{+}^{c} \leq \theta_2 \text{ and } \bar{y}^2 > a_c \quad (7.5)$$

Equalities in Equation 7.5 can be interpreted as follows: if the 100(1 − 2 $\alpha$) percent FCS for $\beta$ has finite length, it is given by the interval $I_F^c = (\theta_{-}^{c}, \theta_{+}^{c})$. Furthermore, FCS is an interval if and only if $\bar{y}^2 > a_c$ holds true.

Of the TOSTs proposed by Sasabuchi and CI based on the Fieller theorem, the former compares $T_1^c$ ($T_2^c$) with critical $t$-value under a prespecified value of $\theta_1$ ($\theta_2$), whereas the latter treats $\theta$ as an unknown random variable and compares its range of plausible values with the margins $(\theta_1, \theta_2)$.

#### *7.2.1.3 Proposed Likelihood Function*

The likelihood approach focuses on showing the statistical evidence instead of making a decision to choose between equivalence and nonequivalence. The likelihood function based on model Equation 7.1 is in the form of

$$L(\beta, \mu, \rho, \gamma, \sigma \mid X, Y) \propto \frac{1}{\gamma^n \sigma^{2n} (1-\rho^2)^{n/2}} \exp\left(-\frac{1}{2\sigma^2(1-\rho^2)} A\right) \quad (7.6)$$

where

$$A = \frac{\sum_{i=1}^{n} (x_i - \beta\mu)^2}{\gamma^2} + \sum_{i=1}^{n} (y_i - \mu)^2 - \frac{2\rho}{\gamma} \sum_{i=1}^{n} (x_i - \beta\mu)(y_i - \mu) = \frac{S_x}{\gamma^2} + S_y$$

$$+ \frac{n(\bar{x} - \beta\mu)^2}{\gamma^2} + n(\bar{y} - \mu)^2 - \frac{2\rho}{\gamma} \sum_{i=1}^{n} (x_i - \beta\mu)(y_i - \mu)$$

Without the knowledge of true $\mu$ and $\sigma$, a likelihood function of $\beta$, $\gamma$, and $\rho$ can be constructed by replacing $\mu$ in Equation 7.6 with its restricted maximum likelihood estimator (rMLE) $\hat{\mu}_{rM}(\beta, \gamma, \rho) = \dfrac{(\beta - \rho\gamma)\bar{x} + \gamma(\gamma - \rho\beta)\bar{y}}{(\beta^2 - 2\rho\beta\gamma + \gamma^2)}$, followed by replacing $\sigma^2$ with its rMLE $\hat{\sigma}_{rM}^2 = \dfrac{B}{2n(1-\rho^2)}$, where $B = \left[\dfrac{S_x}{\gamma^2} + S_y + \dfrac{n(\bar{x} - \beta\bar{y})^2 (1-\rho^2)}{(\beta^2 - 2\rho\beta\gamma + \gamma^2)} - \dfrac{2\rho}{\gamma} S_{xy}\right]$ and $S_{xy} = \sum_{i=1}^{n} (x_i - \bar{x})(y_i - \bar{y})$. That is,

## 7.3 Bayesian Approach

### 7.3.1 Crossover Design

A reparameterization is needed to derive the Bayesian posterior distribution. Rather than using Equation 7.1 we employ the following form of distribution for $x_i$ and $y_i$:

$$\begin{pmatrix} x_i \\ y_i \end{pmatrix} \sim \text{BVN}\left(\begin{pmatrix} \mu_1 \\ \mu \end{pmatrix}, \begin{pmatrix} \gamma^2\sigma^2 & \rho\gamma\sigma^2 \\ \rho\gamma\sigma^2 & \sigma^2 \end{pmatrix}\right) \tag{7.15}$$

Under the BVN model, Equation 7.15, as the likelihood function for $\mu_1, \mu, \gamma, \sigma,$ and $\rho$, can be expressed as

$$L(\mu_1, \mu, \gamma, \sigma, \rho \mid X, Y) \propto \frac{1}{\gamma^n \sigma^{2n}(1-\rho^2)^{n/2}} \exp\left(-\frac{1}{2\sigma^2(1-\rho^2)} C\right) \tag{7.16}$$

where $C = \dfrac{S_x}{\gamma^2} + S_y + \dfrac{n(\bar{x}-\mu_1)^2}{\gamma^2} + n(\bar{y}-\mu)^2 - \dfrac{2\rho}{\gamma}\sum_{i=1}^{n}(x_i-\mu_1)(y_i-\mu)$.

According to Berger et al. (2009) and Rubio and Pérez-Elizalde (2009), the independence Jeffreys prior in Equation 7.17 is a suitable prior.

$$\begin{aligned} \pi_{IJ}(\mu_1, \mu, \gamma, \sigma, \rho) &\propto (\mu_1\mu)^{-\frac{1}{2}} \frac{1}{\gamma\sigma^2 (1-\rho^2)^{\frac{3}{2}}} \\ &= (\mu_1\mu)^{-1/2}\sigma^{-2}\gamma^{-1}(1-\rho^2)^{-\frac{3}{2}} \end{aligned} \tag{7.17}$$

The posterior distribution of the parameters $(\mu_1, \mu, \gamma, \sigma, \rho)$ will have the form

$$\begin{aligned} \pi(\mu_1, \mu, \gamma, \sigma, \rho \mid X, Y) &\propto (\mu_1\mu)^{-1/2}\gamma^{-n-1}\sigma^{-2n-2} \\ &(1-\rho^2)^{-\frac{n}{2}-\frac{3}{2}} \exp\left(-\frac{1}{2\sigma^2(1-\rho^2)} C\right) \end{aligned} \tag{7.18}$$

After some algebra and integrating out parameters other than $\beta$, the marginal posterior distribution of $\beta$ has the form

$$\pi(\beta|X,Y) \propto \int_{-1}^{1}\int_{0}^{1} \beta^{-\frac{1}{2}} u^{\frac{n-1}{2}} (1-u)^{\frac{n-2}{2}} \left(1-\rho^2\right)^{\frac{n-2}{2}}$$
$$\times\left[(1-u)\beta^2 + u - 2\rho\sqrt{(1-u)u}\beta\right]^{-1}$$
$$\cdot\left[S(u,\rho)^2 + \frac{(1-u)u(1-\rho^2)(\beta\bar{y}-\bar{x})^2}{(1-u)\beta^2 + u - 2\rho\sqrt{(1-u)u}\beta}\right]^{-(n-\frac{1}{2})} \tag{7.19}$$
$$\cdot\left[1 - F(t(\beta,u,\rho))\right]^2 \cdot du\,d\rho$$

The derivation of Equation 7.19 is similar to Appendix B in Xu et al. (2014).

### 7.3.2 Parallel Design

In a parallel design where samples $x_i$, $i = 1,\ldots,n$ and $y_j$, $j = 1,\ldots,m$ are independent ($\rho = 0$), the likelihood function for $\mu_1$, $\mu$, $\gamma$, and $\sigma$ can be expressed as

$$L(\mu_1, \mu, \gamma, \sigma \mid X, Y) \propto \frac{1}{\gamma^n \sigma^{n+m}} \exp\left(-\frac{1}{2\sigma^2} D\right) \tag{7.20}$$

where $D = \dfrac{\sum_{i=1}^{n}(x_i-\mu_1)^2}{\gamma^2} + \sum_{j=1}^{m}\left(y_j-\mu\right)^2 = \dfrac{S_x}{\gamma^2} + S_y + \dfrac{n(\bar{x}-\mu_1)^2}{\gamma^2} + m(\bar{y}-\mu)^2.$

According to Berger et al. (2009) and Rubio and Pérez-Elizalde (2009), the independence Jeffreys prior in Equation 7.21 is a suitable prior.

$$\pi_{IJ}(\mu_1, \mu, \gamma, \sigma) \propto (\mu_1\mu)^{-\frac{1}{2}} \frac{1}{\gamma\sigma^2} = (\mu_1\mu)^{-1/2}\sigma^{-2}\gamma^{-1} \tag{7.21}$$

The posterior distribution of the parameters ($\mu_1$, $\mu$, $\gamma$, $\sigma$) will have the form

$$\pi(\mu_1, \mu, \gamma, \sigma \mid X, Y) \propto (\mu_1\mu)^{-1/2}\gamma^{-n-1}\sigma^{-n-m-2}\exp\left(-\frac{1}{2\sigma^2} D\right) \tag{7.22}$$

After some algebraic manipulation and integrating out parameters $\mu$, $u$, and $v$, the marginal posterior distribution of $\beta$ has the form

$$\pi(\beta|X,Y) \propto \int_0^1 \beta^{-\frac{1}{2}} u^{\frac{m-1}{2}} (1-u)^{\frac{n-2}{2}} \left[(1-u)\beta^2 + u\right]^{-\frac{1}{2}}$$

$$\cdot\left[(1-u)S_x^2 + uS_y^2 + \frac{(1-u)u(\beta\bar{y}-\bar{x})^2}{(1-u)\beta^2+u}\right]^{-\frac{n+m}{2}} \tag{7.23}$$

$$\cdot\left[1 - F(t(\beta,u))\right]\cdot du$$

where $F(t(\beta,u))$ is the student's $t$-distribution function with $(m + n)$ df evaluated at

$$t(\beta,u) = \sqrt{\frac{(n+m)\cdot\left[(1-u)\beta^2+u\right]}{\left[(1-u)S_x^2 + uS_y^2 + \frac{(1-u)u(\beta\bar{y}-\bar{x})^2}{(1-u)\beta^2+u}\right]}}\left[-\frac{(1-u)\beta\bar{x}+u\bar{y}}{(1-u)\beta^2+u}\right]$$

The derivation of Equation 7.23 follows similarly to that of Equation 7.19.

## 7.4 Inference on Equivalence Affected by Unspecified Variances

In this section, we illustrate the proposed likelihood method using data from a published crossover study to assess the impact of unspecified variances on the inference about equivalence. The unspecified variances are characterized by $\gamma^2$ (the ratio of two variances), $\sigma^2$ (variance for the reference drug), and $\rho$ (correlation coefficient). To do so, we construct a likelihood function of $\beta$ by retaining one of the three parameters in the model while replacing the other two with sample estimates in the likelihood function Equation 7.8.

### 7.4.1 Normal Dataset and Likelihood Ratio Test Result

Data came from the published crossover study Balthasar (1999).

Test drug $C_{max}$: {140, 13.6, 78.8, 88.0, 54.7, 76.4, 310, 110, 182, 192, 364, 112}.

Reference drug $C_{max}$: {226, 20.1, 51.8, 105, 40.6, 52.6, 175, 135, 337, 326, 346, 126}.

Data came from a simulated cyclosporine bioequivalence study with 12 subjects, for a two-treatment, crossover study of 300 mg of cyclosporine administered orally. Data were assumed having the same parameter values and variances for both study periods; consequently, there was no "true" difference between the formulations on their rate and extent of absorption. For illustration purposes, we take the square root of original data as shown above (they are still normally distributed) and use the transformed data for analysis. Using the notations in Section 7.2.1, the observed mean values of $C_{max}$ are $\bar{x}$ = 11.25 and $\bar{y}$ = 11.81 for test and reference treatments; $S_x$ = 202.34, $S_y$ = 268.52, $S_{xy}$ = 197.22, and correlation is $\hat{\rho}$ = 0.85. Results of the likelihood ratio test are summarized in Table 7.1.

The 90% FCS of $\hat{\beta} = \frac{\bar{x}}{\bar{y}}$ is (0.8496, 1.0781), which falls within the equivalence margins (0.8, 1.25), and overall $p$-value in rejecting the two one-sided null hypotheses in Equation 7.2, $p$ = 0.0101 is significant at 0.05 level. These results suggest sufficient evidence to conclude equivalence.

### 7.4.2 Standardized Profile Likelihood

Figure 7.1 shows the plot of the standardized profile likelihood (SPL) for $L_{max}(\beta,\rho,\gamma \mid X,Y)$ of $\beta$ in Equation 7.8 with $\hat{\gamma}$ = 0.87 and $\hat{\rho}$ = 0.85 (sample estimates) and $\beta$ in the range of (0.6, 1.4). The standardization was taken to have the maximum value of 1 for the vertical scale of the plot: $\text{SPL} = L_{max}\left(\beta| X,Y,\rho=0.85,\gamma=0.87\right) / L_{max}\left(\beta=\frac{\bar{x}}{\bar{y}}| X,Y,\rho=0.85,\gamma=0.87\right)$ and because both $\rho$ and $\gamma$ are specified, the component $L_F(\rho,\gamma)$ in Equation 7.8 is cancelled out in the SPL. According to Royall (1997), SPL = 1/8 and 1/32 are two common reference lines, values that fall into the likelihood interval (LI) corresponding to SPL = 1/8 and 1/32 (namely, 1/8 LI and 1/32 LI) indicate "moderate strong" and "strong" evidence supported by the data, respectively. Two vertical solid lines represent equivalence margins 0.8 and 1.25. The horizontal dashed line, SPL = 0.194, was obtained by inserting one-sided critical value of $t$ distribution, $t$(0.95,11) = 1.796, into the SPL. The two points on the SPL curve intersecting with SPL = 0.194 are 0.8496 and 1.0781. Thus using SPL, the limits are the same as FCS. To avoid the confusion with

**TABLE 7.1**

Likelihood Ratio Test Results, Fieller Confidence Set (FCS), and Equivalence Assessment for Example Data

| | |
|---|---|
| $N$ | 12 |
| Ratio: $\frac{\bar{x}}{\bar{y}}$ | 0.9530 |
| 95% FCS ratio | 0.8275, 1.1118 |
| 90% FCS ratio | 0.8496, 1.0781 |
| Likelihood ratio test ($\alpha$ = 0.05) | |
| $P$ value (upper) | 0.0101 |
| $P$ value (lower) | 0.0023 |
| $P$ value (overall) | 0.0101 |
| Assessment | Equivalent |

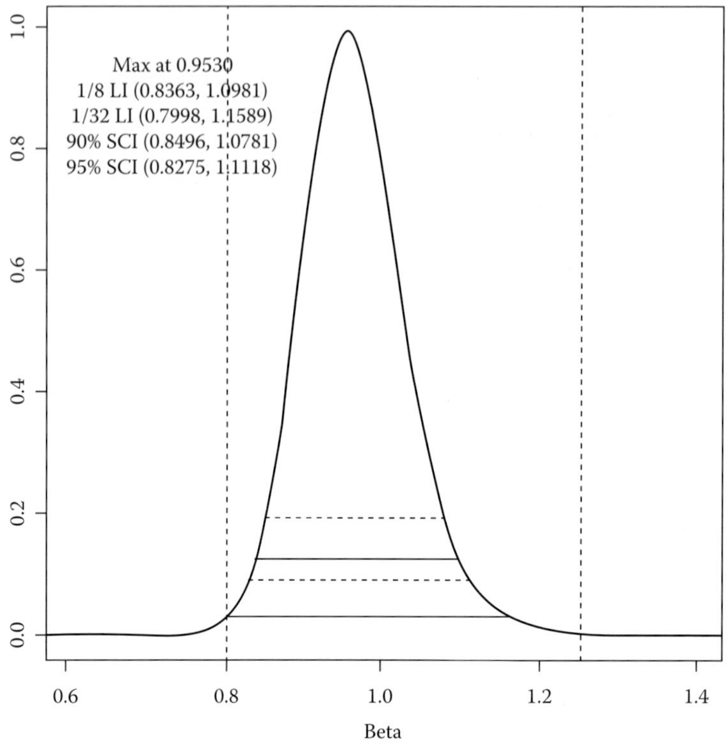


**FIGURE 7.1**
Plot of standardized profile likelihood (SPL) of Beta for Example 1 data. Two vertical dashed lines: $\beta = 1.25$. Horizontal lines, from bottom to top: 1/32 likelihood interval (LI), 95% standardized confidence interval (SCI), 1/8 LI, and 90% SCI. (Solid lines are for LIs, and dashed lines are for SCIs.)

FCS, we name these two limits on the SPL curve as SPL CI and SPL CI with $t(0.95, \text{df})$ as 90% standardized confidence interval (SCI). Hence, with $\gamma$ and $\rho$ taking values given above, the $(1-2\alpha)$% SCI matches the $(1-2\alpha)$% CI using FCS. This can be proven by letting $t^2 = \left(\dfrac{\bar{x}-\beta\bar{y}}{\hat{\sigma}_{(\bar{x}-\beta\bar{y})}}\right)^2 = t^2(1-\alpha, \upsilon)$ in Equation 7.10 and solving for $\beta$. The two values $\beta_{1,2}$ (on SPL) are the same as $\theta_{\pm}^{c}$ given in Equation 7.4.

In Figure 7.1, all 90% SCI, 95% SCI, 1/8 LI, and 1/32 LI are comprised within the equivalence margins, suggesting strong evidence in favor of equivalence. Note that 1/8 LI is very close to 95% SCI (counterpart of 95% CI in SPL setting), which is expected, as Royall (2000) showed for normally distributed random variables, that 1/8 and 1/32 LIs are approximately the same as the 95% and 99% CIs, though 1/32 LI appears to be excessive in the equivalence setting.

Note that the width of $(1 - 2\alpha)\%$ SCI equating to $w = \theta_+^c - \theta_-^c$, according to Equation 7.4 is a function of $\sigma$, in which estimate containing the parameters $\gamma$ and $\rho$. Figure 7.2 is contour plots to characterize how widths of 90% and 95% SCIs are related to $\gamma$ and $\rho$ using example data. The solid thick line represents the width of 90% SCI = 0.2285 (on left panel) and 95% SCI = 0.2843 (on right panel), which are both narrower than the width of the equivalence margins (=0.45). The data suggest adequate evidences of equivalence. Given that there are a range of pairs of $\gamma$ and $\rho$ associated with the same width of a SCI, it should help identify the source of the variability due to heterogeneity, weak correlation, or large variances of the two samples that could reduce the probability in achieving equivalence.

### 7.4.3 Inference about Equivalence Affected by $\gamma$

In this section, we show the impact unspecified variances have on equivalence inference. To do so, we retain $\gamma$ in the likelihood function Equation 7.8 but replace $\rho$ with its sample estimate $\hat{\rho} \approx 0.85$. The use of the sample estimate for $\rho$ allows us to explore how inference about equivalence (based on $\beta$) can be affected by $\gamma$. The distances between the upper and lower margins are considered in demonstrating the sensitivities of the inferences to $\gamma$. Sample estimator $\hat{\gamma} = \sqrt{S_x / S_y} \approx 0.87$ is chosen as the base value. Alternative values of $\gamma$ can be obtained by certain CIs or other meaningful justification. Figure 7.3 presents ratios of $\gamma$ at its alternative values against its base value (take reciprocal if ratio is less than 1). It also shows the ratios of lengths between the upper and lower margins observed at the alternative over the base value of $\gamma$. The ratios of lengths are presented at three levels of SPL, those corresponding to 90% and 95% confidence intervals (SCIs) and those at 1/8 LI.

The ratios of margin lengths, and therefore the sensitivities, are dependent of the level of SPL. Moreover, the sensitivity relationship between margin length and $\gamma$ is more complicated. An exact calculation based on Equation 7.8 gives us a range of $\gamma$, where equivalence is achieved using example data $0.558 \le \gamma \le 1.305$ at 90% SCI level. The 90% SCI when $\gamma = 0.558$ is (0.811, 1.200), when $\gamma = 1.305$ is (0.800, 1.093). Even though the 90% SCI is still within the equivalence margins, the variances of the two drugs are no longer homogeneous, raising concerns that one of the drugs carries more variability in rate of absorption than the other one. From this we have shown by methods replacing $\gamma$ with its rMLE or sample estimate, it may conceal the extent to which inference about equivalence is affected by $\gamma$. This experience was also noted in Blume (2005). We believe that, in the presence of unspecified variances and when the extent of heterogeneity is a concern, the proposed model $L_{\max}(\beta, \rho, \gamma | X, Y)$, Equation 7.8, could help determine a range of $\beta$, where equivalence is more likely to be achieved.

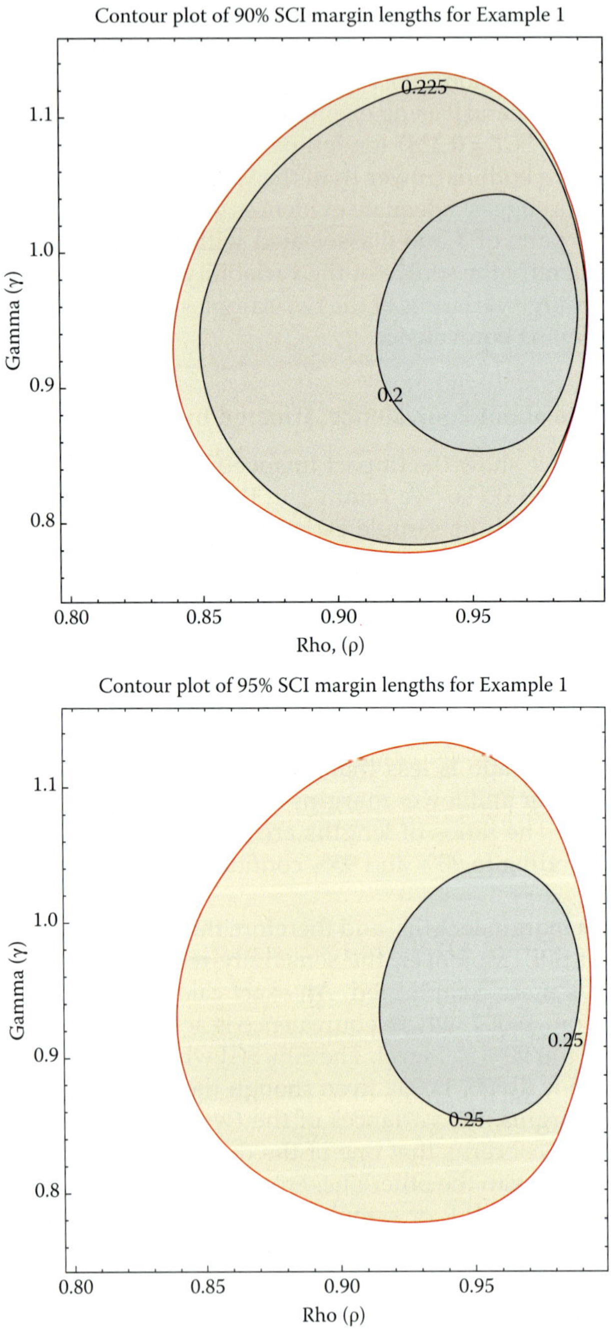


**FIGURE 7.2**
Contour plots for the widths of 90% and 95% SCIs.

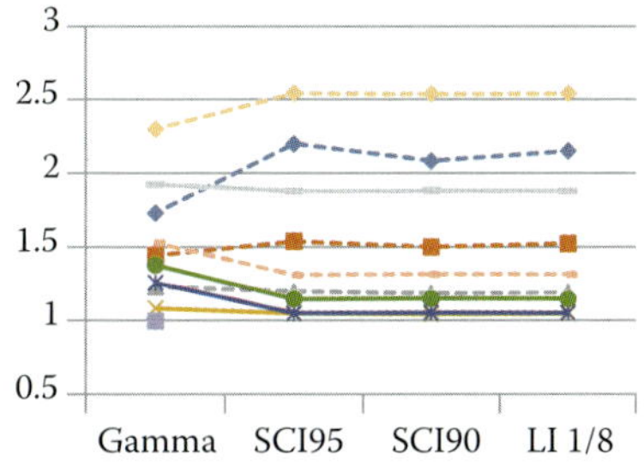


**FIGURE 7.3**
Ratios of $\gamma$ and length of margin at the alternative values against base value.

### 7.4.4 Inference about Equivalence Affected by $\sigma$ and $\rho$

Similarly we refer to two more sensitivity plots to see inference about equivalence affected by $\sigma$ and $\rho$. Sample estimate of each parameter is chosen as the base value. Alternative values of that parameter can be obtained by certain CIs. Figure 7.4 presents ratio of $\sigma$ at its alternative values against its base value (take reciprocal if ratio is less than 1). It also shows the ratios of margin lengths observed at the alternative over the base value of $\sigma$. Three levels of margin are considered, as for $\gamma$. Since the margin length is proportional to $\sigma$, the ratio of $\sigma$ at alternative values and the corresponding ratios at three levels of SPL are constant (Figure 7.4). The sensitivity relationship between margin length and $\rho$ is more complicated (Figure 7.5). Exact calculation by the maximum likelihood function gives range of $\sigma$ and $\rho$, where equivalence is more likely to be achieved at 90% SCI level: $\sigma \leq 7.38$ (0.800, 1.158); $\rho \geq 0.538$ (0.800, 1.142).

## 7.5 Comparison of Different Approaches in Crossover Design

In this section, we compare results based on the proposed likelihood method, likelihood ratio test (operationally equivalent to FCS), and Bayesian approach using the above dataset. Here, we also use the highest posterior density (HPD) interval, which is frequently referred to as the shortest Bayesian credible interval. Due to the partition, when the ratio of two variances is directly proportional to the ratio of two means, or the correlation between two drugs is directly proportional to the ratio of two means, $L_F$ also can be used for equivalence inference based on the ratio of two means. We will lose information if inference of equivalence is based on either one component only.

In general case, i.e., $\gamma$, $\sigma$ ,and $\rho$ are independent (Table 7.2).

One special case, $\gamma = b\beta$, where $b$ is a known constant (Table 7.3).

One special case, $\rho = c\beta$, where $c$ is a known constant (Table 7.4).

Results of different approaches are listed in Tables 7.5 through 7.7.

FCS (See Table 7.5).

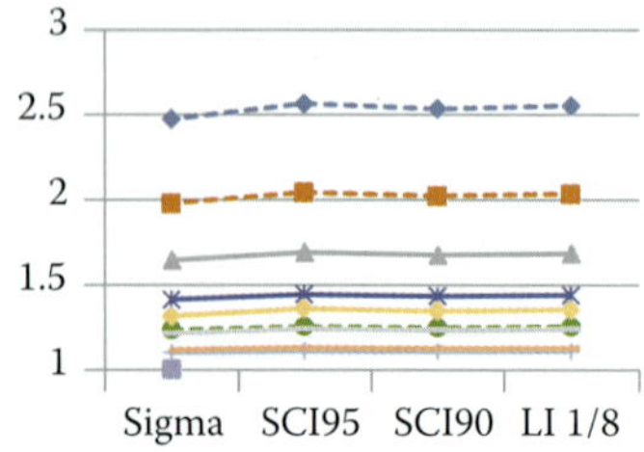


**FIGURE 7.4**
Ratios of σ and length of margin.

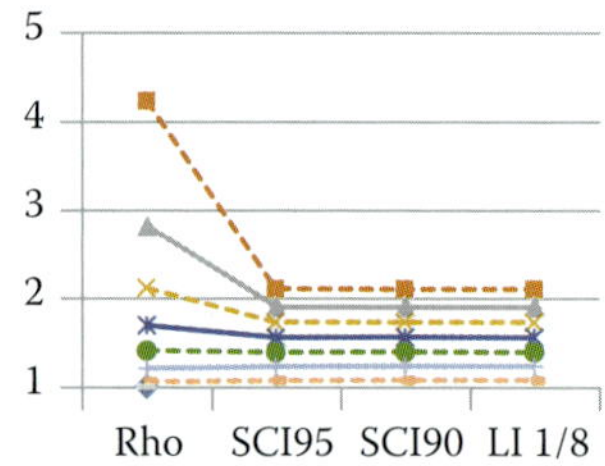


**FIGURE 7.5**
Ratios of ρ and length of margin at the alternative values against base value.

**TABLE 7.2**

In General Case, i.e., γ, σ, and ρ Are Independent

| | Crossover Design | Parallel Design |
|---|---|---|
| $L_F$ | $\frac{(1-\rho^2)^{\frac{n}{2}}}{\gamma^n}\left[\frac{S_x}{\gamma^2}+S_y-\frac{2\rho}{\gamma}S_{xy}\right]^{-n}$ | $\frac{1}{\gamma^n}\left[\frac{S_x}{\gamma^2}+S_y\right]^{-\frac{n+m}{2}}$ |
| $L_t$ | $\left(1+\frac{n(\bar{x}-\beta\bar{y})^2(1-\rho^2)}{\left(\frac{S_x}{\gamma^2}+S_y-\frac{2\rho}{\gamma}S_{xy}\right)(\beta^2-2\rho\gamma\beta+\gamma^2)}\right)^{-n}$ | $\left(1+\frac{nm(\bar{x}-\beta\bar{y})^2}{\left(\frac{S_x}{\gamma^2}+S_y\right)(n\beta^2+m\gamma^2)}\right)^{-\frac{n+m}{2}}$ |

**TABLE 7.3**

One Special Case, γ = bβ, Where *b* Is a Known Constant

| | Crossover Design | Parallel Design |
|---|---|---|
| $L_F$ | $\frac{(1-\rho^2)^{\frac{n}{2}}}{(b\beta)^n}\left[\frac{S_x}{b^2\beta^2}+S_y-\frac{2\rho}{b\beta}S_{xy}\right]^{-n}$ | $\frac{1}{(b\beta)^n}\left[\frac{S_x}{b^2\beta^2}+S_y\right]^{-\frac{n+m}{2}}$ |
| $L_t$ | $\left(1+\frac{n(\bar{x}-\beta\bar{y})^2(1-\rho^2)}{\left(\frac{S_x}{b^2\beta^2}+S_y-\frac{2\rho}{b\beta}S_{xy}\right)(\beta^2-2\rho b\beta^2+b^2\beta^2)}\right)^{-n}$ | $\left(1+\frac{nm(\bar{x}-\beta\bar{y})^2}{\left(\frac{S_x}{b^2\beta^2}+S_y\right)(n\beta^2+mb^2\beta^2)}\right)^{-\frac{n+m}{2}}$ |

**TABLE 7.4**

One Special Case, $\rho = c\beta$, Where $c$ Is a Known Constant

| | Crossover Design | Parallel Design |
|---|---|---|
| $L_F$ | $\frac{(1-c^2\beta^2)^{\frac{n}{2}}}{\gamma^n}\left[\frac{S_x}{\gamma^2}+S_y-\frac{2c\beta}{\gamma}S_{xy}\right]^{-n}$ | Not applicable |
| $L_t$ | $\left(1+\frac{n(\bar{x}-\beta\bar{y})^2(1-c^2\beta^2)}{\left(\frac{S_x}{\gamma^2}+S_y-\frac{2c\beta}{\gamma}S_{xy}\right)(\beta^2-2c\beta^2\gamma+\gamma^2)}\right)^{-n}$ | Not applicable |

**TABLE 7.5**

Likelihood Ratio Test (Equivalent to FCS)

| | General Case | Special Case $\gamma = \beta$ | Special Case $\rho = 0.8 * \beta$ |
|---|---|---|---|
| 95% FCS of $\beta$ | 0.8275, 1.1118 | 0.8277, 1.1048 | 0.7854, 1.1037 |
| 90% FCS of $\beta$ | 0.8496, 1.0781 | 0.8496, 1.0738 | 0.8184, 1.0754 |

*Note:* FCS, Fieller confidence set.

**TABLE 7.6**

Proposed Likelihood Method

| | General Case | Special Case $\gamma = \beta$ | Special Case $\rho = 0.8 * \beta$ |
|---|---|---|---|
| 95% SCI of $\beta$ | $L_{max}$ (0.8275, 1.1118)<br>$L_t$ (0. 8275, 1.1118) | $L_{max}$ (0.8249, 1.0732)<br>$L_t$ (0.8277, 1.1048) | $L_{max}$ (0.8251, 1.1083)<br>$L_t$ (0.7854, 1.1037) |
| 90% SCI of $\beta$ | $L_{max}$ (0.8496, 1.0781)<br>$L_t$ (0.8496, 1.0781) | $L_{max}$ (0.8451, 1.0476)<br>$L_t$ (0.8496, 1.0738) | $L_{max}$ (0.8536, 1.0850)<br>$L_t$ (0.8184, 1.0754) |

*Note:* SCI, standardized confidence interval.

**TABLE 7.7**

Bayesian Method

| | General Case | Special Case $\gamma = \beta$ | Special Case $\rho = 0.8 * \beta$ |
|---|---|---|---|
| 95% HPD of $\beta$ | 0.8001, 1.1184 | 0.8244, 1.0633 | 0.8421, 1.1268 |
| 90% HPD of $\beta$ | 0.8301, 1.0779 | 0.8444, 1.0393 | 0.8683, 1.1033 |
| Probability of $\beta$ falls within (0.8, 1.25) | 0.9707 | 0.9905 | 0.9900 |

*Note:* HPD, highest posterior density.

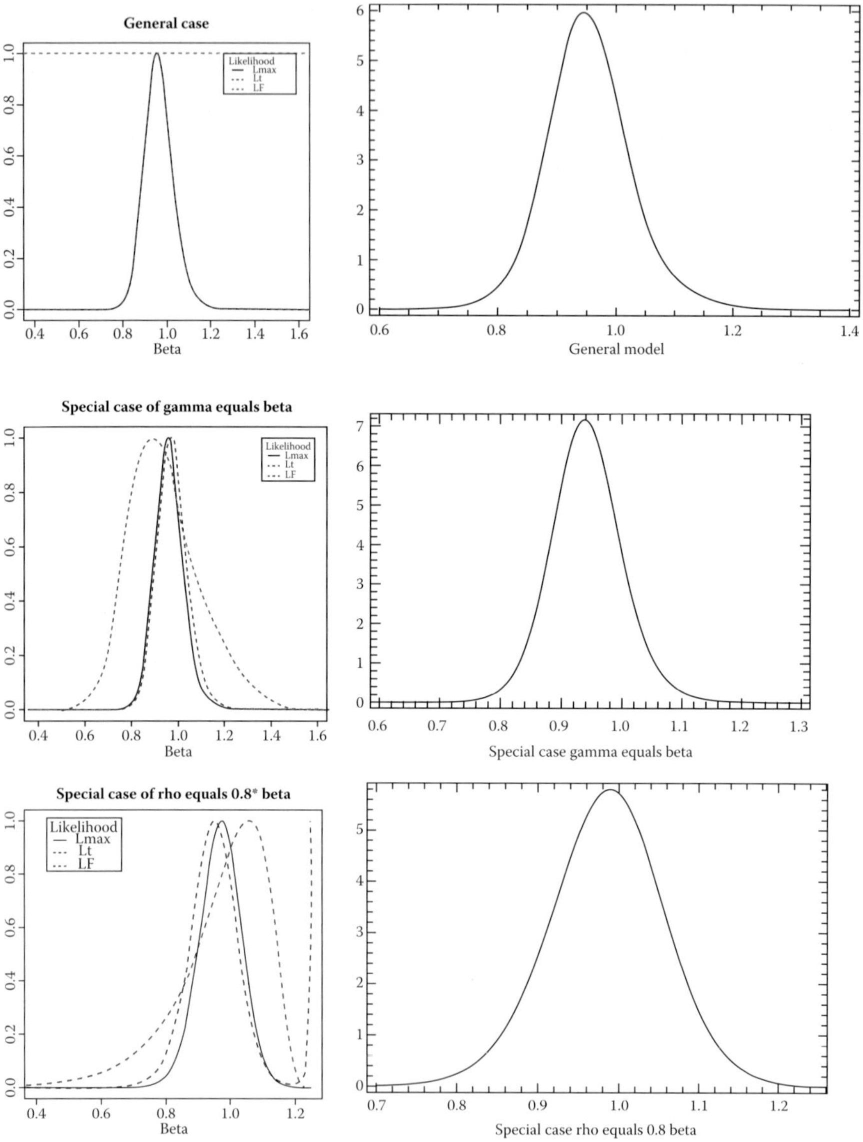


**FIGURE 7.6**
Comparison plots of SPL (left panel) and posterior density of β (right panel).

Proposed likelihood method (See Table 7.6).
Bayesian method (See Table 7.7).

We show that in general case, results of the proposed likelihood method are the same as likelihood ratio test (operationally equivalent to FCS) and comparable with Bayesian methods. In special case, however, the proposed likelihood method produces narrower CI than the likelihood ratio test (operationally equivalent to FCS). Hence, the proposed likelihood method is better than FCS or likelihood ratio test for equivalence inference. While Bayesian method gives similar length of HPD as the proposed method, both 90% and 95% HPDs of $\beta$ are shifted to the left when $\gamma = \beta$ and shifted to the right when $\rho = 0.8 * \beta$. Such an overestimate or underestimate is due to marginalizing out the unspecified variances. The results of the special case are presented in Tables 7.5 through 7.7 and Figure 7.6.

## 7.6 Conclusion and Discussion

Ideally, equivalence of two treatments is achieved on the basis of homogeneity ($\gamma$ close to 1), small variability (small $\sigma$), and strong correlation ($\rho$ close to 1) in addition to $\beta$ close to 1, but as illustrated in Sections 7.4 and 7.5, these conditions are not usually met in practice. In the presence of unspecified variances, unlike other methods that either replace them with sample estimates (likelihood-ratio test) or remove through integration (Bayesian model), the proposed likelihood method retains these variances via $\gamma$, $\sigma$, and $\rho$ in the model. It is shown to better characterize the extent that equivalence is affected by those variances and help identify a range where the equivalence is more likely to be achieved. Our findings confirm that probability of achieving equivalence could be diminished when (1) variances of the two treatments are heterogeneous, (2) variances are large even when homogeneousness is maintained, and (3) data from the two drugs are less correlated in a crossover study. By incorporating the parameters $\gamma$, $\sigma$, and $\rho$ in the proposed likelihood function, these relationships can be easily quantified. For example, when data failed to demonstrate equivalence using the likelihood ratio test or FCS, following our proposed method one could see whether it was attributable to one or more factors, e.g., $\gamma$ much larger than 1 (suggesting heterogeneity) and/or large $\sigma$ (high variability treatment). This information could signal the drug developer or trial sponsor to find ways to reduce the variability of the new treatment or seek an acceptable widened equivalence margins.

Section 7.5 shows that, in general cases, the proposed likelihood method produces results that are same as the likelihood ratio test and comparable to Bayesian analysis. In the special case where the ratio of two means determines the ratio of variances, the proposed method yields better results (narrower CIs) in inference about equivalence than does the likelihood ratio test. The length of HPD interval derived from Bayesian method is almost the same as the SCI from the proposed likelihood method, regardless of whether under the general case or special case. However, the HPD interval is either shifted to the left or right relative to SCI, an indication of over- or underestimate by the Bayesian method due to marginalizing out the unspecified variances. Since equivalence studies place the focus of statistics inference on whether the parameter of interest falls within the predetermined margins even more rigorously than estimating the parameter itself, it is important to find the "confidence limits" as narrow and precise as possible.

Our research results show that the proposed likelihood method is a better alternative than current analysis methods for equivalence inference. We believe that when it comes to establish equivalence, one should look beyond just relying on simple hypothesis testing to reach a final conclusion. Lastly, sample programs used to perform all the calculations, including R codes for likelihood methods and *Wolfram* Mathematica® 7 code for Bayesian model, are available from the authors Siyan Xu and Steven Ye Hua.

## References

Balthasar J.P. (1999). Bioequivalence and bioequivalency testing. *American Journal of Pharmaceutical Education* 63: 194–198.

Berger J.O., Bernardo J.M., Sun D. (2009). The formal definition of reference priors. *Annals of Statistics* 37: 905–938.

Berger R.L., Hsu J.C. (1996). Bioequivalence trials, intersection-union tests and equivalence confidence sets. *Statistical Science* 11: 283–302.

Blume J.D. (2005). How to choose a working model for measuring the statistical evidence about a regression parameter. *International Statistical Review* 73: 351–363.

Díaz-Francés E., Sprott, D.A. (2004). Inference for the ratio of two normal means with unspecified variances. *Biometrical Journal* 46: 83–89.

Food and Drug Administration. (2003). Guidance for Industry Bioavailability and Bioequivalence Studies for Orally Administered Drug Products—General Considerations. http://www.fda.gov/ohrms/dockets/ac/03/briefing/3995B1_07_GFI-BioAvail-BioEquiv.pdf.

Fieller E.C. (1954). Some problems in interval estimation. *Journal of Royal Statistical Society Series B* 16: 175–185.

Hauschke D., Kieser M., Diletti E., Burke, M. (1999). Sample size determination for proving equivalence based on the ratio of two means for normally distributed data. *Statistics in Medicine* 18: 93–105.

Hua S.Y., Hawkins D.L., Zhou J. (2013). Statistical considerations in bioequivalence of two area under the concentration–time curves obtained from serial sampling data. *Journal of Applied Statistics* 40 (5): 1140–1154.

Liu J.-P., Weng C.-S. (1994). Evaluation of log-transformation in assessing bioequivalence. *Communications in Statistics—Theory and Methods* 23: 421–434.

Royall R.M. (1997). *Statistical Evidence: A Likelihood Paradigm.* Chapman & Hall/CRC: London/Boca Raton, FL.

Royall R.M. (2000). On the probability of observing misleading statistical evidence (C/R: P768-780). *Journal of the American Statistical Association* 95: 760–768.

Rubio F.J., Pérez-Elizalde S. (2009). Letter to the editor. *Biometrical Journal* 51: 736–738.

Sasabuchi S. (1988a). A multivariate one-sided test with composite hypotheses determined by linear inequalities when the covariance matrix has an unknown scale factor. *Memoirs of the Faculty of Science, Kyushu University Series A, Mathematics* 42: 9–19.

Sasabuchi S. (1988b). A multivariate one-sided test with composite hypotheses when the covariance matrix is completely unknown. *Memoirs of the Faculty of Science, Kyushu University Series A, Mathematics* 42: 37–46.

Xu S., Hua S.Y., Menton R., Barker K., Menon S., D'Agostino R.B. (2014). Inference of bioequivalence for log-normal distributed data with unspecified variances. *Statistics in Medicine* 33: 2924–2938.

# 8

# *Multiplicity Adjustments in Testing for Bioequivalence*

**Steven Ye Hua, Siyan Xu, and Ralph B. D'Agostino**

**CONTENTS**



**ABSTRACT** Bioequivalence (BE) of two drugs is usually demonstrated by rejecting two one-sided null hypotheses using the two one-sided tests (TOSTs) for the primary metrics: area under the concentration–time curve (AUC) and maximum concentration ($C_{max}$). The decision rule for BE often requires equivalence to be achieved on both metrics that contain four one-sided null hypotheses together; without adjusting for multiplicity, the family-wise error rate (FWER) could rise above the nominal type I error rate $\alpha$. In this chapter, we propose two multiplicity adjustments in testing for BE, including a closed-test procedure that controls FWER by treating the two metrics as a coprimary endpoint problem and an alpha-adaptive sequential testing (AAST) that controls FWER by prespecifying the significance level on AUC ($\alpha_1$) and obtaining it for $C_{max}(\alpha_2)$ adaptively after testing of AUC. Illustrated with published data, the two approaches, although they operate differently, lead to the same substantive conclusion and are better than a traditional method like Bonferroni adjustment.

## 8.1 Introduction

### 8.1.1 Motivation

The U.S. Food and Drug Administration (FDA) guidance document [1] requires that, in order to prove a generic equivalent of an established drug, the sponsors need to provide evidence of the equivalence in average bioavailability of its generic drug product measured by the two pharmacokinetic (PK) parameters, area under the concentration–time curve (AUC) and peak concentration ($C_{max}$), to that of the established drug. These two parameters usually follow log-normal distribution, as such a logarithmic transformation is performed prior to analysis and inference about BE is made on the difference in mean ln(AUC) and mean $\ln(C_{max})$.

Traditionally, BE is demonstrated if 90% two-sided confidence intervals (CIs) for both ln(AUC) and $\ln(C_{max})$ fall within the equivalence margins $(-\theta,\theta)$, $\theta = \ln(1.25) \approx 0.223$, or the two one-sided null hypotheses are rejected using TOSTs [2] at $\alpha = 0.05$ for each parameter. Although equivalence of each parameter is assessed by two tests, there is no need for multiplicity adjustment thanks to the intersection–union test (IUT) process [3]. However, the decision rule for BE often requires equivalence to be achieved on both parameters where the null hypothesis for the treatment differences is defined by the area outside the central square $(-\theta,\theta)\times(-\theta,\theta)$, with the boundaries belonging to the null hypothesis. Without adjusting for multiplicity, the FWER $\alpha_F$ could be inflated above the nominal type I error rate $\alpha$. The multiplicity issue for BE in this regard is barely discussed in the literature. Our research was motivated by a randomized PK trial to demonstrate BE of human–murine monoclonal antibody drugs for the treatment of rheumatoid arthritis. This trial, after the establishment of BE, is to be followed by a late-phase therapeutic equivalence trial of the same drugs, which itself is subject to the multiplicity issue. Since both trials will be submitted for regulatory reviews where multiplicity issues are rigorously scrutinized, the need for multiplicity adjustments is apparent even though it is less common in BE trials. In this chapter, we focus on multiplicity issues related to BE studies.

Multiplicity in equivalence trials is mostly considered in pairwise comparisons of multiple treatments measured by one parameter. A conservative option to adjust multiplicity of two parameters is to follow the recommendation from the Committee for Proprietary Medicinal Products (CPMP) guidance [4] using one-sided $\alpha$ of 0.025 or 95% two-sided CIs for assessments, which is more restrictive than the usual approach for BE where, in contrast, 90% two-sided CIs are applied. A Bonferroni-based method proposed by Lauzon and Caffo [5] controls FWER for equivalence by dividing the nominal error rate $\alpha$ by 2 in pairwise comparisons of three treatments. Röhmel [6] proposed a $p$-value-based approach based on the closure test principle for pairwise comparisons of multiple treatments [7–9]. These approaches do not address the multiplicity issue caused by two parameters in BE trials.

A closure test has a certain appeal as it is $p$-value based and controls FWER by rejecting all intersection null hypotheses (defined by this approach) at $\alpha$, so it does not require a priori deduction in the nominal error rate $\alpha$ for each test. It also treats the two parameters with the same importance. However, a large number of intersection null hypotheses could increase the chance of failing to reject at least one null hypothesis. Also, calculation of $p$-values for these intersection null hypotheses usually relies on a complex distribution of bivariate TOSTs in our case, which is not provided in these articles. On the other hand, we noticed in some BE studies that equivalence to be achieved in AUC takes a higher priority over that of $C_{max}$, which is frequently more variable than AUC. In this case, AUC and $C_{max}$ are ranked as primary and secondary metrics. A literature search led to recently published methods, such as Adaptive Alpha Allocation Approach (4A) by Li and Mehrotra [10], alpha-adaptive strategy for sequential testing by Alosh and Huque [11], and an extension of 4A by Li et al. [12]. These approaches allow the significance level for testing the secondary endpoint to adapt in a specific function form to the $p$-value of the primary endpoint. However, these published approaches are limited to demonstrating only superiority rather than BE, and they assume the test statistics for the two endpoints follow a bivariate normal density that cannot be applied to BE data, which are tested using two TOSTs that are correlated.

### 8.1.2 Outline

In this chapter, we propose two multiplicity adjustments in testing for BE. A $p$-value-based closed test approach that carries out tests for eight intersection sets of the four null hypotheses (each at $\alpha$ level) can be applied to BE trials, where AUC and $C_{max}$ are coprimary metrics. $P$-values are calculated using a numerical method based on a bivariate noncentral $t$-distribution. According to Grechanovsky and Hochberg [13], testing at full $\alpha$ (or $\alpha$ exhaustive) is uniformly more powerful than not $\alpha$ exhaustive. We also propose AAST procedure to allow control of FWER by prespecifying a significant level $\alpha_1$ for ln(AUC) and obtaining $\alpha_2$ for $\ln(C_{max})$ after testing of ln(AUC). An AAST approach can be applied to BE trials where AUC and $C_{max}$ are primary and secondary metrics, and we show that AAST fully controls FWER. A general power function is presented for the closed test and AAST methods. These methods are illustrated using the published data.

## 8.2 Closed Test Procedure in Bioequivalence Using Two One-Sided Test

The equivalence hypothesis is given by:

$$\begin{aligned} &\text{Null hypothesis} \quad H_{01}: \Delta u \le -\theta \text{ or } H_{02}: \Delta u \ge \theta \\ &\text{Alternative hypothesis} \quad H_a: -\theta < \Delta u < \theta \end{aligned} \tag{8.1}$$

The hypotheses given in Equation 8.1 can be tested using TOST [2] compared with critical values of $t$-distribution. The pair of null hypotheses $H_{01}$ and $H_{02}$ are rejected at the significance level of $\alpha$ if and only if:

$$T_l = \frac{\Delta\bar{X} + \theta}{\hat{\sigma}_{\Delta\bar{X}}} > t_{1-\alpha,\,\nu} \text{ and } T_u = \frac{\theta - \Delta\bar{X}}{\hat{\sigma}_{\Delta\bar{X}}} > t_{1-\alpha,\,\nu} \tag{8.2}$$

The parameters in Equations 8.1 and 8.2 are $\Delta u = u_T - u_R$ (T, R: test and reference) and $\Delta\bar{X} = \bar{X}_T - \bar{X}_R$, $u_T = E(\ln(\text{AUC}_T))$, $u_R = E(\ln(\text{AUC}_R))$, $\bar{X}_T = \overline{\ln(\text{AUC})}_T$, $\bar{X}_T = \overline{\ln(\text{AUC})}_R$, and $\hat{\sigma}_{\Delta\bar{X}}$ is the estimated standard deviation (SD) of $\Delta\bar{X}$; the same notations can be written for $C_{max}$ by replacing $\Delta u$ with $\Delta v$ and $\Delta\bar{X}$ with $\Delta\bar{Y}$, where $v_T = E(\ln(C_{max\,T}))$, $v_R = E(\ln(C_{max\,R}))$, $\bar{Y}_T = \overline{\ln(C_{max})}_T$, and $\bar{Y}_R = \overline{\ln(C_{max})}_R$. We use BE acceptance limits $\theta = \ln(1.25) \approx 0.223$ and $-\theta \approx -0.223$ as the upper and lower equivalence margins, respectively.

We define following notations to be used throughout this chapter: $T_{A,l} = \frac{\Delta\bar{X} + \theta}{\hat{\sigma}_{\Delta\bar{X}}}$ and $T_{A,u} = \frac{\theta - \Delta\bar{X}}{\hat{\sigma}_{\Delta\bar{X}}}$ are TOST for ln(AUC) with the corresponding $p$-values $p_{A,l}$ and $p_{A,u}$, respectively; $T_{C,l} = \frac{\Delta\bar{Y} + \theta}{\hat{\sigma}_{\Delta\bar{Y}}}$ and $T_{C,u} = \frac{\theta - \Delta\bar{Y}}{\hat{\sigma}_{\Delta\bar{Y}}}$ are TOST for ln($C_{max}$) with $p$-values of $p_{C,l}$ and $p_{C,u}$. In addition, $T_A = \frac{\Delta\bar{X} - \Delta u}{\sigma_{\Delta\bar{X}}}$,

$T_C = \frac{\Delta\bar{Y} - \Delta v}{\sigma_{\Delta\bar{Y}}}$, $T_A^* = \frac{\Delta\bar{X}}{\hat{\sigma}_{\Delta\bar{X}}} = \frac{T_A + \delta_A}{\frac{\hat{\sigma}_{\Delta\bar{X}}}{\sigma_{\Delta\bar{X}}}}$, $T_C^* = \frac{\Delta\bar{Y}}{\hat{\sigma}_{\Delta\bar{Y}}} = \frac{T_C + \delta_C}{\frac{\hat{\sigma}_{\Delta\bar{Y}}}{\sigma_{\Delta\bar{Y}}}}$, $\delta_A = \frac{\Delta u}{\sigma_{\Delta\bar{X}}}$, $\delta_C = \frac{\Delta v}{\sigma_{\Delta\bar{Y}}}$; $T_A^{mx} = \max(T_{A,l}, T_{A,u})$, $T_A^{mi} = \min(T_{A,l}, T_{A,u})$, $T_C^{mx} = \max(T_{C,l}, T_{C,u})$, and $T_C^{mi} = \min(T_{C,l}, T_{C,u})$.

The hypothesis sets for both ln(AUC) and ln($C_{max}$) can be expressed as:

Null sets: $H_{A,01} = \{\Delta u \le -\theta\}$, $H_{A,02} = \{\Delta u \ge \theta\}$, $H_{C,01} = \{\Delta v \le -\theta\}$, and $H_{C,02} = \{\Delta v \ge \theta\}$.

$$\text{Alternative sets: } H_{A,a} = \{-\theta < \Delta u < \theta\} \text{ and } H_{C,a} = \{-\theta < \Delta v < \theta\} \tag{8.3}$$

The intersection and union are two common operations: $\bigcap$ and $\bigcup$, meaning "and" and "or" of two sets, respectively. There are $2^4 - 1 = 15$ possible intersection sets of the four null hypotheses given in Equation 8.3, because $H_{A,01} \bigcap H_{A,02} = H_{C,01} \bigcap H_{C,02} = \phi$, where only eight intersection sets are nonempty. Figure 8.1 shows the relative locations and sizes of these intersection hypotheses in two dimensions.

$$
\begin{array}{l}
H_{A,01} \bigcap H_{C,a}, H_{A,02} \bigcap H_{C,a}, H_{A,a} \bigcap H_{C,01}, H_{A,a} \bigcap H_{C,02} \\
H_{A,01} \bigcap H_{C,01}, H_{A,01} \bigcap H_{C,02}, H_{A,02} \bigcap H_{C,01}, H_{A,02} \bigcap H_{C,02}
\end{array} \tag{8.4}
$$

It follows from the closure test principle, and the probability of false rejection of each null hypothesis in Equation 8.4 must be $< \alpha$.

$$
\Pr\left(T_A^{mi} > t_{1-\alpha,v} \mid H_{A,01} \bigcup H_{A,02}\right) \le \alpha \tag{8.5}
$$

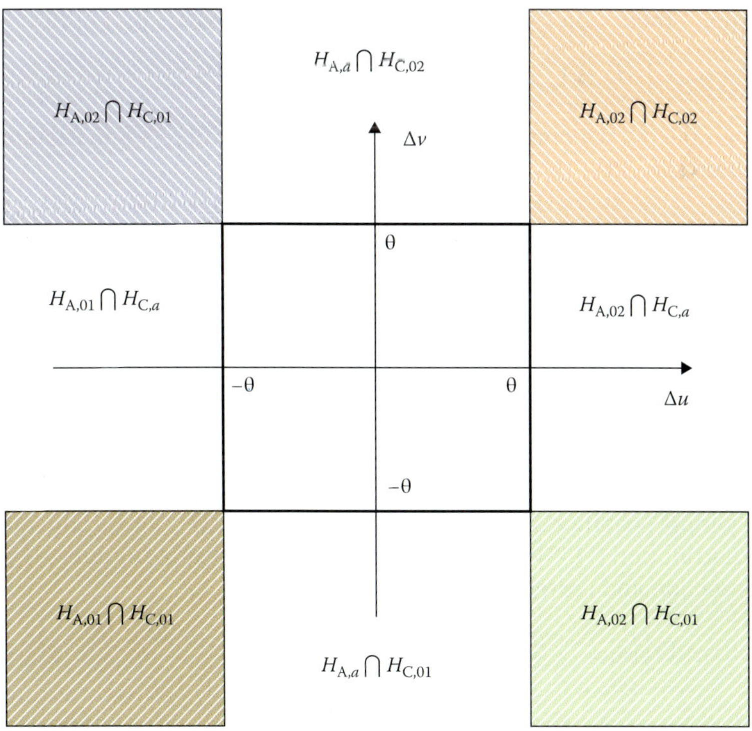


**FIGURE 8.1**
Intersection null hypotheses for the closure test procedure.

$$\Pr\left(T_{\mathrm{C}}^{\mathrm{mi}} > t_{1-\alpha,v} \mid H_{\mathrm{C},01} \bigcup H_{\mathrm{C},02}\right) \le \alpha \tag{8.6}$$

$$\Pr\left(T_{\mathrm{A}}^{\mathrm{mi}} > t_{1-\alpha,v} \text{ and } T_{\mathrm{C}}^{\mathrm{mi}} > t_{1-\alpha,v} \mid \text{null in Equation 8.4}\right) \le \alpha \tag{8.7}$$

The inequalities in Equations 8.5 and 8.6 are implied when the null hypotheses in Equation 8.1 are rejected for both $\Delta u$ and $\Delta v$, and we show that in the following equation by applying Equation 8.5:

$$\begin{aligned} &\Pr\left(T_{\mathrm{A}}^{\mathrm{mi}} > t_{1-\alpha,v} \mid H_{\mathrm{A},01} \bigcup H_{\mathrm{A},02}\right) \\ &= \Pr\left(\frac{-\theta-\Delta u}{\hat{\sigma}_{\Delta\bar{X}}} + t_{1-\alpha,v} < \frac{\Delta\bar{X}-\Delta u}{\hat{\sigma}_{\Delta\bar{X}}} < \frac{\theta-\Delta u}{\hat{\sigma}_{\Delta\bar{X}}} - t_{1-\alpha,v} \mid H_{\mathrm{A},01} \bigcup H_{\mathrm{A},02}\right) \end{aligned} \tag{8.8}$$

If $H_{\mathrm{A},01}$ is true, then $\Delta u \le -\theta$ implies $\frac{\Delta\bar{X}-\Delta u}{\hat{\sigma}_{\Delta\bar{X}}} > t_{1-\alpha,v}$; if $H_{\mathrm{A},02}$ is true, then $\Delta u \ge \theta$ means $\frac{\Delta\bar{X}-\Delta u}{\hat{\sigma}_{\Delta\bar{X}}} < -t_{1-\alpha,v}$. In either case, $\Pr\left(T_{\mathrm{A}}^{\mathrm{mi}} > t_{1-\alpha,v} \mid H_{\mathrm{A},01} \bigcup H_{\mathrm{A},02}\right) \le \alpha$.

For simplicity, we omit $v$ in $t_{1-\alpha,v}$, and the probability in Equation 8.7 can be written as

$$\begin{aligned} &\Pr\left(T_{\mathrm{A}}^{\mathrm{mi}} > t_{1-\alpha} \text{ and } T_{\mathrm{C}}^{\mathrm{mi}} > t_{1-\alpha} \mid \text{null in Equation 8.4}\right) \\ &= \Pr\left[\begin{array}{l} \left(\frac{-\theta}{\hat{\sigma}_{\Delta\bar{X}}} + t_{1-\alpha} < T_{\mathrm{A}}^{*} < \frac{\theta}{\hat{\sigma}_{\Delta\bar{X}}} - t_{1-\alpha}\right), \\ \left(\frac{-\theta}{\hat{\sigma}_{\Delta\bar{Y}}} + t_{1-\alpha} < T_{\mathrm{C}}^{*} < \frac{\theta}{\hat{\sigma}_{\Delta\bar{Y}}} - t_{1-\alpha}\right) \mid \text{null in Equation 8.4} \end{array}\right] \end{aligned} \tag{8.9}$$

The joint probability of $(T_{\mathrm{A}}^{*}, T_{\mathrm{C}}^{*})$ in Equation 8.9 follows a bivariate noncentral $t$-distribution [14,15] with noncentrality parameters $\delta_{\mathrm{A}}$, $\delta_{\mathrm{C}}$ defined earlier in this section and correlation coefficient $\rho_{AC}$ given later.

$$\begin{aligned} &\Pr\left[\left(a_1 < T_{\mathrm{A}}^{*} \le a_2\right), \ \left(c_2 < T_{\mathrm{C}}^{*} < c_2\right)\right] \\ &= \frac{1}{2^{\frac{v}{2}-1}\Gamma(\frac{v}{2})} \int_0^{\infty} x^{v-1} e^{-\frac{x^2}{2}} \Phi_2\left(\frac{\boldsymbol{a}\cdot x}{\sqrt{\nu}} - \delta_{\mathrm{A}}, \ \frac{\boldsymbol{c}\cdot x}{\sqrt{\nu}} - \delta_{\mathrm{C}}; \rho_{AC}\right) dx \end{aligned} \tag{8.10}$$

where $\Phi_2\left(\frac{\boldsymbol{a}\cdot x}{\sqrt{\nu}}-\delta_A,\ \frac{c\cdot x}{\sqrt{\nu}}-\delta_C;\rho_{AC}\right)$ is a bivariate normal integral, $\boldsymbol{a}=\begin{pmatrix}a_2\\a_1\end{pmatrix}$, $\boldsymbol{c}=\begin{pmatrix}c_2\\c_1\end{pmatrix}$.

In parallel designs, if two drug groups are independent of each other, then $\hat{\rho}_{AC}=\hat{\rho}_{X_T,Y_T}\cdot\frac{\hat{\sigma}_{\bar{X}_T}\hat{\sigma}_{\bar{Y}_T}}{\hat{\sigma}_{\Delta\bar{X}}\hat{\sigma}_{\Delta\bar{Y}}}+\hat{\rho}_{X_R,Y_R}\cdot\frac{\hat{\sigma}_{\bar{X}_R}\hat{\sigma}_{\bar{Y}_R}}{\hat{\sigma}_{\Delta\bar{X}}\hat{\sigma}_{\Delta\bar{Y}}}$, in which $\hat{\rho}_{X_T,Y_T}$, $\hat{\rho}_{X_R,Y_R}$ are estimated correlation coefficients between $\ln(AUC_T)$ and $\ln(C_{max\,T})$, and $\ln(AUC_R)$ and $\ln(C_{max\,R})$, respectively; $\hat{\sigma}_{\bar{X}_T}$, $\hat{\sigma}_{\bar{X}_R}$, $\hat{\sigma}_{\bar{Y}_T}$, $\hat{\sigma}_{\bar{Y}_R}$, $\hat{\sigma}_{\Delta\bar{X}}$, and $\hat{\sigma}_{\Delta\bar{Y}}$ are sample SDs. In the case of equal variances, if $\sigma_{\bar{X}_T}=\sigma_{\bar{X}_R}$ and $\sigma_{\bar{Y}_T}=\sigma_{\bar{Y}_R}$, then $\hat{\rho}_{AC}=\frac{1}{2}\left(\hat{\rho}_{X_T,Y_T}+\hat{\rho}_{X_R,Y_R}\right)$.

In crossover designs, data are correlated between parameters and within each parameter, and thus

$$\hat{\rho}_{A,C}=\hat{\rho}_{X_T,Y_T}\cdot\frac{\hat{\sigma}_{\bar{X}_T}\hat{\sigma}_{\bar{Y}_T}}{\hat{\sigma}_{\Delta\bar{X}}\hat{\sigma}_{\Delta\bar{Y}}}+\hat{\rho}_{X_R,Y_R}\cdot\frac{\hat{\sigma}_{\bar{X}_R}\hat{\sigma}_{\bar{Y}_R}}{\hat{\sigma}_{\Delta\bar{X}}\hat{\sigma}_{\Delta\bar{Y}}}-\hat{\rho}_{X_T,Y_R}\cdot\frac{\hat{\sigma}_{\bar{X}_T}\hat{\sigma}_{\bar{Y}_R}}{\hat{\sigma}_{\Delta\bar{X}}\hat{\sigma}_{\Delta\bar{Y}}}-\hat{\rho}_{X_R,Y_T}\cdot\frac{\hat{\sigma}_{\bar{X}_R}\hat{\sigma}_{\bar{Y}_T}}{\hat{\sigma}_{\Delta\bar{X}}\hat{\sigma}_{\Delta\bar{Y}}} \quad (8.11)$$

where $\hat{\sigma}_{\Delta\bar{X}}=\sqrt{\frac{1}{n}\left(\hat{\sigma}^2_{X_T}+\hat{\sigma}^2_{X_R}-2\hat{\rho}_{X_T,X_R}\cdot\hat{\sigma}_{X_T}\hat{\sigma}_{X_R}\right)}$ and

$$\hat{\sigma}_{\Delta\bar{Y}}=\sqrt{\frac{1}{n}\left(\hat{\sigma}^2_{Y_T}+\hat{\sigma}^2_{Y_R}-2\hat{\rho}_{Y_T,Y_R}\cdot\hat{\sigma}_{Y_T}\hat{\sigma}_{Y_R}\right)}.$$

Calculations of the probabilities in Equation 8.9 can be performed by a numerical method like R package "mvtnorm" available in Comprehensive R Archive Network (CRAN) and references [14–16]. One should check to avoid invalid calculations that might otherwise arise, for example, $\min\left\{\frac{2\theta}{\hat{\sigma}_{\Delta\bar{X}}},\frac{2\theta}{\hat{\sigma}_{\Delta\bar{Y}}}\right\}>2t_{1-\alpha}$ in Equation 8.9.

## 8.3 Analysis of Two Datasets

We illustrate the closed test procedure described in Section 8.2 using the data presented by Marzo et al. [17; Table II]. In this trial, 24 subjects were treated with a new formulation of ticlopidine hydrochloride (test) and the reference Tiklid in a crossover design. The drug works by preventing excessive blood clotting and is used to reduce the risk of stroke and treat intermittent claudication, a condition generally affecting the blood vessels in the legs. The PK data were assumed to follow a log-normal distribution; thus logarithmic transformation of individual $AUC_{0-t}$ and $C_{max}$ data was performed prior to data analysis. We consider two scenarios: S1 represents the published data, which shows a sufficient consistency between the two parameters; we then modified the S1 data to generate S2, a case of insufficient consistency of the two parameters.

S1: $n = 24$, $\bar{X}_T = 6.6388$, $\bar{X}_R = 6.7191$, $\bar{Y}_T = 5.6665$, $\bar{Y}_R = 5.7607$; $\Delta\bar{X} = -0.0803\,(\ln(0.9238))$, $\Delta\bar{Y} = -0.0963(\ln(0.9102))$, $\hat{\sigma}_{\Delta\bar{X}} = 0.0588$, $\hat{\sigma}_{\Delta\bar{Y}} = 0.0657$, and $\hat{\rho}_{A,C} = 0.8076$; $H_{A,01}$, $H_{A,02}$, $H_{C,01}$, $H_{C,02}$ are each rejected with $p$-values of $p_{A,u} < .0001$, $p_{A,l} = .0116$ for $\ln(AUC_{0-t})$, and $p_{C,u} < .0001$, $p_{C,l} = .0309$ for $\ln(C_{max})$.

S2: $n = 24$, $\bar{X}_T = 6.6537$, $\bar{X}_R = 6.5178$, $\bar{Y}_T = 5.6665$, $\bar{Y}_R = 5.7766$; $\Delta\bar{X} = 0.1359\,(\ln(1.1456))$, $\Delta\bar{Y} = -0.11\,(\ln(0.8957))$, $\hat{\sigma}_{\Delta\bar{X}} = 0.0490$, $\hat{\sigma}_{\Delta\bar{Y}} = 0.0657$, and $\hat{\rho}_{A,C} = 0.6794$; $H_{A,01}$, $H_{A,02}$, $H_{C,01}$, $H_{C,02}$ are each rejected with $p$-values of $p_{A,u} = .0442$, $p_{A,l} < .0001$ for $\ln(AUC_{0-t})$, and $p_{C,u} < .0001$, $p_{C,l} = .0492$ for $\ln(C_{max})$.

### 8.3.1 Test of Equivalence for Each Parameter Using Two One-Sided Test

As previously stated, BE is commonly declared either by showing that 90% CIs of $\Delta\bar{X}$ and $\Delta\bar{Y}$ are comprised in (−0.223, 0.223) or by rejecting the null hypotheses in Equation 8.1 for each parameter using TOST. These analyses can be easily performed using the SAS© PROC TTEST (with dist=normal TOST(−0.223, 0.223) options), and results are presented in Table 8.1. For S1, one may find the $p$-values for which the four one-sided null hypotheses are rejected slightly differ than those presented by the authors. The differences, although negligible, may be attributable to rounding or use of pooled SD instead of using $\hat{\sigma}_{\Delta\bar{X}}$ and $\hat{\sigma}_{\Delta\bar{Y}}$ provided in Equation 8.11 to generate TOST. As indicated by Hua et al. [18], the control of type I error rate could be inflated if pooled variance is used even when pooling of two variances is unjustifiable. Table 8.1 further suggests that although equivalence is achieved for each parameter based on 90% CIs, they would have failed if 95% two-sided CIs or one-sided $\alpha$ of 0.025 were considered.

### 8.3.2 Bayesian Analysis

The authors of this chapter have developed a Bayesian posterior distribution to describe BE data. In which, they presented a posterior probability distribution of $\delta$ ($\delta = \Delta u$ or $\Delta v$), which is determined by the prior probability distribution of $\delta$ and likelihood function (probability model for the observed data based on a bivariate normal distribution). It focuses on inference in $\delta$ changing from prior, through observed data

**TABLE 8.1**

Marginal Results—TOST, 90% CIs, and Equivalence Assessments for S1 and S2 Data

| | S1 | | S2 | |
|---|---|---|---|---|
| | **ln(AUC)** | **ln($C_{max}$)** | **ln(AUC)** | **ln($C_{max}$)** |
| *N* | 24 | 24 | 24 | 24 |
| Difference in mean | −0.0803 | −0.0942 | 0.1359 | −0.1100 |
| 90% CI of mean | −0.1810, 0.0205 | −0.2067, 0.0184 | 0.0519, 0.2199 | −0.2226, 0.0025 |
| 95% CI of mean | −0.2018, 0.0413 | −0.2300, 0.0417 | 0.0345, 0.2373 | −0.2459, 0.0258 |
| SD/SE | 0.2879/0.0588 | 0.3217/0.0657 | 0.2401/0.0490 | 0.3217/0.0657 |
| TOST ($\alpha = 0.05$) | | | | |
| *P*-value (upper[a]) | 0.0116 | 0.0309 | <0.0001 | 0.0492 |
| *P*-value (lower[a]) | <0.0001 | <0.0001 | 0.0442 | <0.0001 |
| *P*-value (overall) | 0.0116 | 0.0309 | 0.0442 | 0.0490 |
| Equivalence assessment | Equivalent for 90% and 95% CIs | Equivalent for 90% CI only | Equivalent for 90% CI only | Equivalent for 90% CI only |

*Notes:* CI, confidence interval; TOST, two one-sided test; SD, standard deviation; SE, standard error.

[a] The upper *p*-values corresponds to $p_{A,l}$ and $p_{C,l}$; lower *p*-values correspond to $p_{A,u}$ and $p_{C,u}$ in the text.

(via likelihood function) to posterior. Details of this Bayesian analysis method, which are readily available in Xu et al. [19] are thus omitted. Posterior density plots of $\delta = \Delta u$ and $\Delta v$ for ln(AUC) and ln($C_{max}$) for both scenarios are shown in Figures 8.2 and 8.3 for the two examples. In Figures 8.2a and 8.3a, $\pi(\delta,| X_T, X_R)$ is the posterior probability density for ln(AUC) that $\delta = E(\ln(AUC_T)) - E(\ln(AUC_R))$, while in Figures 8.2b and 8.3b, $\pi(\delta,| Y_T, Y_R)$ is the posterior probability density for ln($C_{max}$) such that $\delta = E(\ln(C_{max\,T})) - E(\ln(C_{max\,R}))$. Although equivalence in ln(AUC) and ln($C_{max}$) can be declared individually for either scenario, consistency of the two PK parameters is shown only in S1. Lack of consistency between ln(AUC) and ln($C_{max}$) in S2 as evident by $\Delta\bar{X}$ and $\Delta\bar{Y}$ in opposite directions, difference between $\hat{\sigma}_{\Delta\bar{X}}$ and $\hat{\sigma}_{\Delta\bar{Y}}$ ($\hat{\sigma}^2_{\Delta\bar{Y}} / \hat{\sigma}^2_{\Delta\bar{X}} = 1.8$) and smaller $\hat{\rho}_{A,C}$ may have contributed to pushing FWER above the 0.05 level.

### 8.3.3 Closed Test

Data are further analyzed using the closed test described in Section 8.2, and *p*-values for the eight intersection null hypotheses in Equation 8.4 are presented in Table 8.2. Those *p*-values were calculated numerically using R package "mvtnorm," and each value corresponds to the largest value across

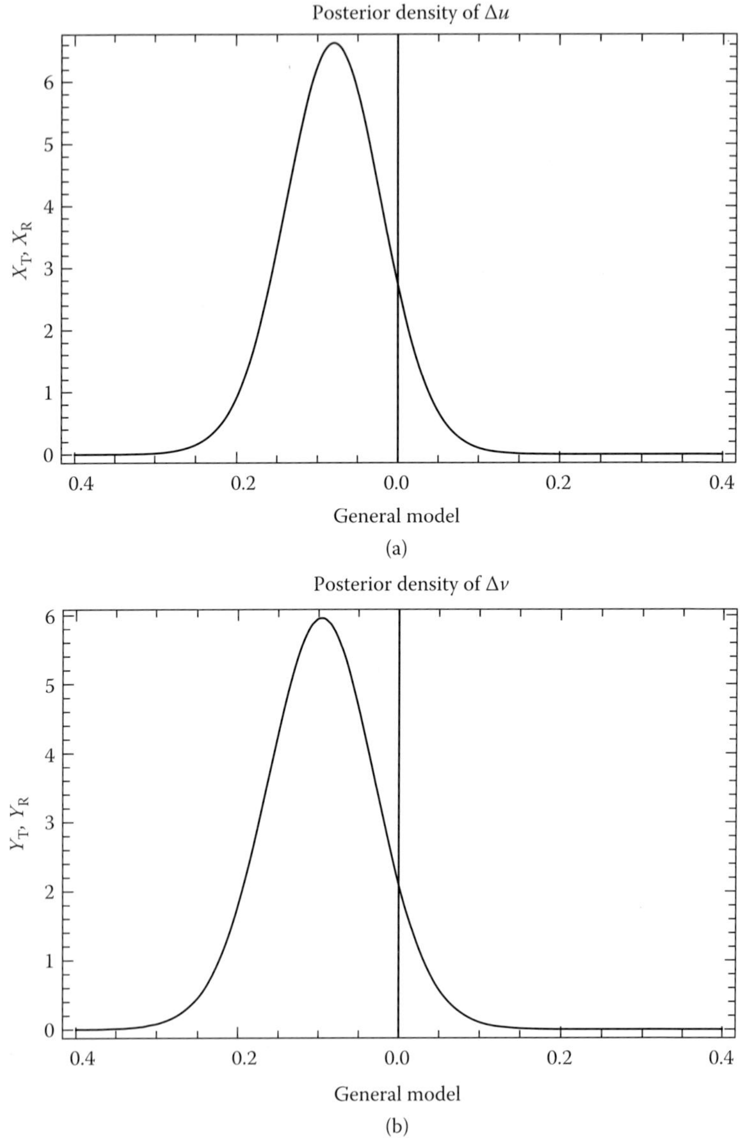


**FIGURE 8.2**

Posterior density of $\Delta u = u_T - u_R$ (ln(AUC) and $\Delta v = v_T - v_R$ (ln(Cmax) for S1. (a) S1—posterior density of $\Delta u$ (ln(AUC)). (b) S1—posterior density of $\Delta v$ (ln($C_{max}$)).

the respective ranges of $\Delta u$ and $\Delta v$. For example, 0.4789891, the $p$-value corresponding to $\Delta u = \ln(0.8)$ and $\Delta v = \ln(0.8936)$ is the largest of all $p$-values in the area of $\Delta u \leq \ln(0.8)$ and $\ln(0.8) < \Delta v < \ln(1.25)$. Based on these results, we conclude that BE can be declared with FWER controlled at $\alpha_F = 0.05$ for S1 for which all eight intersection null hypotheses are rejected at $\alpha = 0.05$. In

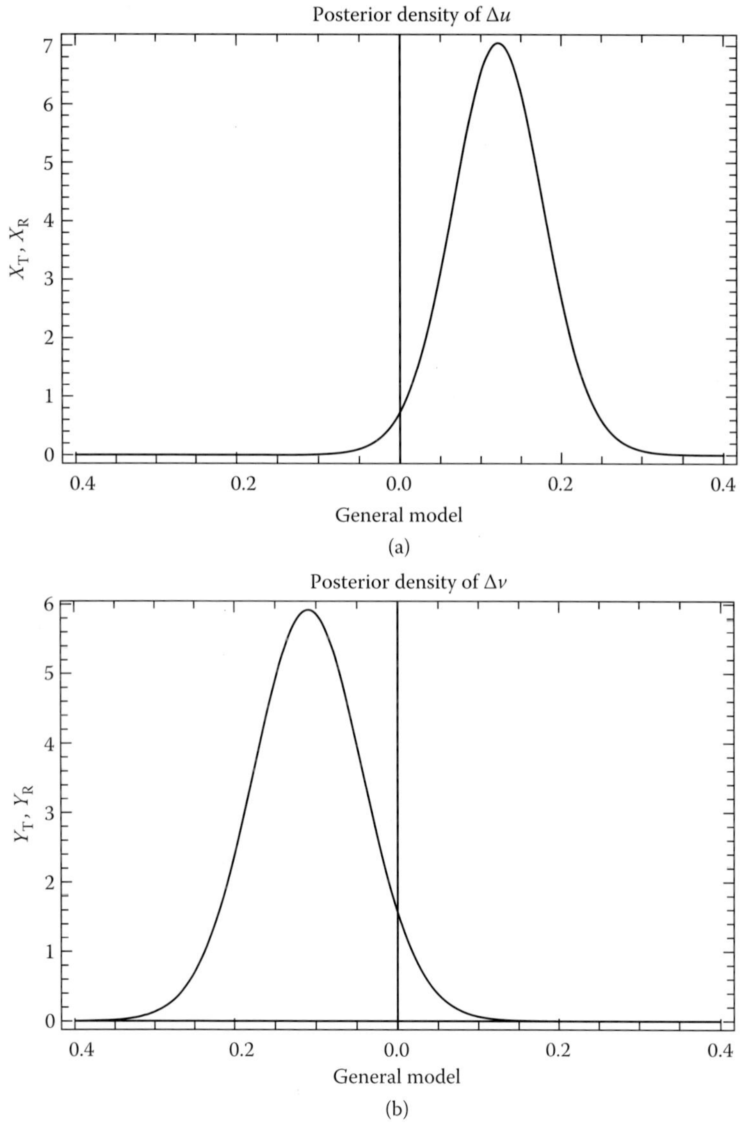


**FIGURE 8.3**

Posterior density of $\Delta u = u_T - u_R$ (ln(AUC) and $\Delta v = v_T - v_R$ (ln($C_{max}$)) for S2. (a) S2—Posterior density of $\Delta u$ (ln(AUC)). (b) S2—Posterior density of $\Delta v$ (ln($C_{max}$)).

S2, although equivalence is achieved at $\alpha = 0.05$ for each parameter, two of the eight intersection null hypotheses failed to be rejected at $\alpha = 0.05$. Hence, BE cannot be declared with FWER controlled at 0.05. A precision rate of $10^{-5}$ or higher was achieved in the calculation of these *p*-values by numerical integration.

**TABLE 8.2**

Probabilities of Rejecting Intersect Null Hypotheses with At Least One True Null Hypothesis

| | Scenario 1 | | Scenario 2 | |
|---|---|---|---|---|
| **Intersection** | **Probability of Rejecting Intersection Hypothesis** | **$\Delta u$ and $\Delta v$ Led to the Largest $p$-Value** | **Probability of Rejecting Intersection Hypothesis** | **$\Delta u$ and $\Delta v$ Led to the Largest $p$-Value** |
| $H_{A,01} \cap H_{C,a}$ | 0.04789891 | $\Delta u \le \ln(0.8)$, $\Delta v = \ln(0.8936)$ | 0.05244283 | $\Delta u \le \ln(0.8)$, $\Delta v = \ln(0.9098)$ |
| $H_{A,02} \cap H_{C,a}$ | 0.04790242 | $\Delta u \ge \ln(1.25)$, $\Delta v = \ln(1.12445)$ | 0.05243202 | $\Delta u \ge \ln(1.25)$, $\Delta v = \ln(1.09925)$ |
| $H_{A,a} \cap H_{C,01}$ | 0.04626713 | $\Delta u = \ln(0.89675)$, $\Delta v \le \ln(0.8)$ | 0.04637270 | $\Delta u = \ln(0.9188)$, $\Delta v \le \ln(0.8)$ |
| $H_{A,a} \cap H_{C,02}$ | 0.04627075 | $\Delta u = \ln(1.12085)$, $\Delta v \ge \ln(1.25)$ | 0.04636811 | $\Delta u = \ln(1.0844)$ $\Delta v \ge \ln(1.25)$ |
| $H_{A,01} \cap H_{C,01}$ | 0.02445466 | $\Delta u \le \ln(0.8)$, $\Delta v \le \ln(0.8)$ | 0.01965423 | $\Delta u \le \ln(0.8)$, $\Delta v \le \ln(0.8)$ |
| $H_{A,01} \cap H_{C,02}$ | $1.31893 \times 10^{-6}$ | $\Delta u \le \ln(0.8)$, $\Delta v \ge \ln(1.25)$ | $5.718305 \times 10^{-5}$ | $\Delta u \le \ln(0.8)$, $\Delta v \ge \ln(1.25)$ |
| $H_{A,02} \cap H_{C,01}$ | $1.380019 \times 10^{-6}$ | $\Delta u \ge \ln(1.25)$, $\Delta v \le \ln(0.8)$ | $5.582486 \times 10^{-5}$ | $\Delta u \ge \ln(1.25)$, $\Delta v \le \ln(0.8)$ |
| $H_{A,02} \cap H_{C,02}$ | 0.02443862 | $\Delta u \ge \ln(1.25)$, $\Delta v \ge \ln(1.25)$ | 0.01963947 | $\Delta u \ge \ln(1.25)$, $\Delta v \ge \ln(1.25)$ |
| Conclusion | FWER $\le$ 0.05 | | FWER > 0.05 | |

## 8.4 Alpha-Adaptive Sequential Testing Procedure Using Two One-Sided Test

In this section, we propose an AAST that controls FWER by prespecifying the significance level $\alpha_1$ for ln(AUC) in advance. The significance level $\alpha_2$ for ln($C_{max}$) is obtained adaptively after testing of ln(AUC). The following steps, which are also shown in Figure 8.4, give an outline.

Step 1: Prespecify a significance level $\alpha_1 < \alpha = 0.05$ to test $H_{A,01}$ and $H_{A,02}$ for ln(AUC). Let $p_{A,l}$, $p_{A,u}$ be the two $p$-values of TOST for ln(AUC), if both $H_{A,01}$ and $H_{A,02}$ are rejected with $p_A^{mx} = \max\{p_{A,l}, p_{A,u}\} \le \alpha_1$, then test $H_{C,01}$ and $H_{C,02}$ each at $\alpha$ for ln($C_{max}$). If both $H_{C,01}$ and $H_{C,02}$ are rejected at $\alpha$ for ln($C_{max}$), then BE is declared with FWER controlled at $\alpha$.

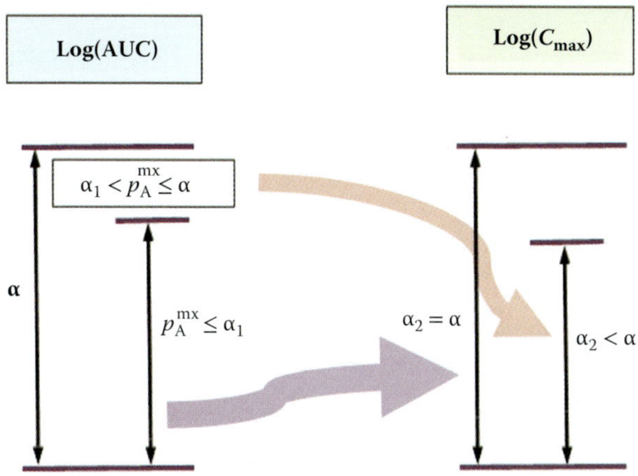


**FIGURE 8.4**
Alpha-adaptive sequential testing procedure.

Step 2. If $\alpha_1 \leq p_A^{mx} < \alpha$, then test $H_{C,01}$ and $H_{C,02}$ for $C_{max}$ at $\alpha_2 = f_2(g, p_A^{mx})$ as described in Equation 8.13. If the two $p$-values of TOST satisfy $p_C^{mx} = \max\{p_{C,I}, p_{C,II}\} \leq \alpha_2$, then BE can be declared with FWER controlled at $\alpha$.

When either parameter fails to meet the equivalence criteria, BE cannot usually be declared except for highly variable generic drug products for which widened equivalence margins such as (ln(0.7), ln(1/0.7 $\approx$ 1.43)) or the reference-scaled average BE (RSABE) approach might be considered acceptable [20,21]. When widened equivalence margins are considered, both closed test in Section 8.2 and AAST as described in Steps 1 and 2 are appropriate since the inference of BE can still be made by TOST, though the widened equivalence margins will need to be applied in all calculations. On the other hand, to achieve RSABE, the two drugs are considered bioequivalent if the 95% upper confidence bound for $(\mu_T - \mu_R)^2 - \theta_s \cdot \sigma_{WR}^2$ is $\leq 0$, in which $\mu$ is the population mean for ln(AUC) or ln($C_{max}$), $\sigma_{WR}^2$ is the population within-subject variance of the reference formulation and $\theta_s = (\ln(1.25))^2 / (0.25^2)$. The within-subject variability is determined using a partial replicate (three-way crossover: RTR, RRT, or TRR) or full replicate (four-way crossover: RTRT or TRTR) design. However, the decision to declare RSABE cannot be simply accomplished by TOST, and as a result, the two TOST-based methods proposed in this chapter may not be sufficient to address the multiplicity issues associated with RSABE.

The significant levels $\alpha, \alpha_1$, and $\alpha_2$ for the proposed AAST are related in the following probability equation:

$$\alpha - \alpha_1 = Pr\left[\left(t_{1-\alpha,v} < T_A^{mi} \leq t_{1-\alpha_1,v}\right), \left(t_{1-\alpha_2,v} < T_C^{mi}\right) | \text{null}\right] \tag{8.12}$$

in which

$$\alpha_2 = \begin{cases} \alpha & \text{if } 0 < p_A^{mx} < \alpha_1 \\ f_2\left(g, p_A^{mx}\right) = 1 - T^{-1}\left[t_{1-\alpha,v} + \dfrac{g - t_{1-\alpha,v}}{t_{1-\alpha_1,v} - t_{1-\alpha,v}}\left(t_{1-\alpha_1,v} - T_A^{mi}\right), v\right] & \text{if } \alpha_1 \le p_A^{mx} < \alpha \end{cases} \tag{8.13}$$

The "null" in Equation 8.12 consists of three distinctive scenarios: null hypotheses true for both ln(AUC) and ln($C_{max}$), null hypotheses true for ln(AUC) and false for ln($C_{max}$), and null hypotheses false for ln(AUC) and true for ln($C_{max}$). It can be expressed by the sets defined in Equations 8.3 and 8.4 as

$$\begin{aligned} \text{null} &= [(H_{A,01} \bigcup H_{A,02}) \bigcap (H_{C,01} \bigcup H_{C,02})] \bigcup [(H_{A,01} \bigcup H_{A,02}) \bigcap H_{C,a}] \bigcup [H_{A,a} \bigcap (H_{C,0} \bigcup H_{C,02})] \\ &= (H_{A,01} \bigcup H_{A,02}) \bigcup [H_{A,a} \bigcap (H_{C,01} \bigcup H_{C,02})] \\ &= [(H_{A,01} \bigcup H_{A,02}) \bigcap H_{C,a}] \bigcup (H_{C,01} \bigcup H_{C,02}) \end{aligned}$$

When $\alpha_2 \neq \alpha$, $\alpha_2$ in Equation 8.12 is a function of $g$ and $p_A^{mx}$ that $g$ can be solved by a numerical method, which will be discussed later, $\alpha_1 \le p_A^{mx} < \alpha$ is defined above while $t_{1-\alpha,v} < T_A^{mi} \le t_{1-\alpha_1,v}$ is its corresponding $t$-statistic. We further express $g$ in the form of $t$-statistic: $g = t_{1-w,v}$.

Under $t_{1-\alpha,v} < T_A^{mi} \le t_{1-\alpha_1,v}$, since $T_C^{mi} > t_{1-\alpha_2,v}$ is equivalent to

$$\frac{-\theta}{\hat{\sigma}_{\Delta\bar{Y}}} + t_{1-\alpha_2,v} < \frac{\Delta\bar{Y}}{\hat{\sigma}_{\Delta\bar{Y}}} < \frac{\theta}{\hat{\sigma}_{\Delta\bar{Y}}} - t_{1-\alpha_2,v} \tag{8.14}$$

we omit $v$ in $t$-critical values for simplicity and further express $\alpha - \alpha_1$ in Equation 8.12 as follows:
when $T_A^{mi} = T_{A,L}$, Equation 8.12 can be written as

$$\begin{aligned} \alpha - \alpha_1 &= \Pr\left[\left(\frac{-\theta}{\hat{\sigma}_{\Delta\bar{X}}} + t_{1-\alpha} < \frac{\Delta\bar{X}}{\hat{\sigma}_{\Delta\bar{X}}} \le \frac{-\theta}{\hat{\sigma}_{\Delta\bar{X}}} + t_{1-\alpha_1}\right), \left(\frac{-\theta}{\hat{\sigma}_{\Delta\bar{Y}}} + t_{1-\alpha_2} < \frac{\Delta\bar{Y}}{\hat{\sigma}_{\Delta\bar{Y}}} < \frac{\theta}{\hat{\sigma}_{\Delta\bar{Y}}} - t_{1-\alpha_2}\right)\right] \\ &= \Pr\left[\left(\frac{-\theta}{\hat{\sigma}_{\Delta\bar{X}}} + t_{1-\alpha} < T_A^* \le \frac{-\theta}{\hat{\sigma}_{\Delta\bar{X}}} + t_{1-\alpha_1}\right), \left(\frac{-\theta}{\hat{\sigma}_{\Delta\bar{Y}}} + t_{1-\alpha_2} < T_C^* < \frac{\theta}{\hat{\sigma}_{\Delta\bar{Y}}} - t_{1-\alpha_2}\right) \middle| \text{ null}\right] \end{aligned} \tag{8.15}$$

when $T_{\text{A}}^{\text{mi}} = T_{\text{A,u}}$, Equation 8.12 can be expressed as

$$\alpha - \alpha_1 = \Pr\left[\left(\frac{\theta}{\hat{\sigma}_{\Delta\bar{X}}} - t_{1-\alpha_1} < T_{\text{A}}^{*} \leq \frac{\theta}{\hat{\sigma}_{\Delta\bar{X}}} - t_{1-\alpha}\right), \left(\frac{-\theta}{\hat{\sigma}_{\Delta\bar{Y}}} + t_{1-\alpha_2} < T_{\text{C}}^{*} < \frac{\theta}{\hat{\sigma}_{\Delta\bar{Y}}} - t_{1-\alpha_2}\right) \middle| \text{null}\right] \tag{8.16}$$

According to Equation 8.10, the joint probability of $(T_{\text{A}}^{*}, T_{\text{C}}^{*})$ in Equations 8.15 and 8.16 follows a bivariate noncentral $t$-distribution with noncentrality parameters $\delta_{\text{A}}$ and $\delta_{\text{C}}$. We further denote if $a_1 = \frac{-\theta}{\hat{\sigma}_{\Delta\bar{X}}} + t_{1-\alpha}$, $a_2 = \frac{-\theta}{\hat{\sigma}_{\Delta\bar{X}}} + t_{1-\alpha_1}$, $b_1 = \frac{\theta}{\hat{\sigma}_{\Delta\bar{X}}} - t_{1-\alpha_1}$, $b_2 = \frac{\theta}{\hat{\sigma}_{\Delta\bar{X}}} - t_{1-\alpha}$, $c_1 = \frac{-\theta}{\hat{\sigma}_{\Delta\bar{Y}}} + t_{1-\alpha_2}$, and $c_2 = \frac{\theta}{\hat{\sigma}_{\Delta\bar{Y}}} - t_{1-\alpha_2}$, then Equation 8.15 can be written as

$$\begin{aligned}\alpha - \alpha_1 &= Pr\left[\left(a_1 < T_{\text{A}}^{*} \leq a_2\right),\quad \left(c_2 < T_{\text{C}}^{*} < c_2\right)\right] \\ &= \frac{1}{2^{\frac{v}{2}-1}\Gamma(\frac{v}{2})} \int_0^{\infty} x^{v-1} e^{-\frac{x^2}{2}} \Phi_2\left(\frac{\boldsymbol{a}\cdot x}{\sqrt{\text{v}}} - \delta_{\text{A}},\ \frac{\boldsymbol{c}\cdot x}{\sqrt{\text{v}}} - \delta_{\text{C}}; \rho_{\text{AC}}\right) \text{d}x\end{aligned} \tag{8.17}$$

in which $\Phi_2\left(\frac{\boldsymbol{a}\cdot x}{\sqrt{\text{v}}} - \delta_{\text{A}},\ \frac{c\cdot x}{\sqrt{\text{v}}}\ \delta_{\text{C}}, \rho_{\text{AC}}\right)$ is a bivariate normal integral, $\boldsymbol{a} = \begin{pmatrix} a_2 \\ a_1 \end{pmatrix}$, $\boldsymbol{c} = \begin{pmatrix} c_2 \\ c_1 \end{pmatrix}$, and $\rho_{\text{AC}}$ is the correlation between $T_{\text{A}}^{*}$ and $T_{\text{C}}^{*}$. We express this bivariate normal integral as a conditional density function so that $\alpha_2$ is conditional on $p_{\text{A}}^{\text{mx}}$.

$$\begin{aligned}\Phi_2\left(\frac{\boldsymbol{a}\cdot x}{\sqrt{\text{v}}} - \delta_{\text{A}},\ \frac{c\cdot x}{\sqrt{\text{v}}} - \delta_{\text{C}}; \rho_{\text{AC}}\right) &= \frac{1}{2\pi\sqrt{(1-\rho_{\text{AC}}^2)}} \int_{\frac{a_1\cdot x}{\sqrt{\text{v}}}-\delta_{\text{A}}}^{\frac{a_2\cdot x}{\sqrt{\text{v}}}-\delta_{\text{A}}} \int_{\frac{c_1\cdot x}{\sqrt{\text{v}}}-\delta_{\text{C}}}^{\frac{c_2\cdot x}{\sqrt{\text{v}}}-\delta_{\text{C}}} \phi(t_{\text{A}}, t_{\text{C}}) \text{d}t_{\text{C}} \text{d}t_{\text{A}} \\ &= \frac{1}{2\pi\sqrt{(1-\rho_{\text{AC}}^2)}} \int_{\frac{a_1\cdot x}{\sqrt{\text{v}}}-\delta_{\text{A}}}^{\frac{a_2\cdot x}{\sqrt{\text{v}}}-\delta_{\text{A}}} \int_{\frac{c_1\cdot x}{\sqrt{\text{v}}}-\delta_{\text{C}}}^{\frac{c_2\cdot x}{\sqrt{\text{v}}}-\delta_{\text{C}}} \phi(t_{\text{C}} \mid t_{\text{A}}) \phi(t_{\text{A}}) \text{d}t_{\text{C}} \text{d}t_{\text{A}}\end{aligned}$$

$$= \frac{1}{2\pi\sqrt{(1-\rho_{AC}^2)}} \int_{\frac{a_1 \cdot x}{\sqrt{v}}-\delta_A}^{\frac{a_2 \cdot x}{\sqrt{v}}-\delta_A} \exp\left(-\frac{t_A^2}{2}\right) \int_{\frac{c_1 \cdot x}{\sqrt{v}}-\delta_C}^{\frac{c_2 \cdot x}{\sqrt{v}}-\delta_C} \exp\left[-\frac{(t_C - \rho_{AC} \cdot t_A)^2}{2(1-\rho_{AC}^2)}\right] dt_C dt_A \quad (8.18)$$

Hence, by applying Equations 8.17 and 8.18, the probability in Equation 8.15 can be written as

$$\alpha - \alpha_1 = \frac{1}{2^{\frac{v}{2}-1}\Gamma(\frac{v}{2})} \int_0^{\infty} x^{v-1} e^{-\frac{x^2}{2}} \Phi_2\left(\frac{\boldsymbol{a} \cdot x}{\sqrt{v}} - \delta_A, \frac{\boldsymbol{c} \cdot x}{\sqrt{v}} - \delta_C; \rho_{AC}\right) dx \quad (8.19)$$

$$\Phi_2\left(\frac{\boldsymbol{a} \cdot x}{\sqrt{v}} - \delta_A, \frac{c \cdot x}{\sqrt{v}} - \delta_C; \rho_{AC}\right)$$

$$= \frac{1}{2\pi\sqrt{(1-\rho_{AC}^2)}} \int_{\frac{a_1 \cdot x}{\sqrt{v}}-\delta_A}^{\frac{a_2 \cdot x}{\sqrt{v}}-\delta_A} \exp\left(\frac{-t_A^2}{2}\right) \int_{\frac{c_1 \cdot x}{\sqrt{v}}-\delta_C}^{\frac{c_2 \cdot x}{\sqrt{v}}-\delta_C} \exp\left[\frac{-(t_C - \rho_{AC} \cdot t_A)^2}{2(1-\rho_{AC}^2)}\right] dt_C dt_A$$

By analogy, the probability in Equation 8.16 can be written as follows:

$$\alpha - \alpha_1 = Pr\left[\left(b_1 < T_A^* \le b_2\right) \cap \left(c_2 < T_C^* < c_2\right)\right]$$
$$= \frac{1}{2^{\frac{v}{2}-1}\Gamma(\frac{v}{2})} \int_0^{\infty} x^{v-1} e^{-\frac{x^2}{2}} \Phi_2\left(\frac{\boldsymbol{b} \cdot x}{\sqrt{v}} - \delta_A, \frac{\boldsymbol{c} \cdot x}{\sqrt{v}} - \delta_C; \rho_{AC}\right) dx \quad (8.20)$$

$$\Phi_2\left(\frac{\boldsymbol{b} \cdot x}{\sqrt{v}} - \delta_A, \frac{\boldsymbol{c} \cdot x}{\sqrt{v}} - \delta_C; \rho_{AC}\right)$$

$$= \frac{1}{2\pi\sqrt{(1-\rho_{AC}^2)}} \int_{\frac{b_1 \cdot x}{\sqrt{v}}-\delta_A}^{\frac{b_2 \cdot x}{\sqrt{v}}-\delta_A} \exp\left(\frac{-t_A^2}{2}\right) \int_{\frac{c_1 \cdot x}{\sqrt{v}}-\delta_C}^{\frac{c_2 \cdot x}{\sqrt{v}}-\delta_C} \exp\left[\frac{-(t_C - \rho_{AC} \cdot t_A)^2}{2(1-\rho_{AC}^2)}\right] dt_C dt_A$$

Therefore, numerical methods can be applied leading to the determination of $\alpha_2$. For example, when $t_{1-\alpha,v} < T_A^{mi} \le t_{1-\alpha_1,v} (\alpha_1 \le p_A^{mx} < \alpha)$, by replacing $\alpha_2$ with $f_2\left(g, p_A^{mx}\right)$ in both $c_1$ and $c_2$ in Equations 8.19 or 8.20, one can solve $g$ iteratively by a numerical procedure like SAS PROC IML.

To illustrate this method, we consider a crossover BE study of two drugs with $n = 60$ or degrees of freedom $v = 59$. The observed difference in mean ln(AUC) is $\Delta\bar{X} = 0.0583$ (approximately $\ln(1.06)) = 0.3217/\sqrt{60}$ $\hat{\sigma}_{\Delta\bar{X}}$ and we assume $T_A^{mi} = T_{A,l}$. We assume $\hat{\sigma}_{\Delta\bar{Y}} = 0.2879/\sqrt{60}$ in regard to $\ln(C_{max})$. Since the calculation of $\alpha_2$ requires a set of true null hypotheses, we choose $(H_{A,a1} \cap H_{A,a2}) \cap (H_{C,01} \cup H_{C,02})$ and set $\Delta u = \ln(1.06)$ and $\Delta v \le -\theta = \ln(0.8)$. According to Equation 8.13, the value $g$ in the function $\alpha_2 = f_2\left(g, p_A^{mx}\right)$ needs to be determined prior to obtaining $\alpha_2$. To do so, let $\alpha_1 = 0.040 - 0.048$ and $\rho_{AC} = 0.5 - 0.9$, then we obtain $g$ values by iteratively solving Equation 8.19, and the results are shown in Table 8.3. Figure 8.5 shows the relationship of $\alpha_2$ for $\ln(C_{max})$ and $p$-values of ln(AUC) or $p_A^{mx}$, for the case where $n = 60$, $v = 59$,

**TABLE 8.3**

Values of $g$ and $w$ Obtained from Equation 8.19 by Varying $\alpha_1 = 0.040 - 0.048$ and $\rho_{AC} = 0.5 - 0.9$

| | g (w) | | | | |
|---|---|---|---|---|---|
| | AC | | | | |
| 1 | 0.5 | 0.6 | 0.7 | 0.8 | 0.9 |
| 0.040 | 1.895737 (0.031448) | 1.882312(0.032364) | 1.872539 (0.033045) | 1.869149 (0.033284) | 1.877957 (0.032666) |
| 0.041 | 1.873849 (0.032953) | 1.862025 (0.033791) | 1.853491 (0.034407) | 1.850706 (0.034610) | 1.858712 (0.0340290) |
| 0.042 | 1.851802 (0.034530) | 1.841505 (0.035288) | 1.834164 (0.035837) | 1.831909 (0.036007) | 1.83907 (0.0354691) |
| 0.043 | 1.829611 (0.036181) | 1.820796 (0.036855) | 1.814562 (0.037338) | 1.812780 (0.037477) | 1.819071 (0.0369881) |
| 0.044 | 1.807291 (0.037908) | 1.799886 (0.038496) | 1.794716 (0.038911) | 1.793340 (0.0390221) | 1.7987357 (0.038588) |
| 0.045 | 1.784842 (0.039714) | 1.778802 (0.040212) | 1.774630 (0.040559) | 1.773589 (0.040646) | 1.778091 (0.040271) |
| 0.046 | 1.762278 (0.041601) | 1.757558 (0.042005) | 1.754321 (0.042284) | 1.753580 (0.042348) | 1.757174 (0.042038) |
| 0.047 | 1.739623 (0.043570) | 1.736145 (0.043879) | 1.733793 (0.044089) | 1.733301 (0.044133) | 1.735988 (0.043893) |
| 0.048 | 1.716864 (0.045625) | 1.714597 (0.045834) | 1.713073 (0.045975) | 1.712781 (0.046002) | 1.714570 (0.0458365) |

*Note:* Data source: a crossover study with $n = 60$, $\hat{\sigma}_{\Delta\bar{X}} = 0.2879/\sqrt{60}$, $\hat{\sigma}_{\Delta\bar{Y}} = 0.3217/\sqrt{60}$, degrees of freedom (df) $v = 59$ and assume $T_A^{mi} = T_{A,l}$, $\Delta u = \ln(1.06)$, and $\Delta v = \ln(0.8)$.

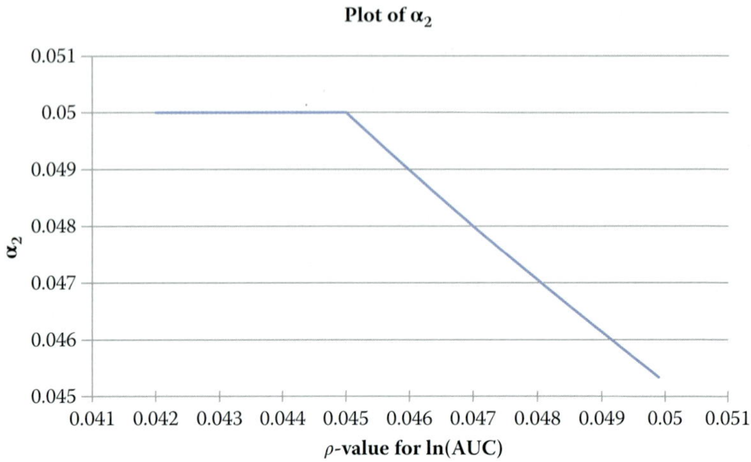


**FIGURE 8.5**
Plot of type I error rate ($\alpha_2$) for ln($C_{max}$) versus $p$-values of ln(AUC).

$\alpha = 0.05$, $\alpha_1 = 0.045$, and $g = 1.773589$ (the entry in Table 8.3 with $\alpha_1 = 0.045$ and $\rho_{AC} = 0.8$). For example, when $p_A^{mx} = 0.046$, by applying $g$ and $p_A^{mx}$ to Equation 8.13, we have $\alpha_2 = 0.0489836$.

It is quite obvious that BE can be declared for S1 in Section 8.3 with FWER controlled by AAST. For S2, only if $\alpha_1$ were prespecified at $\alpha_1 \geq 0.045$, then $\alpha_2 = 0.05$ since $p_A^{mx} = 0.0442$ is $< \alpha_1$, and BE would be declared with FWER controlled at $\alpha = 0.05$. By maintaining a sizable value in $\alpha_1$, it may prevent $\alpha_2$ from adaptation. For example, if $\alpha_1 = 0.043$, assuming $\Delta u = \ln(1.1456)$ (observed value), since $\alpha_1 < p_A^{mx} = 0.0442 < \alpha$, it results in $\alpha_2 = 0.047864$ under $\Delta v = \ln(0.8)$ or $\alpha_2 = 0.047996$ under $\Delta v = \ln(1.25)$. In either case, FWER is not controlled at $\alpha = 0.05$ since $p_C^{mx} = 0.0492 > \alpha_2$. Whether $\Delta v$ should be ln(0.8) or ln(1.25) depends on how close is $\Delta v$ to $\Delta \bar{Y}$ (observed).

## 8.5 Control of Family-Wise Error Rate in Alpha-Adaptive Sequential Procedure

In this section, we show the alpha-adaptive sequential approach controls FWER. We first define the following single and union sets to describe BE hypotheses, then calculate probabilities of false rejection of null hypotheses for either or both ln(AUC) and ln($C_{max}$) when null hypotheses are true for one or both parameters.

$$R_{11} = [T_A^{mi} = \min(T_{A,l}, T_{A,u}) > t_{1-\alpha_1}],\ R_{12} = [t_{1-\alpha,v} < T_A^{mi} \leq t_{1-\alpha_1}]$$

$$R_{21} = [T_C^{mi} = \min(T_{C,l}, T_{C,u}) > t_{1-\alpha}],\ R_{22} = [t_{1-\alpha_2} < T_C^{mi}]$$

$A_1 = R_{11} \bigcap R_{21}$ [$H_{01}$ and $H_{02}$ are rejected for ln(AUC) at $\alpha_1$ and rejected for ln($C_{\max}$) at $\leq \alpha$]

$A_2 = R_{11} \bigcap \bar{R}_{21}$ [$H_{01}$ and $H_{02}$ are rejected for ln(AUC) at $\alpha_1$ and failed to be rejected for ln($C_{\max}$) at $\leq \alpha$]

$A_3 = R_{12} \bigcap R_{22}$ [$H_{01}$ and $H_{02}$ are rejected for ln(AUC) at $\alpha^* \in [\alpha_1, \alpha)$ and rejected for ln($C_{\max}$) at $\alpha_2$].

### 8.5.1 Null Hypotheses Are True for Both ln(AUC) and ln($C_{max}$)

In this case, the null hypothesis is $\text{null}_1 = (H_{A,01} \bigcup H_{A,02}) \bigcap (H_{C,01} \bigcup H_{C,02})$. The probability of falsely rejecting the null hypothesis for either or both ln (AUC) and ln($C_{\max}$), which is the probability of the union of $A_1$, $A_2$, and $A_3$, is as follows:

$$\begin{aligned}\Pr(A_1 \bigcup A_2 \bigcup A_3 \mid \text{null}_1) &= \Pr[R_{11} \bigcup (R_{12} \bigcap R_{22}) \mid \text{null}_1] \\ &= \Pr(R_{11} \mid \text{null}_1) + \Pr(R_{12} \bigcap R_{22} \mid \text{null}_1)\end{aligned} \tag{8.21}$$

According to Equation 8.12, we have Pr

$$(R_{12} \bigcap R_{22} \mid \text{null}_1) = Pr\left[\left(t_{1-\alpha} < T_A^{\text{mi}} \leq t_{1-\alpha_1}\right), \left(t_{1-\alpha_2} < T_C^{\text{mi}}\right) \mid \text{null}_1\right] \leq \alpha - \alpha_1.$$

But for

$$\Pr(R_{11} \mid \text{null}_1) = \Pr\left(\frac{-\theta - \Delta u}{\hat{\sigma}_{\Delta\bar{X}}} + t_{1-\alpha_1} < T_A = \frac{\Delta\bar{X} - \Delta u}{\hat{\sigma}_{\Delta\bar{X}}} < \frac{\theta - \Delta u}{\hat{\sigma}_{\Delta\bar{X}}} - t_{1-\alpha_1} \mid \text{null}_1\right)\begin{pmatrix} a_1 & & 0 \\ & \ddots & \\ 0 & & a_n \end{pmatrix}$$

$$\leq \Pr\left(\frac{-\theta - \Delta u}{\hat{\sigma}_{\Delta\bar{X}}} + t_{1-\alpha_1} < T_A = \frac{\Delta\bar{X} - \Delta u}{\hat{\sigma}_{\Delta\bar{X}}} < \frac{\theta - \Delta u}{\hat{\sigma}_{\Delta\bar{X}}} - t_{1-\alpha_1} \mid (H_{A,01} \bigcup H_{A,02})\right)$$

if $H_{A,01}$ for ln(AUC) is true, then $\Delta u \leq -\theta$, so $T_A > t_{1-\alpha_1}$ or $\Pr(R_{11} \mid \text{null}) < \alpha_1$ holds. If $H_{A,02}$ is true, then $\Delta u \geq \theta$, so we have $T_A < -t_{1-\alpha_1}$ or $\Pr(R_{11} \mid \text{null}) < \alpha_1$. As a result, we have

$$\Pr(A_1 \bigcup A_2 \bigcup A_3 \mid \text{null}_1) = \Pr(R_{11} \mid \text{null}_1) + \Pr(R_{12} \bigcap R_{22} \mid \text{null}_1) < \alpha_1 + (\alpha - \alpha_1) = \alpha \tag{8.22}$$

### 8.5.2 Null Hypotheses Are True for ln(AUC) but False for ln($C_{max}$)

In this case, the true null hypotheses can be expressed as: $\text{null}_2 = (H_{A,01} \bigcup H_{A,02}) \bigcap H_{C,a}$, the probability of false rejection of ln(AUC) is

$$\Pr(R_{11} \mid \text{null}_2) + \Pr(R_{12} \bigcap R_{22} \mid \text{null}_2) \leq \alpha_1 + (\alpha - \alpha_1) = \alpha \tag{8.23}$$

### 8.5.3 Null Hypotheses Are False for ln(AUC) but True for ln($C_{max}$)

In this case, the true null hypotheses can be presented as: $\text{null}_3 = H_{A,a} \cap (H_{C,01} \cup H_{C,02})$, and the probability of false rejection of ln($C_{max}$) is

$$\Pr(A_1 \cup A_3 \mid \text{null}_3) = \Pr[(R_{11} \cap R_{21}) \cup (R_{12} \cap R_{22}) \mid \text{null}_3]$$
$$\leq \Pr(R_{11} \cap R_{21} \mid \text{null}_3) + \Pr(R_{12} \cap R_{22} \mid \text{null}_3)$$

We know from Equation 8.12 that $\Pr(R_{12} \cap R_{22} \mid \text{null}_3) \leq \alpha - \alpha_1$, since

$$\Pr(R_{11} \cap R_{21} \mid \text{null}_3) = \Pr\left[\left(t_{1-\alpha_1} < T_A^{mi}\right), \left(t_{1-\alpha} < T_C^{mi}\right) \mid \text{null}_3\right]$$
$$\leq \Pr[\left(t_{1-\alpha_1} < T_A^{mi}\right)] = \alpha_1 \tag{8.24}$$

hence we have $\Pr(A_1 \cup A_3 \mid \text{null}_3) \leq \alpha$.

## 8.6 Power Calculation

The power is essentially the probability of rejecting the null hypotheses when $H_{A,a}$ and $H_{C,a}$ are true. Power functions for the closed test procedure and alpha-adaptive sequential approach for the desired type I and type II error rates α and β can be characterized in three categories:

1. Reject $H_{01}$ and $H_{02}$ for ln(AUC) at α and for ln($C_{max}$) at α

$$1-\beta = Pr\left[\left(t_{1-\alpha} < T_A^{mi}\right) \cap \left(t_{1-\alpha} < T_C^{mi}\right) \mid \{-\theta \leq \Delta u \leq \theta\} \cap \{-\theta \leq \Delta v \leq \theta\}\right]$$
$$= \Pr\left[\left(\frac{-\theta}{\hat{\sigma}_{\Delta \bar{X}}} + t_{1-\alpha} < T_A^* \leq \frac{\theta}{\hat{\sigma}_{\Delta \bar{X}}} - t_{1-\alpha}\right) \cap \left(\frac{-\theta}{\hat{\sigma}_{\Delta \bar{Y}}} + t_{1-\alpha} < T_C^* < \frac{\theta}{\hat{\sigma}_{\Delta \bar{Y}}} - t_{1-\alpha}\right) \mid \{-\theta \leq \Delta u \leq \theta\} \cap \{-\theta \leq \Delta v \leq \theta\}\right] \tag{8.25}$$

2. Reject $H_{01}$ and $H_{02}$ for ln(AUC) at $\alpha_1$ and for ln($C_{max}$) at α

$$1-\beta = Pr\left[\left(t_{1-\alpha_1} < T_A^{mi}\right) \cap \left(t_{1-\alpha} < T_C^{mi}\right) \mid \{-\theta \leq \Delta u \leq \theta\} \cap \{-\theta \leq \Delta v \leq \theta\}\right]$$
$$= \Pr\left[\left(\frac{-\theta}{\hat{\sigma}_{\Delta \bar{X}}} + t_{1-\alpha_1} < T_A^* \leq \frac{\theta}{\hat{\sigma}_{\Delta \bar{X}}} - t_{1-\alpha_1}\right) \cap \left(\frac{-\theta}{\hat{\sigma}_{\Delta \bar{Y}}} + t_{1-\alpha} < T_C^* < \frac{\theta}{\hat{\sigma}_{\Delta \bar{Y}}} - t_{1-\alpha}\right) \mid \{-\theta \leq \Delta u \leq \theta\} \cap \{-\theta \leq \Delta v \leq \theta\}\right] \tag{8.26}$$

3. Reject $H_{01}$ and $H_{02}$ for ln(AUC) with $p_A^{mx} \in [\alpha_1, \alpha)$ and for ln($C_{max}$) at $\alpha_2$

$$1-\beta = Pr\left[\left(t_{1-\alpha} < T_A^{mi} \leq t_{1-\alpha_1}\right) \cap \left(t_{1-\alpha_2} < T_C^{mi}\right) \mid \{-\theta \leq \Delta u \leq \theta\} \cap \{-\theta \leq \Delta v \leq \theta\}\right]$$

when $T_A^{mi} = T_{A,l}$, we have

$$1-\beta = \Pr\left[\begin{array}{l}\left(\frac{-\theta}{\hat{\sigma}_{\Delta\bar{X}}} + t_{1-\alpha} < T_A^* \le \frac{-\theta}{\hat{\sigma}_{\Delta\bar{X}}} + t_{1-\alpha_1}\right), \left(\frac{-\theta}{\hat{\sigma}_{\Delta\bar{Y}}} + t_{1-\alpha_2} < T_C^* < \frac{\theta}{\hat{\sigma}_{\Delta\bar{Y}}} - t_{1-\alpha_2}\right) | \\ \{-\theta \le \Delta u \le \theta\} \cap \{-\theta \le \Delta v \le \theta\}\end{array}\right]$$

when $T_A^{mi} = T_{A,u}$, then

$$1-\beta = \Pr\left[\begin{array}{l}\left(\frac{\theta}{\hat{\sigma}_{\Delta\bar{X}}} - t_{1-\alpha_1} < T_A^* \le \frac{\theta}{\hat{\sigma}_{\Delta\bar{X}}} - t_{1-\alpha}\right), \left(\frac{-\theta}{\hat{\sigma}_{\Delta\bar{Y}}} + t_{1-\alpha_2} < T_C^* < \frac{\theta}{\hat{\sigma}_{\Delta\bar{Y}}} - t_{1-\alpha_2}\right) | \\ \{-\theta \le \Delta u \le \theta\} \cap \{-\theta \le \Delta v \le \theta\end{array}\right] \quad (8.27)$$

According to Equation 8.10, the joint probability of $(T_A^*, T_C^*)$ follows a bivariate noncentral $t$-distribution with noncentrality parameters $\delta_A$ and $\delta_C$ with correlation coefficient $\rho_{AC}$ defined in Section 8.2. These powers can be calculated numerically by R package "mvtnorm" available in CRAN. Table 8.4 shows the power calculations based on Equation 8.25 for a crossover design, in which $n = 24$, $\alpha = 0.05$, $\hat{\sigma}_{\Delta\bar{X}} = \frac{0.288}{\sqrt{24}}$, $\hat{\sigma}_{\Delta\bar{Y}} = \frac{0.322}{\sqrt{24}}$, $\rho_{AC} = (0.5, 0.7, 0.9)$, $\Delta u$ and $\Delta v$ vary from ln(0.85) to ln(1.25). Also based on Equation 8.25, the post hoc power is around 55.8% for S1 when using the observed differences $\Delta\bar{X} = \ln(0.9238)$, $\Delta\bar{Y} = \ln(0.9102)$ for the expected values $\Delta u$ and $\Delta v$; and 16.75% for S2 when $\Delta\bar{X} = \ln(1.1456)$, $\Delta\bar{Y} = \ln(0.8957)$ are used for $\Delta u$ and $\Delta v$. These power values are relatively low because of the use of observed differences for expected differences (usually unobservable). For study planning, the expected values $\Delta u$ and $\Delta v$ are usually set to ln(0.95), ln(1.05), or other values. For example, the power for S1 would be about 74.6% when choosing $\Delta u = \Delta v = \ln(0.95)$ and $\hat{\rho}_{A,C} = 0.8076$; and power for S2 would be 75.5% and 59.9% corresponding to $(\Delta u = \ln(1.05), \Delta v = \ln(0.95))$ and $(\Delta u = \ln(1.1), \Delta v = \ln(0.95))$, respectively, with $\hat{\rho}_{A,C} = 0.6794$. Clearly, the low post hoc power for S2, resulting from inconsistent results between ln(AUC) and ln($C_{max}$), further explains why the FWER could not be controlled at 0.05 level for S2 based on the closed test procedure in Section 8.2. Note that in Equation 8.27, $\alpha_2$ must be obtained from Equation 8.13 conditional on a $p$-value $p_A^{mx} \in [\alpha_1, \alpha)$ for ln(AUC), instead of an arbitrary value.

**TABLE 8.4**

Power Calculations Using Formula in Equation 8.25 for a Crossover Design, Where $n = 24$, $\alpha = 0.05$, $\hat{\sigma}_{\Delta\bar{X}} = \frac{0.288}{\sqrt{24}}$, $\hat{\sigma}_{\Delta\bar{Y}} = \frac{0.322}{\sqrt{24}}$, $\rho_{AC} = (0.5, 0.7, 0.9)$, $\Delta u$ and $\Delta v$ take the values from ln(0.85) to ln(1.25)

| | | Power (%) | | | | | | | | |
|---|---|---|---|---|---|---|---|---|---|---|
| | | $\Delta u$ | | | | | | | | |
| $\Delta v$ | $\rho$ | ln(0.85) | ln(0.9) | ln(0.95) | ln(1) | ln(1.05) | ln(1.1) | ln(1.15) | ln(1.2) | ln(1.25) |
| ln(0.85) | 0.5 | 11.2 | 19.9 | 23.4 | 22.0 | 16.6 | 9.5 | 3.9 | 1.2 | 0.21 |
| | 0.7 | 14.0 | 22.4 | 24.0 | 21.1 | 14.4 | 6.8 | 2.1 | 0.42 | 0.048 |
| | 0.9 | 17.8 | 24.6 | 24.2 | 20.3 | 11.7 | 3.8 | 0.7 | 0.05 | 0.0015 |
| ln(0.90) | 0.5 | 18.7 | 40.0 | 53.7 | 54.6 | 45.0 | 28.9 | 13.9 | 4.5 | 1.02 |
| | 0.7 | 20.5 | 43.7 | 56.1 | 54.8 | 43.4 | 25.9 | 10.8 | 2.7 | 0.44 |
| | 0.9 | 21.6 | 48.6 | 58.7 | 54.8 | 42.0 | 22.5 | 7.2 | 10.3 | 0.075 |
| ln(0.95) | 0.5 | 21.1 | 49.8 | 73.1 | 79.1 | 68.9 | 47.7 | 25.2 | 9.7 | 2.52 |
| | 0.7 | 21.3 | 51.2 | 75.1 | 80.1 | 68.7 | 46.5 | 23.4 | 7.85 | 1.68 |
| | 0.9 | 21.4 | 52.1 | 77.9 | 81.5 | 68.7 | 45.7 | 21.5 | 5.5 | 0.75 |
| ln(1.0) | 0.5 | 20.2 | 50.0 | 76.9 | 86.2 | 77.6 | 55.8 | 30.9 | 13.7 | 3.90 |
| | 0.7 | 19.8 | 50.0 | 77.3 | 87.2 | 78.2 | 55.8 | 30.6 | 12.8 | 3.35 |
| | 0.9 | 19.3 | 50.0 | 77.9 | 88.7 | 78.8 | 55.8 | 30.3 | 11.8 | 2.54 |
| ln(1.05) | 0.5 | 16.3 | 43.0 | 68.7 | 79.8 | 74.3 | 55.3 | 31.7 | 15.0 | 4.55 |
| | 0.7 | 14.6 | 41.7 | 68.6 | 80.9 | 76.2 | 56.8 | 32.2 | 15.2 | 4.41 |
| | 0.9 | 12.6 | 40.7 | 68.5 | 82.2 | 78.9 | 57.9 | 32.4 | 15.0 | 4.15 |
| ln(1.1) | 0.5 | 9.8 | 28.8 | 49.5 | 60.3 | 58.9 | 46.6 | 28.4 | 13.9 | 4.50 |
| | 0.7 | 7.3 | 25.9 | 48.1 | 60.7 | 61.4 | 50.1 | 30.7 | 15.2 | 4.73 |
| | 0.9 | 4.4 | 22.4 | 47.0 | 61.0 | 64.3 | 54.7 | 32.5 | 15.8 | 4.74 |
| ln(1.15) | 0.5 | 3.93 | 13.9 | 25.2 | 30.9 | 31.7 | 28.45 | 20.4 | 10.5 | 3.76 |
| | 0.7 | 2.13 | 10.8 | 23.4 | 30.6 | 32.2 | 30.7 | 23.8 | 12.8 | 4.46 |
| | 0.9 | 0.66 | 7.2 | 21.5 | 30.3 | 32.4 | 32.5 | 28.5 | 15.3 | 4.83 |
| ln(1.2) | 0.5 | 1.17 | 4.9 | 9.9 | 13.0 | 13.8 | 13.0 | 10.3 | 6.1 | 2.5 |
| | 0.7 | 0.44 | 3.1 | 8.4 | 12.5 | 13.8 | 13.8 | 12.2 | 8.0 | 3.4 |
| | 0.9 | 0.06 | 1.3 | 6.5 | 12.0 | 13.8 | 14.0 | 13.8 | 10.9 | 4.57 |
| ln(1.25) | 0.5 | 0.26 | 1.27 | 2.9 | 4.13 | 4.53 | 4.45 | 3.83 | 2.58 | 1.2 |
| | 0.7 | 0.06 | 0.61 | 2.16 | 3.78 | 4.48 | 4.60 | 4.40 | 3.50 | 1.9 |
| | 0.9 | 0.0016 | 0.135 | 1.2 | 3.26 | 4.40 | 4.62 | 4.63 | 4.47 | 3.05 |

## 8.7 Conclusions

Because BE is declared on the equivalence of two PK parameters that are correlated with each other, regardless of the means of rejecting the two one-sided null hypotheses or using 90% CIs, the need to account for multiplicity should not be ignored. It was demonstrated by Scenario 2 in Section 8.3

that FWER for the two parameters could exceed 0.05 even if the four one-sided null hypotheses for the two parameters are each rejected at $\alpha = 0.05$. The two scenarios in Section 8.3 suggest that by maintaining a consistency between the two parameters, it increases the chance of controlling FWER at $\alpha = 0.05$. The two proposed approaches serve different purposes. The closure test procedure is $p$-value based and controls FWER by rejecting eight nonempty null hypotheses. It does not require a prespecified significance level for each parameter and both parameters are equally important. AAST controls FWER by prespecifying $\alpha_1$ for ln(AUC) and then obtaining $\alpha_2$ for ln($C_{max}$) conditional on the result of AUC, although corresponding $p$-values are determined by the traditional TOST method. Both methods lead to the same conclusion on S1: in regard to S2, FWER is failed to be controlled by the closed test and controlled only by AAST if the prespecified $\alpha_1 \geq 0.045$ was considered. Such a discrepancy may be attributable to the fact that $p$-values $p_A^{mx}$ and $p_C^{mx}$ are barely below their respective significance levels. Nevertheless, the two proposed approaches offer a better alternative to a traditional method that controls FWER by using 95% two-sided CIs in BE assessment.

Both proposed methods are computationally intensive; the proposed closure test procedure relies on numerical integration based on a bivariate noncentral $t$-distribution for the calculation of $p$-values. For the alpha-adaptive sequential procedure, we showed that numerical integration based on a conditional bivariate normal density function can be used to calculate $\alpha_2$ for ln($C_{max}$), conditional on the $p$-values of ln(AUC). Numerical method is also provided for power calculations for both proposed methods. Sample programs used to perform all the calculations including R codes, SAS PROC IML program, and *Wolfram* Mathematica® 7 code are available from Steven Ye Hua.

Through simple modification of the equivalence margins, both methods can be applied to therapeutic equivalence trials where the equivalence of the two treatments is required at two different time points of the same parameter or on two efficacy endpoints. Both proposed methods can be applied to parallel and crossover designs.

## References

1. FDA, FDA Guidance for Industry Bioavailability and Bioequivalence Studies for Orally Administered Drug Products—General Considerations, 2003 (http://www.fda.gov/downloads/Drugs/GuidanceComplianceRegulatoryInformation/Guidances/ucm070124.pdf).
2. Schuirmann DJ, A comparison of the two one-sided tests procedure and the power approach for assessing the equivalence of average bioavailability. *Journal of Pharmacokinetics and Biopharmaceutics*, 1987, 15, 657–680.

3. Berger RL and Hsu JC, Bioequivalence trials, intersection-union tests and equivalence confidence sets (with discussion). *Statistical Science*, 1996, 11, 283–319.
4. CPMP, Points to consider on multiplicity issues in clinical trials. *Biometrical Journal*, 2001, 43, 1039–1048.
5. Lauzon C and Caffo B, Easy multiplicity control in equivalence testing using two one sided tests. *The American Statistician*, 2009, 63, 147–154.
6. Röhmel J, On familywise type I error control for multiplicity in equivalence trials with three or more treatments. *Biometrical Journal*, 2011, 53(6), 914–926.
7. Marcus R, Peritz E, and Gabriel KR, On closed testing procedures with special reference to ordered analysis of variance. *Biometrika*, 1976, 63, 655–660.
8. Hommel G, A stagewise rejective multiple test procedure based on modified Bonferroni test. *Biometrika*, 1988, 5, 383–386.
9. Sonnemann E and Allgemeine L, Sungen multipler Testprobleme. *EDV in Medizin und Biologie* 13, 120–128; translated into English 2008 by H. Finner: General solutions to multiple testing problems. *Biometrical Journal*, 1983, 50, 641–656.
10. Li J and Mehrotra D, An efficient method for accommodating potentially underpowered primary endpoints. *Statistics in Medicine*, 2008, 27, 5377–5391.
11. Alosh M and Huque MF, A consistency-adjusted alpha-adaptive strategy for sequential testing. *Statistics in Medicine*, 2010, 29(15), 1559–1571.
12. Li H, Sankoh AJ, and D'Agostino RB Sr., Extension of adaptive alpha allocation methods for strong control of the family-wise error rate. *Statistics in Medicine*, 2013, 32(2), 181–195.
13. Grechanovsky E and Hochberg Y, Closed procedures are better and often admit a shortcut. *Journal of Statistical Planning and Inference*, 1999, 76, 79–91.
14. Genz A and Bretz F, Numerical computation of multivariate t-probabilities with application to power calculation of multiple contrasts. *Journal of Statistical Computation and Simulation* 1999, 63, 361–378.
15. Genz A and Bretz F, Methods for the computation of multivariate t-probabilities. *Journal of Computational and Graphical Statistics*, 2002, 11, 950–971.
16. Hothorn T, Bretz F, and Genz A, On multivariate t and Gauss probabilities in R. *R News*, 2001, 1/2, 27–29.
17. Marzo A, Bo DL, Rusca A, and Zini P, Bioequivalence of ticlopidine hydrochloride administered in single dose to healthy volunteers. *Pharmacology Research* 2002, 46(5), 401–447.
18. Hua SY, Hawkins DL, and Zhou J, Statistical considerations in bioequivalence of two area under the concentration–time curves obtained from serial sampling data. *Journal of Applied Statistics*, 2013, 40, 5, 1140–1154.
19. Xu S, Hua SY, Menton R, Barker K, Menon S, and D'Agostino RB, Inference of bioequivalence for log-normal distributed data with unspecified variances. *Statistics in Medicine*, 2014, 33, 2924–2938.
20. Davit BM, Chen M-L, Conner DP, Haidar SH, Kim S, Lee CH, Lionberger RA, Makhlouf FT, Nwakam PE, Patel DT, Schuirmann DJ, and Yu LX, Implementation of a reference-scaled average bioequivalence approach for highly variable generic drug products by the US Food and Drug Administration. *AAPS Journal*, 2012, 14: 915–924.

21. FDA, FDA Draft Guidance for Industry, Bioequivalence Recommendations for Progesterone Oral Capsules. U.S. Department of Health and Human Services, Food and Drug Administration Center for Drug Evaluation and Research, Silver Spring, MD, 2011. Available at http://www.fda.gov/downloads/Drugs/GuidanceComplianceRegulatoryInformation/Guidances/UCM209294.pdf (Accessed on 20 June, 2016).

# 9

# *Bayesian Methods to Assess Bioequivalence and Biosimilarity with Case Studies*

**Steven Ye Hua, Siyan Xu, Kerry B. Barker, Shan Mei Liao, and Shujie Li**

**CONTENTS**



**ABSTRACT** In this chapter, we present two case studies using Bayesian methods. In the first case study, a Bayesian approach was taken to assess average bioequivalence and biosimilarity by conducting an interim analysis of a pharmacokinetic similarity trial to determine probability of success. The second case study describes derivation of a margin, which is used to demonstrate similarity of two versions of a biologic drug in a Phase 3 biosimilar clinical trial for the treatment of rheumatoid arthritis disease.

## 9.1 Introduction

There are two major paradigms in making statistical inference: *frequentist* (sometimes called classical or traditional) and *Bayesian*. In this chapter, we take a Bayesian approach to assess average bioequivalence (ABE) and biosimilarity (noted as *bios* in some equations of Section 9.2.4). As described in the finalized Food and Drug Administration (FDA) guidance,[1] biosimilar or biosimilarity means that "the biological product is highly similar to the reference product notwithstanding minor differences in clinically inactive components" and that "there are no clinically meaningful differences between the biological product and the reference product in terms of the safety, purity, and potency of the product."

The key advantage of using a Bayesian approach for ABE and biosimilar trials is the ability of the Bayesian inferential paradigm to generate a posterior probability distribution of the parameter of interest (e.g., δ: difference or ratio of two means), which is determined by the prior probability distribution of that parameter combined with a likelihood function (probability model for the observed data). In other words, it focuses on inference in δ changing from prior, through observed data (via likelihood function) to posterior (distribution), with the available prior information coherently incorporated into the statistical model. Also there is no need for a large sample size with a Bayesian approach.

According to the Bayesian paradigm, the unobservable parameters in a statistical model are treated as random variables. When no data are available, a *prior distribution* is used to quantify our knowledge about the parameter. When data are available, the prior knowledge can be updated using the conditional distribution of parameters. The transition from the prior to the posterior is possible via the Bayes theorem.

With the elements including the likelihood function: Likelihood = P(data|parameters) and a *prior* probability model for the parameters, P(parameters), Bayes theorem gives a prescription for posterior inference:

$$P(\text{parameters}|\text{data}) \propto \text{constant} * \text{Likelihood} * \text{prior}$$

While methods to establish ABE arose historically due to the development of the generic version of a small-molecule drug, their applications in seeking regulatory approval of generic copies of large-molecule drugs have drastically increased, which resulted in the rapid development of biologic drugs. Biologic drugs with their ability to treat many unmet and critical needs are frequently viewed as miracle drugs that can transform patients' lives and provide cure and treatment for diseases that would otherwise be labeled *hopeless*. But due to their high costs, many biologics are off-limits in areas and regions facing large, aging populations and increase in chronic diseases such as rheumatoid arthritis (RA) and cancer. These and other reasons (e.g., high revenue generation) make good cases for biopharmaceutical companies to develop generic copies of biologic drugs known as biosimilars.

Biosimilars must be *highly similar* to the reference drug. While there can be minor differences in clinically inactive components under U.S. law (Public Health Service [PHS] Act), there can be no *clinically meaningful differences* between the biosimilar and the reference drug in terms of safety, purity, and potency. Regulatory agencies including U.S. FDA, European Medicines Agency, and others support a stepwise approach in developing the evidence to support a demonstration of biosimilarity. Such approach requires similarities established in the chemistry, manufacturing, and controls (CMC) process, where the drug quality attributes are analytically measured and compared. Since a biosimilar relies on prior findings of efficacy and safety for the reference product, it has to demonstrate similarity to the reference product in head-to-head trials, including pharmacokinetic (PK) and comparative clinical trials.

The level of similarity required may differ from country to country and product to product, as such, the demonstration of similarity in various aspects of biosimilar drug development often posts challenging tasks to statistical applications, especially in a global clinical trial setting. Some of these tasks call for standardization in the assessment of drug quality attributes, variability, stability testing, methodology for PK/pharmacodynamics (PD) similarity, immunogenicity, establishing equivalence margins that exclude clinical meaningful differences, statistical study design, and biosimilar interchangeability. Without standards, it seems to leave drug makers to make their own cases on less desirable positions.

A literature review provided decades-long development in the applications of Bayesian paradigm on the topics of bioequivalence (BE); for example, Breslow[2] argued that BE is a perfectly natural concept to be subjected to Bayesian analysis. Several authors have also advocated a Bayesian approach to ABE inference.[3–7] The main idea of all the above methods is to find the posterior distribution of the parameter of interest based on noninformative prior distributions for the parameters. Ghosh and Khattree[8] used an intrinsic Bayes factor approach to test ABE. In recent articles by Xu et al.,[9,10] the authors present a Bayesian inference of ABE for log-normal distributed data with unspecified variances, as well as inference of equivalence for the ratio of two normal means with unspecified variances. Gubbiotti and Santis[11] derived two criteria based on Bayesian predictive approach to select optimal sample size in equivalence trials. We have found a few literatures applying Bayesian paradigm on biosimilars, which are relatively recent and evolving. Hsieh et al.[12] proposed a biosimilar index deriving on the basis of estimated reproducibility probability approach and Bayesian approach. Combest et al.[13] stated that in some cases, Bayesian method could result in 26%–29% reduction in sample sizes in clinical biosimilar trials compared to traditional approach. Bayesian mixed treatment comparison method were used to compare the efficacy and safety of infliximab biosimilar with other biological drugs (Baji et al.[14]). To be clear, although Bayesian approaches to facilitate design and analysis of biosimilar trials and data are evolving and appealing, they seem to have yet to be considered to be definitive approaches by regulatory authorities for biosimilar approvals. Among others, it requires more collaboration between industry and regulatory agencies, better understanding of Bayesian approaches, and accumulation of real-case trial applications to promote the use of Bayesian approaches in biosimilar approvals.

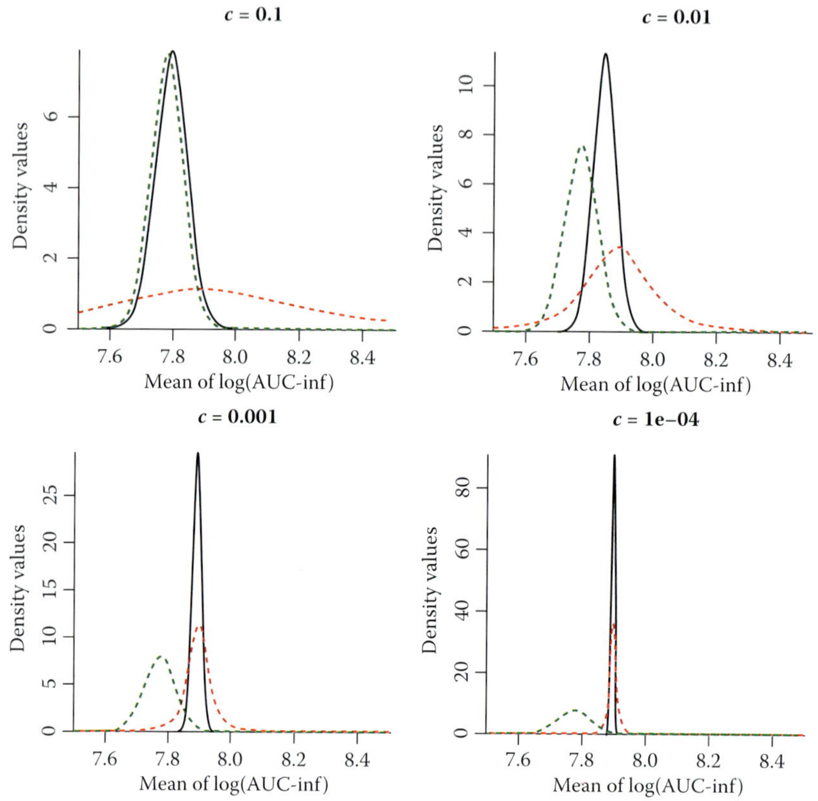


**FIGURE 9.1**
Comparison of prior, interim analysis (IA) data, and posterior distribution for different values of $c$ (a measure of the spread or variability of the prior mean value) for log(AUC-inf). Plot legend: dashed dotted line (green) represents the sample distribution of mean log(AUC-inf) at IA, solid line (black) represents the posterior distribution of $u$, and dashed line (red) denotes prior distribution of $u$.

The reason we choose the low-information prior also is that we have low beliefs in the Study A data and want to let Study B interim data *speak for itself.* On the other hand, a *high-information* case means we strongly believe that the prior is true and then the variability of the prior distribution becomes smaller, resulting in the posterior distribution being more influenced by the prior distribution than by the IA data.

The NIG prior is a conjugate prior that allows estimating the joint distribution of the posterior mean and precision of variance as shown in Figure 9.2.

Besides the conjugate prior as suggested above, we will also consider a nonconjugate prior that uses simulation-based techniques. The nonconjugate prior has a simpler form of the distribution; it can be used to compare with the results obtained by the conjugate prior, while the calculations to estimate posterior parameters can be implemented using the OpenBUGS package.

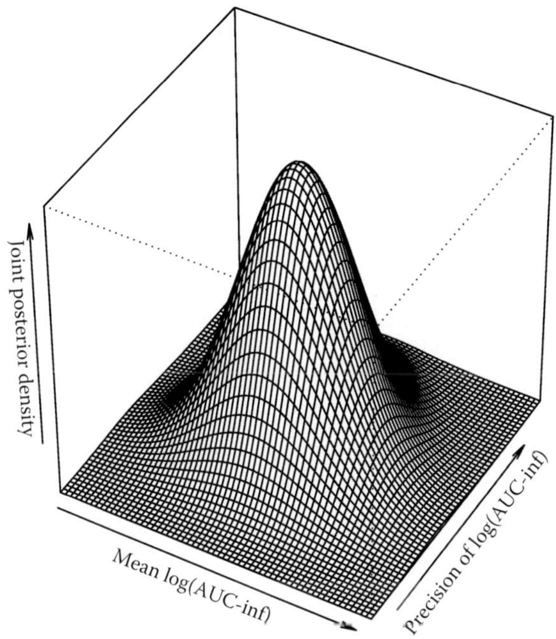


**FIGURE 9.2**
Joint posterior density of $u$ (expectation) and $\sigma^2$ ( precision) of log(AUC-inf).

The nonconjugate prior takes the following generic form for the $u$ (expectation) and $\sigma^2$ ( precision) of log(AUC-inf):

$$u \sim N(\mu_0, \sigma_0^2) \text{ and } \sigma^2 \sim \text{IG}(a_0, b_0)$$

where $N$ stands for normal distribution and IG stands for inverse-gamma distribution.

The nonconjugate prior uses an independent distribution for $u$ (expectation) and $\sigma^2$ (variance) rather than a correlated distribution function for $u$ and $\sigma^2$ used for a conjugate prior.

Technical details of the Bayesian analysis methods can be found in Ntzoufras[15] and Gelman et al.[16]

### 9.2.4 Simulate Datasets for Comparative Analysis

Once the posterior distribution of $u$ (expectation) and $\sigma^2$ (variance) of log(AUC-inf) for each of the three treatment groups are estimated based on the procedures described previously, we will simulate 10,000 sets of data (depending on the time needed to generate these data) with each set containing three treatment groups (biosimilar, innovator-EU, and innovator-US) as one simulated study. Each simulated dataset is the size of the Study B study (324 evaluable subjects or by addition 10% loss to reach $N = 360$). The PoS or percent of times that all the geometric mean ratios of biosimilar versus innovator-EU and biosimilar versus innovator-US and their 90% CIs for AUC-inf fall within (80%, 125%) will be calculated.

The following outlines the algorithm for the simulation and PoS.

1. For the biosimilar group,
   a. We will generate a pair of $(u_{bios},\sigma_{bios})$ from the posterior distribution of biosimilar: $f_{bios}$ $(u,\sigma|$Study A data and Study B IA data) as described in Section 9.2.3.
   b. For the pair of $(u_{bios},\sigma_{bios})$ in (a), we will generate log(AUC-inf) with a sample size of $n = 108$ from $N(u_{bios},\sigma_{bios})$.
2. For EU reference and US reference groups, we repeat (a) and (b) above similarly with corresponding parameters.
3. Combine $n = 108$ log(AUC-inf) samples from $N(u_{bios},\sigma_{bios})$ for biosimilar arm, $N(u_{EU},\sigma_{EU})$ for innovator-EU arm, and $N(u_{US},\sigma_{US})$ for innovator-US arm, respectively. This forms one simulated study.
4. For each simulated study, comparative PK analyses will be performed (using ratios and 90% CIs).
5. Repeat steps 1–4 M times (M = 10,000 times, depending on computing time).
6. PoS will be calculated. (PoS = proportion of the simulated studies meeting the BE criteria for AUC-inf for both biosimilar versus innovator-EU and biosimilar versus innovator-US groups.)

### 9.2.5 Go or No-Go Decision and Operating Characteristics

As discussed previously, one of the advantages of conducting an IA data is to allow an early determination of PoS for the final outcome. In this section, we illustrate in an example in Table 9.1, using simulated data, to describe some operating characteristics of a decision process. The percentages in Table 9.1 represent percentage of positive and/or negative results at both IA and final analyses. There are four possible pairs for IA and final outcomes: (+, –), (–, +), (+, +), and (–, –), with first and second signs indicating the outcome of the IA and final outcome in Study B, respectively. A positive outcome means the two drugs achieved BE, while a negative outcome means the two drugs failed to achieve BE. The probability of positive at IA, positive at final, and conditional probabilities such as false positive at IA and false negative at IA are also provided. These results were based on simulations assuming common coefficient of variance (CV, with values as 30%, 35%, and 40%) across all three treatment groups.

**TABLE 9.1**

Operating Characteristics of Go and No-Go Decision Rules

**CV = 30%**

| | Ratios[a] of AUC-inf between $u_{bios}$ and $u_{EU}$ | | | | |
|---|---|---|---|---|---|
| **Outcomes of IA and final** | **1.0** | **1.05** | **1.1** | **1.15** | **1.2** |
| (+, −) | 0% | 0% | 1% | 3% | 6% |
| (−, +) | 5% | 12% | 29% | 31% | 17% |
| (+, +) | 95% | 87% | 65% | 36% | 11% |
| (−, −) | 0% | 0% | 5% | 30% | 67% |
| Best scenario − worst scenario | **95%** (+, +) − (+, −) | **87%** (+, +) − (+, −) | **64%** (+, +) − (+, −) | **33%** (+, +) − (+, −) | **5%** (+, +) − (+, −) |
| *Overall probability* | | | | | |
| Positive at IA | 95% | 87% | 66% | 39% | 17% |
| Positive at final | 100% | 99% | 94% | 67% | 28% |
| *Conditional probability*[b] | | | | | |
| False positive at IA | 0% | 0% | 2% | 8% | 35% |
| False negative at IA | 100% | 98% | 85% | 51% | 20% |

**CV = 35%**

| | Ratios[a] of AUC-inf between $u_{bios}$ and $u_{EU}$ | | | | |
|---|---|---|---|---|---|
| **Outcomes of IA and final** | **1.0** | **1.05** | **1.1** | **1.15** | **1.2** |
| (+, −) | 0% | 0% | 1% | 5% | 6% |
| (−, +) | 14% | 22% | 32% | 29% | 13% |
| (+, +) | 86% | 76% | 55% | 26% | 9% |
| (−, −) | 0% | 2% | 12% | 40% | 72% |
| Best scenario − worst scenario | **86%** (+, +) − (−, −) | **76%** (+, +) − (−, −) | **54%** (+, +) − (−, −) | **21%** (+, +) − (−, −) | **3%** (−, −) − (−, +) |
| *Overall probability* | | | | | |
| Positive IA | 86% | 76% | 56% | 31% | 15% |
| Positive final | 100% | 98% | 87% | 55% | 22% |
| *Conditional probability*[b] | | | | | |
| False positive at IA | 0% | 0% | 2% | 16% | 40% |
| False negative at IA | 99% | 92% | 73% | 42% | 15% |

*(Continued)*

**TABLE 9.1** ***(Continued)***

Operating Characteristics of Go and No-Go Decision Rules

**CV = 40%**

| | **Ratios[a] of AUC-inf between $u_{bios}$ and $u_{EU}$** | | | | |
|---|---|---|---|---|---|
| **Outcomes of IA and final** | **1.0** | **1.05** | **1.1** | **1.15** | **1.2** |
| (+, −) | 0.1% | 1% | 3% | 5% | 4% |
| (−, +) | 26% | 31% | 34% | 26% | 12% |
| (+, +) | 73% | 65% | 44% | 22% | 8% |
| (−, −) | 0.7% | 4% | 19% | 47% | 76% |
| Best scenario − worst scenario | **73%** (+, +) − (−, −) | **64.4%** (+, +) − (−, −) | **41%** (+,+) − (−, −) | **21%** (+, +) − (−, −) | **4%** (−, −) − (−, +) |
| *Overall probability* | | | | | |
| Positive IA | 73% | 66% | 47% | 27% | 12% |
| Positive final | 99% | 96% | 78% | 48% | 20% |
| *Conditional probability[b]* | | | | | |
| False positive at IA | **0%** | 1% | 6% | 19% | 33% |
| False negative at IA | **97%** | 89% | 64% | 36% | 14% |

*Notes:* AUC-inf, area under the concentration–time curve infinity; CV, coefficient of variance; IA, interim analysis.

a *Assume the ratio between $u_{EU}$ and $u_{US}$ is 1. These ratios are assumed as true values for the entire study.*

b *Conditional probability of false positive at IA = (+, −)/[(+, −) + (+, +)]; conditional probability of false negative at IA = (−, +)/[(−, +) + (−, −)].*

**Color code:**

Go decision: probability >50%

Inconclusive: ≤10% probability ≤50%

No-go decision: probability <10%

Best scenario

Worst scenario

The decision criteria and level of decision are color-coded for differentiation. The decisions made based on the high probability of (+, +) are desirable. In a decision process, we also greatly value the high probabilities of "best scenario – worst scenario" with ((+, +) – (+, –)) to assure that a decision can be reached not only with a high probability of (+, +) but also with a low probability of (+, –). In reality, how well such a prediction is to be served also depends on the unobservable true ratio of the two treatment groups for the parameter of interest (e.g., AUC-inf). For example, when the true ratio is at 1.15, the value of ((+, +) – (+, –)) is only about 33%, which could lead to a risky decision. So when the observed ratio at IA is at ≥1.15, one suggestion is to accrue additional data and further evaluate before making a decision.

## 9.3 Case Study 2: Equivalence Margin to Demonstrate Equivalence in Efficacy of a Biosimilar Drug versus Innovative (Original) Biologic Drug for the Treatment of Rheumatoid Arthritis Disease

This case describes derivation of a margin, which is used to demonstrate similarity of two versions of a biologic drug in a Phase 3 biosimilar clinical trial for the treatment of RA disease: infliximab biosimilar versus infliximab (Ramicade®) EU. The primary efficacy endpoint is American College of Rheumatology 20% improvement (ACR20) response rates at 3 months after the initial treatment.

To help construct a margin to demonstrate similarity between infliximab-biosimilar and infliximab-EU, we identified and performed a meta-analysis of five historical randomized, placebo-controlled clinical trials of infliximab in subjects with active RA who had inadequate response to prior methotrexate

**TABLE 9.2**

Summary of Results of Five Randomized Clinical Trials of Infliximab

| Title/Reference | Brief Summary |
|---|---|
| Infliximab (chimeric antitumor necrosis factor alpha monoclonal antibody) versus placebo in RA patients receiving concomitant MTX: a randomized Phase 3 trial. ATTRACT Study Group[17] | Four hundred and twenty-eight patients with active RA despite treatment with MTX were randomized to receive placebo and MTX or one of the four regimens of infliximab and MTX: 3 mg/kg or 10 mg/kg of infliximab at weeks 0, 2, and 6 followed by additional infusions every 4 or 8 weeks. At week 30, a significantly higher percentage of patients achieved an ACR20, ACR50, and ACR70 in all infliximab groups compared to patients in the placebo group. ACR20 responses were achieved by 53%, 50%, 58%, and 52% of patients receiving infliximab 3 mg/kg q 4 or 8 weeks or 10 mg/kg q 4 or 8 weeks, respectively, compared with 20% of patients in the placebo group. |
| Efficacy and safety of abatacept or infliximab versus placebo in ATTEST: a Phase 3, multicenter, randomized, double-blind, placebo-controlled study in patients with RA and an inadequate response to MTX[18] | Efficacy and safety of abatacept (approximately 10 mg/kg) plus MTX or infliximab (3 mg/kg), plus MTX versus placebo plus MTX were evaluated in 431 patients randomized to the three treatment groups. Similar efficacy was seen in abatacept and infliximab groups. At day 197, ACR20, ACR50, and ACR70 responses were significantly greater in the abatacept group compared to the placebo group. ACR20 responses were achieved by 66.7% of patients in the abatacept group compared to 41.8% of patients in the placebo group. ACR20, ACR50, and ACR70 responses were also significantly higher in the infliximab group compared to the placebo group. ACR20 responses were achieved by 59.4% of patients in the infliximab group compared to 41.8% of patients in the placebo group. |

*(Continued)*

**TABLE 9.3**

Summary of Meta-Analysis of Infliximab by Difference Metrics—Parametric Empirical Bayesian Approach

| Historical Trial | Raw Data, ACR20 MTX Only | | | Raw Data, ACR20 Infliximab + MTX | | | RR | | | RD | | | OR | | |
|---|---|---|---|---|---|---|---|---|---|---|---|---|---|---|---|
| | *x* | *N* | % | *x* | *n* | % | Obs'ed RR | RR est | 95% CI | Obs'ed RD | RD est | 95% CI | Obs'ed OR | OR est | 95% CI |
| Westhovens et al.[19] | 87 | 341 | 25.5 | 199 | 343 | 58.0 | 0.44 | 0.45 | 0.38, 0.55 | −0.33 | −0.31 | −0.37, −0.25 | 0.25 | 0.26 | 0.20, 0.35 |
| Schiff et al.[18] | 46 | 110 | 41.8 | 98 | 165 | 59.4 | 0.70 | 0.65 | 0.52, 0.82 | −0.18 | −0.25 | −0.33, −0.18 | 0.49 | 0.37 | 0.26, 0.54 |
| Maini et al.[17] | 18 | 88 | 20.0 | 43 | 86 | 50.0 | 0.41 | 0.47 | 0.33, 0.66 | −0.30 | −0.29 | −0.37, −0.21 | 0.26 | 0.28 | 0.18, 0.43 |
| Zhang et al.[20] | 42 | 86 | 48.8 | 66 | 87 | 75.9 | 0.64 | 0.61 | 0.49, 0.76 | −0.27 | −0.28 | −0.37, −0.20 | 0.30 | 0.30 | 0.19, 0.45 |
| Abe et al.[21] | 11 | 47 | 23.4 | 30 | 49 | 61.2 | 0.38 | 0.47 | 0.32, 0.68 | −0.38 | −0.30 | −0.39, −0.21 | 0.19 | 0.27 | 0.17, 0.43 |
| Overall mean effect | | | | | | | | 0.52 | 0.41, 0.67 | | −0.29 | −0.35, −0.21 | | 0.29 | 0.22, 0.40 |
| Overall heterogeneity | | | | | | | $I^2 = 69\%$, $\tau^2 = 0.05$, $p = .0117$ | | | $I^2 = 27.2\%$, $\tau^2 = 0.0014$, $p = .2402$ | | | $I^2 = 36.4\%$, $\tau^2 = 0.0445$, $p = .1783$ | | |

*Notes:* CI, confidence interval; Obs'ed, observed; OR, odds ratio; OR est, OR study specific estimate; RD, rate difference; RD est, RD study specific estimate; RR, rate ratio; RR est, RR study specific estimate.

**TABLE 9.4**

Treatment Effect Sizes for the RD in ACR20 Response Rates

| Historical Trial | Model 1: Noniterative Weighted Estimate | | Model 2: Parametric Empirical Bayesian Approach | | Model 3: MCMC | |
|---|---|---|---|---|---|---|
| | RD est | CI | RD est | CI | RD est | CI |
| Westhovens et al.[19] | −0.33 | −0.39, −0.26 | −0.31 | −0.37, −0.25 | −0.31 | −0.38, −0.25 |
| Schiff et al.[18] | −0.18 | −0.29, −0.06 | −0.25 | −0.33, −0.18 | −0.24 | −0.33, −0.12 |
| Maini et al.[17] | −0.30 | −0.43, −0.16 | −0.29 | −0.37, −0.21 | −0.29 | −0.39, −0.19 |
| Zhang et al.[20] | −0.27 | −0.41, −0.13 | −0.28 | −0.37, −0.20 | −0.28 | −0.38, −0.18 |
| Abe et al.[21] | −0.38 | −0.56, −0.20 | −0.30 | −0.39, −0.21 | −0.31 | −0.45, −0.21 |
| Overall mean effect | −0.29 | −0.35, −0.23 | −0.29 | −0.35, −0.21 | −0.29 | −0.37, −0.20 |

*Note:* MCMC, Markov chain Monte Carlo.

## References


1. U.S. Food and Drug Administration. U.S. Food and Drug Administration (FDA) Guidance on Scientific Considerations in Demonstrating Biosimilarity to a Reference Product, April 2015.
2. Breslow, N. 1990. Biostatistics and Bayes. *Statistical Science*, 5: 269–298.
3. Rodda, B. E. and Davis, R. L. 1980. Determining the probability of an important difference in bioavailability. *Clinical Pharmacology & Therapeutics*, 28: 247–252.
4. Mandallaz, D. and Mau, J. 1981. Comparison of different methods for decision making in bioequivalence assessment. *Biometrics*, 37: 213–222.
5. Selwyn, M. R., Dempster, A. P., and Hall, N. R. 1981. A Bayesian approach to bioequivalence for the 2 × 2 changeover design. *Biometrics*, 37: 11–21.
6. Grieve, A. P. 1985. A Bayesian analysis of the two-period crossover design in clinical trials. *Biometrics*, 41: 979–990.
7. Racine-Poon, A., Grieve, A. P., Fluhler, H., and Smith, A. F. 1987. A two-stage procedure for bioequivalence studies. *Biometrics*, 43: 847–856.
8. Ghosh, P. and Khattree, R. 2003. Bayesian approach to average bioequivalence using Bayes factor. *Journal of Biopharmaceutical Statistics*, 13: 719–734.
9. Xu, S., Hua, S. Y., Menton, R., Barker, K., Menon, S., and D'Agostino, R.B. 2014. Inference of bioequivalence for log-normal distributed data with unspecified variances. *Statistics in Medicine*, 33(17): 2924–2938.
10. Xu, S., Hua, S. Y., Menton, R., Barker, K., Menon, S., and D'Agostino, R. B. 2014. Inference of equivalence for the ratio of two normal means with unspecified variances. *Journal of Biopharmaceutical Statistics*, 24(6): 1264–1279, doi: 10.1080/10543406.2014.941990.

11. Gubbiotti, S. and Santis, F. D. 2011. A Bayesian method for the choice of the sample size in equivalence trials. *Australian & New Zealand Journal of Statistics*, 53(4): 443–460.
12. Hsieh T., Chow, S., Yang, L., and Chi, E. 2013. The evaluation of biosimilarity index based on reproducibility probability for assessing follow-on biologics. *Statistics in Medicine*, 32(3): 406–414.
13. Combest, A.J., Wang, S., Healey, B.T., and Reitsma, D.J. 2014. Alternative statistical strategies for biosimilar drug development. *Generics and Biosimilars Initiative Journal*, 3(1): 13–20.
14. Baji, P., Pentek, M., Szanto, S., Geher, P., Gulacsi1, L., Balogh, O., and Brodszky, V. 2014. Comparative efficacy and safety of biosimilar infliximab and other biological treatments in ankylosing spondylitis: Systematic literature review and meta-analysis. *The European Journal of Health Economics*, 15(1): 45–52.
15. Ntzoufras, I. *Bayesian Modeling Using WinBUGS, Wiley Series in Computational Statistics*, John Wiley & Sons, Inc., Hoboken, NJ, 2009.
16. Gelman, A., Carlin, J. B., Stern, H. S., and Rubin, D. B. *Bayesian Data Analysis*. Second Edition, Chapman & Hall/CRC, Boca Raton, FL, 2003 (ISBN 10: 158488388X/ISBN 13: 9781584883883).
17. Maini, R., St Clair, E. W., Breedveld, F., Furst, D., Kalden, J., Weisman, M., Smolen, J., Emery, P., Harriman, G., Feldmann, M., and Lipsky, P. 1999. Infliximab (chimeric anti-tumour necrosis factor alpha monoclonal antibody) versus placebo in rheumatoid arthritis patients receiving concomitant methotrexate: A randomised phase III trial. ATTRACT Study Group. *Lancet*, 354 (9194): 1932–1939.
18. Schiff, M., Keiserman, M., Codding, C., Songcharoen, S., Berman, A., Nayiager, S., Saldate, C., Li, T., Aranda, R., Becker, J. C., Lin, C., Cornet, P. L., and Dougados, M. 2008. Efficacy and safety of abatacept or infliximab vs placebo in ATTEST: A phase III, multi-centre, randomised, double-blind, placebo-controlled study in patients with rheumatoid arthritis and an inadequate response to methotrexate. *Annals of the Rheumatic Diseases*, 67 (8): 1096–1103.
19. Westhovens, R., Yocum, D., Han, J., Berman, A., Strusberg, I., Geusens, P., and Rahman, M.U. 2006. The safety of infliximab, combined with background treatments, among patients with rheumatoid arthritis and various comorbidities: A large, randomized, placebo-controlled trial. *Arthritis and Rheumatism*, 54 (4): 1075–1086.
20. Zhang, F.C, Hou, Y., Huang, F., Wu, D.-H., Bao, C.-D., Ni, L.-Q., and Yao, C. 2006. Infliximab versus placebo in rheumatoid arthritis patients receiving concomitant methotrexate: A preliminary study from China. *APLAR Journal of Rheumatology*, 9: 127–130.
21. Abe, T., Takeuchi, T., Miyasaka, N., Hashimoto, H., Kondo, H., Ichikawa, Y., Nagaya, I. 2006. A multicenter, double-blind, randomized, placebo controlled trial of infliximab combined with low dose methotrexate in Japanese patients with rheumatoid arthritis. *The Journal of Rheumatology*, 33: 37–44.
22. Hedges, L. V. 1983. A random effects model for effect size. *Psychological Bulletin*, 93: 388–395.
23. Der Simonian, R. and Laird, N. M. 1983. Evaluating the effect of coaching on SAT scores: A meta-analysis. *Harvard Educational Review*, 53(1): 1–15.

24. Morris, C. N. 1983. Parametric empirical Bayes inference: Theory and applications. *Journal of the American Statistical Association*, 78: 47–59.
25. Gelfand, A. E., Hills, S. E., Racine-Poon, A., and Smith, A. F. M. 1990 Illustration of Bayesian inference in normal data models using Gibbs sampling. *Journal of American Statistical Association*, 85: 972–985.

# 10

# *Average Inferiority Measure and Standardized Margins to Address the Issues in Biosimilar Trials*

**Gang Li and Weichung Joe Shih**

**CONTENTS**



**ABSTRACT** The choice of similarity or inferiority margins is a key design element for biosimilar and noninferiority (NI) studies. There are three major issues with the current practice of margin specifications: the subjectivity in the process of determining the margin, the data variability not considered or only implicitly expressed, and the concern of "biocreep" controversy. In this chapter, an average inferiority measure (AIM) is introduced as a tool for specification of margins to address these issues and the standardized margins derived from AIM reflect naturally the variability of data. AIM is applied to the normal, binary, and the survival data. A general theorem is obtained to establish the asymptotic normality of a test statistic for the NI hypothesis defined by the standardized margin. We also propose an additional requirement on the treatment effect difference for concluding NI to address the concern of biocreep and show that this additional requirement does not reduce the power when the treatment and control are true equivalent.

## 10.1 Introduction

The U.S. Food and Drug Administration (FDA) issued a guidance document for the approval of less-costly biosimilar medicines in 2015 (See U.S. Food and Drug Administration, 2015b), which specifies that a comparative clinical study is necessary to support a demonstration of biosimilarity. One of the key design elements of such a comparative clinical study is the similarity margin. The statistical evidence for biosimilarity is established when the proposed product is neither inferior nor superior to the reference product by more than the margin.

Margin specification in NI trials has been discussed extensively in the literature, e.g., Temple and Ellenberg (2000), D'Agostino (2003), Rothmann et al. (2003), Senn (2000), Hung et al. (2005, 2009), EMEA Committee for Medicinal Products for Human Use (2006, 2015), Ng (2008), Chi et al. (2010), and Peterson et al. (2010). In the last decade, many publications have come out of research on this topic. However, no satisfactory method has surfaced due to problems inherent in the nature of NI trials without a concurrent placebo. Currently, the fixed margin approach and the synthesis approach are commonly used for NI margin specifications, while the fixed margin approach is preferred by the FDA (U.S. Food and Drug Administration, 2010). These two approaches require the availability of historical studies that compare the control to placebo. However, such historical studies may not always be available or may have been conducted decades ago and hence the constancy assumption is doubtful. In this chapter, we address three prominent issues associated with the determination of inferiority/similarity margins in these approaches: subjectivity, variability, and biocreep.

There are several potential sources of subjectivity in the process of determining the margin. These include the selection of historical placebo-controlled studies, the model for meta-analysis to estimate the effect of the control, the choice of confidence threshold for the estimated confidence bounds of the control effect, and the magnitude of the retention fraction. One or more of these potential sources of subjectivity may result in an excessively stringent margin. For instance, in anti-infective trials, historical placebo-controlled studies are often not available. In the FDA draft Guidance to the Industry on Non-Inferiority Clinical Trials (U.S. Food and Drug Administration, 2010), an example was discussed in detail on the determination of an NI margin for complicated urinary tract infection (cUTI) using the fixed margin approach. Since historical placebo-controlled cUTI studies are not available, the guidance derived indirectly the placebo eradication rate from two sets of data. The first set of data was from uncomplicated urinary tract infection (UTI) studies, which is a much less serious condition than cUTI, resulting in a higher estimate for the placebo eradication rate. The second set of data came from studies with inadequate therapies, which again is likely to result in a higher estimate for the placebo eradication rate. The levofloxacin rate was estimated from a third set of studies. The eradication rate of the active control was derived from yet another set of studies.

To alleviate this subjectivity, an inferiority index is proposed by Li and Chi (2011). The inferiority index essentially establishes a standard for measuring the degree of inferiority. It compares the distribution of the treatment to that of the control and finds the worst inferiority level of the former to the latter as the index. However, it is possible that within some portion of the distribution, the treatment is superior to the control. The inferiority index does not take this possibility into consideration. In this chapter, we propose an alternative standard, called AIM, to address this issue.

The second issue with the margin is the data variability. In practice, the variability of data is considered only implicitly in the margin specifications. For example, consider NI trials for diabetes drug development, where HbA1c is the primary endpoint. The U.S. Food and Drug Administration (2008) recommended both 0.3% and 0.4% as possible choices for the margin, depending on the data variability. Another example is NI trials for anti-infective drug development, where the cure rate was the primary endpoint. The FDA guidance specified the margin as a step function of the cure rate of the control group (U.S. Food and Drug Administration, 1992). The closer to 50% the cure rate of the control was, the larger the variance, and thus the bigger the margin recommended. But this recommendation was criticized for its lack of a theoretical basis. The inferiority index of Li and Chi (2011) does not address this criticism satisfactorily (see Section 10.8 and Figure 10.2). On the other hand, the margin derived from AIM relates naturally to the variability of the data. Consequently, AIM provides a theoretical framework to include the data variability in the margin specification.

The third important concern is the so-called biocreep issue. There seemingly is a controversy in the report by the Government Accountability Office (GAO, 2010) regarding the evidence of biocreep as a result of the use of NI trials over time for regulatory approval of new drugs. On one hand, the GAO report examined the materials of 18 approved new drug applications (NDAs) based on NI trials and found no obvious evidence of biocreep. On the other hand, the report identified improper calculation or justification of the NI margin as an issue. This was consonant with FDA's remark that the sponsors used a margin larger than what the FDA had agreed to. Thus the concern of biocreep intertwines with the selection of the NI margin. The GAO report gave a scenario (Clinical Trial C in Figure 1 on page 8) showing that the lower bound of a 95% confidence interval (CI) is above the inferiority bound but the upper bound is less than zero, thus indicating a controversy that the treatment is noninferior to the control but, at the same time, is significantly worse than the control. This example suggested that the controversy may be partially due to the selection of a liberal NI margin. Setting a stringent margin was recommended to tame biocreep by some authors (e.g., Gladstone and Vach, 2014). Thus, in this chapter, we propose a different approach using AIM to handle the biocreep issue.

The structure of this chapter is as follows. In Section 10.2, we describe AIM in relation to the inferiority index of Li and Chi (2011). Subsequently, in Sections 10.3 through 10.5, the relationships between AIM and the usual inferiority/similarity margin are established for the normal, binary, and survival cases, respectively. The notion of the standardized margin is also introduced. In Section 10.6, the NI hypotheses are expressed in terms of the standardized margin, and the asymptotic distribution of the corresponding test statistic is developed. Next, in Section 10.7, we propose an additional requirement on the treatment effect difference for preventing biocreep with the NI claim and show that this additional requirement does not reduce the power in case of true equivalence. We conclude with a discussion and recommendation in Section 10.8.

## 10.2 Average Inferiority Measure

Let $X_C$ and $X_T$ be the response variables of the control and treatment, and $F_C$ and $F_T$ be the corresponding distribution functions, respectively. Suppose a smaller response represents a worse response. Then $F_T(x) - F_C(x) > 0$ (<0) indicates the inferiority (superiority) level of $X_T$ to $X_C$ at $x$. Li and Chi (2011) considered the worst inferiority level of $X_T$ to $X_C$,

$$\rho = \text{Sup}_{-\infty<x<\infty}\left[F_T(x) - F_C(x)\right] \tag{10.1}$$

and discussed its potential application in design and analysis of NI clinical trials. However, it is possible that on some portion the treatment distribution is above (inferior to) the control, while on other portion it is the reverse: for example, when $X_T$ and $X_C$ are normally distributed, with means $\mu_T = -0.4$ and $\mu_C = 0$, and variances $\sigma_T^2 > 1$ and $\sigma_C^2 = 1$, respectively. Their distribution functions are presented in Figure 10.1.

Note that $F_T(x) > F_C(x)$ if $x < 0.55$, $F_T(x) < F_C(x)$ if $x > 0.55$. Obviously, by taking the maximum point (i.e., the worst inferiority) among all $x$, $\rho$ does not take the possible superiority level of T to C into consideration. Therefore, we propose an alternative approach, the AIM. Specifically, when $F_C(x)$ and $F_T(x)$ are continuous, we define the AIM as

$$r = \int_{-\infty}^{\infty}\left(F_T(x) - F_C(x)\right)\mathrm{d}F_C(x) \tag{10.2}$$

When $X_C$ and $X_T$ are independent, the AIM can be written as

$$r = P(X_C > X_T) - 0.5 \tag{10.3}$$

Obviously, $r$ is centered at 0 for identically distributed $X_C$ and $X_T$ and its range is $(-0.5, 0.5)$. A positive (negative) $r$ indicates an average level of

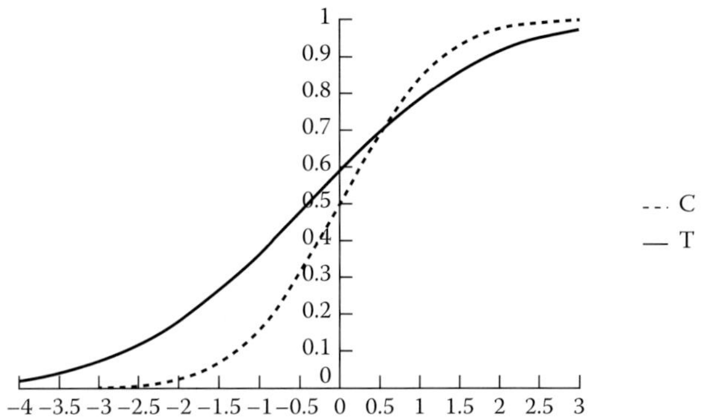


**FIGURE 10.1**
Normal distributions: $\sigma > 1$.

inferiority (superiority) of T to C. We will explore the characteristics of $r$ for the cases of normal, binary, and survival data in Sections 10.3 through 10.5. In the normal and binary cases, we can view $\Phi^{-1}(0.5 - r)$ as the standardized margin.

## 10.3 Average Inferiority Measure for Normal Data

Let $X_T \sim N(\mu_T, \sigma_T^2)$ and $X_C \sim N(\mu_C, \sigma_C^2)$ be independently normally distributed. Let us assume that $\mu_T < \mu_C$. We first standardize both random variables relative to the distributions of $X_C$, i.e., consider the $Z$-scores $X_C' = \dfrac{X_C - \mu_C}{\sigma_C}$ and $X_T' = \dfrac{X_T - \mu_C}{\sigma_C}$. Equivalently, we need only consider $X_C \sim N(0, 1)$ and $X_T \sim N(\delta, \sigma^2)$, where $\delta = \dfrac{\mu_T - \mu_C}{\sigma_C}$ and $\sigma^2 = \dfrac{\sigma_T^2}{\sigma_C^2}$, with $\delta < 0$. The AIM is as follows:

$$
\begin{aligned}
r = P(X_C > X_T) - 0.5 &= P\left(\frac{X_C - (X_T - \delta)}{\sqrt{1+\sigma^2}} > \frac{\delta}{\sqrt{1+\sigma^2}}\right) - 0.5 \\
&= 0.5 - \Phi\left(\frac{\delta}{\sqrt{1+\sigma^2}}\right)
\end{aligned}
\tag{10.4}
$$

Conversely, for a given $r$ in (−0.5, 0.5),

$$
\frac{\delta}{\sqrt{1+\sigma^2}} = \Phi^{-1}(0.5 - r) \tag{10.5}
$$

This shows that $r$ relates to the pair $(\delta, \sigma)$. This relationship suggests that when considering equivalence or nonequivalence, inferiority or NI, it is important to take both the means and the variances of the two groups into consideration. However, in many applications, such as population bioequivalence studies and biosimilar and NI clinical trials, the so-called equivalence, biosimilar or NI margins often ignore the variances. The traditional margins are usually set on the difference of the unstandardized means. If we use the AIM $r$, then Equation 10.5 suggests a way to define the margin in terms of a standardized mean difference. We illustrate this relation with the following example.

**Example 1.** The first biosimilar product approved in the United States is Zarxio, a leukocyte growth factor, which is biosimilar to Amgen Inc.'s Neupogen (filgrastim) (see U.S. Food and Drug Administration, 2015a). The primary endpoint of the pivotal biosimilar clinical trial was duration of severe neutropenia (DNS). A smaller DNS value indicates a better result. The margin for testing the NI hypotheses was –1 day for comparing DSN means between Neupogen and Zarxio. It was chosen in some way without taking into consideration the variability. The standard deviations were 1.11 days and 1.02 day, respectively, for Neupogen Zarxio from the historical data. If we assume reasonably a common standard deviation of 1.06 days for the two groups, then the AIM is $r = 0.5 - \Phi\left(\frac{-1}{\sqrt{2 \times 1.06^2}}\right) = 0.5 - \Phi(-0.667) = 0.246.$ Conversely, suppose we set AIM $r =$ 0.25, then we can justify using $\frac{\delta}{\sqrt{1+\sigma^2}} = \Phi^{-1}(0.5 - 0.25) = -\ 0.674$ as the standardized margin.

## 10.4 Average Inferiority Measure for Binary Data

In the analysis of binary data, the difference in mean rates is used to construct the statistic. The asymptotic normality theory is often applied for hypothesis testing or CIs. Therefore, we will obtain the NI margin for binary data by applying the approach for normal data. Suppose $X_T$ and $X_C$ are binary endpoints, with event rates $p_T$ and $p_C$, respectively. To utilize the result in Equation 10.4, we set the mean $\mu_T = p_T$ and the variance $\sigma_T^2 = p_T(1 - p_T)$ for $X_T$, and similarly for $X_C$. Then the AIM is as follows:

$$r = 0.5 - \Phi\left(\frac{p_T - p_C}{\sqrt{p_T(1 - p_T) + p_C(1 - p_C)}}\right) \tag{10.6}$$

Given $r$, let $\Delta = \Phi^{-1}(0.5 - r)$. Then (10.6) becomes

$$\frac{p_T - p_C}{\sqrt{p_T(1 - p_T) + p_C(1 - p_C)}} = \Delta \tag{10.7}$$

To help the interpretation of $r$, we examine the relationship of $p_T - p_C$ with $p_C$. Note that $p_T(1-p_T) = -(p_T - p_C)^2 + (1-2p_C)(p_T - p_C) + p_C(1-p_C)$. Equation 10.6 is changed to a quadratic equation of $p_T - p_C$: $(1+\Delta^2)(p_T - p_C)^2 - \Delta^2(1-2p_C)(p_T - p_C) - 2\Delta^2 p_C(1-p_C) = 0$.

Its determinant is as follows:

$$\begin{aligned}
&\left[\Delta^2(1-2p_C)\right]^2 + 4(1+\Delta^2)\cdot 2\Delta^2 p_C(1-p_C) \\
&= \Delta^2\left[\Delta^2 - 4\Delta^2 p_C + 4\Delta^2 p_C^2 + 8p_C(1-p_C) + 8\Delta^2 p_C - 8\Delta^2 p_C^2\right] \\
&= \Delta^2\left[\Delta^2 + 4\Delta^2 p_C - 4\Delta^2 p_C^2 + 8p_C(1-p_C)\right] \\
&= \Delta^2\left[\Delta^2 + 4\Delta^2 p_C(1-p_C) + 8p_C(1-p_C)\right] \\
&= \Delta^2\left[\Delta^2 + 4p_C(1-p_C)(2+\Delta^2)\right]
\end{aligned}$$

The solution of $p_T - p_C$ is a function of $p_C$ as

$$p_T - p_C = \frac{\Delta^2(1-2p_C) - \sqrt{\Delta^2[\Delta^2 + 4p_C(1-p_C)(2+\Delta^2)]}}{2(1+\delta_0^2)} \tag{10.8}$$

The margin $p_T - p_C$ is related with $p_C$ and the standardized margin $\Delta$ $(= \Phi^{-1}(0.5 - r))$.

## 10.5 Average Inferiority Measure for Survival Data

Let the cumulative hazard of the control group be $H_C(t) = \int_{-\infty}^{t} h_C(u)\,du$, then its distribution $F_C(t) = 1 - \exp\{-H_C(t)\}$. Under the proportional hazard assumption $\frac{h_T(t)}{h_C(t)} = \delta$, the cumulative hazard and distribution functions of the treatment group are given by $H_T(t) = \delta H_C(t)$ and $F_T(t) = 1 - \exp\{-\delta H_C(t)\}$. The AIM is as follows:

$$\begin{aligned}
r &= P(X_C > X_T) - 0.5 = \int_0^{\infty} \exp\{-H_C(t)\}\, d\left[\exp\{-\delta H_C(t)\}\right] - 0.5 \\
&= \int_0^{\infty} e^{-t}\delta e^{-\delta t}\, dt - 0.5 = \frac{\delta}{1+\delta} - 0.5 = \frac{\delta - 1}{2(1+\delta)}
\end{aligned}$$

For a given $r$, $\Delta = \dfrac{1+2r}{1-2r}$. Note that $\Delta = 1$ corresponds to $r = 0$.

## 10.6 Noninferiority Hypothesis and Asymptotic Distribution

For the normal data, let $\delta_0 = \dfrac{\mu_T - \mu_C}{\sqrt{\sigma_T^2 + \sigma_C^2}}$. The NI hypothesis in term of the standardized margin $\Delta = \Phi^{-1}(0.5 - r)$ is set as:

$$H_0 : \delta_0 \le \Delta \text{ versus } H_1 : \delta_0 > \Delta \tag{10.9}$$

Because the hypothesis involves the standard deviation, the existence of the fourth moments of $X_T$ and $X_C$ is needed. Let us denote the third and fourth moments of $X_T$ by $\mu_T^{(3)} = E(X_T - \mu_T)^3$ and $\mu_T^{(4)} = E(X_T - \mu_T)^4$ and similarly for $X_C$, $\mu_C^{(3)} = E(X_C - \mu_C)^3$, and $\mu_C^{(4)} = E(X_C - \mu_C)^4$. Let $\hat{X}_T$ and $\hat{X}_C$ be the respective sample means. Let us define $\hat{\sigma}_T^2 = \frac{1}{n}\sum_{i=1}^{n}(X_{Ti} - \hat{X}_T)^2$ and $\hat{\sigma}_C^2 = \frac{1}{n}\sum_{i=1}^{n}(X_{Ci} - \hat{X}_C)^2$.

Then, we have $\dfrac{\hat{\sigma}_T^2}{\sigma_T^2} \to 1$ and $\dfrac{\hat{\sigma}_C^2}{\sigma_C^2} \to 1$ in probability.

Now consider the following statistic: $\sqrt{n}\left[\dfrac{(\hat{X}_T - \hat{X}_C)}{\sqrt{\hat{\sigma}_T^2 + \hat{\sigma}_C^2}} - \delta_0\right]$. The asymptotic normality of this statistic is established in the following Theorem 1.

**Theorem 1:** Suppose that $X_T$ and $X_C$ have the first four moments.

Then, $\sqrt{n}\left[\dfrac{(\hat{X}_T - \hat{X}_C)}{\sqrt{\hat{\sigma}_T^2 + \hat{\sigma}_C^2}} - \delta_0\right]$ is asymptotically $N(0, S)$, where

$$S = 1 + \frac{\delta_0^2}{4(\sigma_T^2 + \sigma_C^2)^2}\left[\left(\mu_T^{(4)} - \sigma_T^4\right) + (\mu_C^{(4)} - \sigma_C^4)\right] - \frac{\delta_0}{2(\sigma_T^2 + \sigma_C^2)}\left[\mu_T^{(3)} - \mu_C^{(3)}\right].$$

The proof of Theorem 1 is given in Appendix I. Note that under the true equivalence $\mu_T - \mu_C = 0$, $\delta_0 = 0$, thus $S = 1$.

Let $\hat{S}$ be a consistent estimate of $S$. Then $\sqrt{n/\hat{S}}\left[\frac{(\hat{X}_T - \hat{X}_C)}{\sqrt{\hat{\sigma}_T^2 + \hat{\sigma}_C^2}} - \delta_0\right]$ is approximately $N(0, 1)$ and can be used as a statistic for testing NI. The NI hypothesis Equation 10.6 is rejected if

$$\sqrt{n/\hat{S}}\left[\frac{(\hat{X}_T - \hat{X}_C)}{\sqrt{\hat{\sigma}_T^2 + \hat{\sigma}_C^2}} - \Delta\right] > z_{\alpha/2} \tag{10.10}$$

at two-sided significant level $\alpha$.

For binary data, the mean $\mu_T = p_T$ and the variance $\sigma_T^2 = p_T(1-p_T)$ for $X_T$ and similarly for $X_C$. Then

$$S = 1 + \frac{\delta_0^2}{4\left(p_T(1-p_T) + p_C(1-p_C)\right)^2}\left[p_T(1-p_T)(1-2p_T)^2 + p_C(1-p_C)(1-2p_C)^2\right]$$

$$- \frac{\delta_0}{2\left(p_T(1-p_T) + p_C(1-p_C)\right)}\left[p_T(1-p_T)(1-2p_T) - p_C(1-p_C)(1-2p_C)\right].$$

The test Equation 10.10 applies with $\mu_T$, $\mu_C$, and $\delta_0$ in the form of $p_T$ and $p_C$.

For the survival data case, $\delta_0 = \frac{h_T(t)}{h_C(t)}$ and $\Delta = \frac{1+2r}{1-2r}$. The usual test for the hazard ratio applies directly.

## 10.7 Handling the Concern of Biocreep

The concern of biocreep intertwines with the selection of the NI margin. Some authors (e.g., Gladstone and Vach, 2014) suggest setting a stringent margin to tame biocreep. We propose a different approach using the standardized margin $\Delta = \Phi^{-1}(0.5 - r)$.

In the normal data case, NI of $X_T$ to $X_C$ is concluded if $\sqrt{\frac{n}{S}}\left[\frac{\hat{X}_T - \hat{X}_C}{\sqrt{\hat{\sigma}_T^2 + \hat{\sigma}_C^2}} - \Delta\right] > z_{\alpha/2}$ (see Section 10.6). Under the condition of true equivalence of $X_T$ to $X_C$, i.e., $\mu_T - \mu_C = 0$, a sample size $n = \frac{(z_{\alpha/2} + z_\beta)^2}{\Delta^2}$ per group will have a power of $1-\beta$, where $z_\beta$ is the $(1-\beta)$-quantile of the standard normal. An additional requirement on the mean difference can mitigate the concern of biocreep with the NI claim:

$$\frac{\hat{X}_T - \hat{X}_C}{\sqrt{\hat{\sigma}_T^2 + \hat{\sigma}_C^2}} > \Delta_1 \tag{10.11}$$

for $\Delta_1 = \frac{z_\beta}{z_{\alpha/2} + z_\beta}\Delta$. Note that $0 > \Delta_1 > \frac{\Delta}{2}$ for $\alpha/2 < \beta$. Then we have the following results:

**Theorem 2:** Under the condition of true equivalence that $\mu_T - \mu_C = 0$, the per-group sample size $n = \frac{(z_{\alpha/2} + z_\beta)^2}{\Delta^2}$, and define $\Delta_1 = \frac{z_\beta}{z_{\alpha/2} + z_\beta}\Delta$,

i. $P\left\{\frac{\hat{X}_T - \hat{X}_C}{\sqrt{\hat{\sigma}_T^2 + \hat{\sigma}_C^2}} > \Delta_1\right\} \approx 1 - \beta.$

ii. Equation 10.11 implies that the upper limit of the CI of $\frac{\mu_T - \mu_C}{\sqrt{\sigma_T^2 + \sigma_C^2}}$ is greater than 0, for $\alpha/2 < \beta$.

The proof of Theorem 2 is in Appendix II. The result (i) indicates that the new restriction Equation 10.11 does not reduce the power of the NI test for the hypotheses Equation 10.9 when the true equivalence holds. The result (ii) rules out the controversial scenario of "Clinical Trial C' in the GAO report. Since the upper bound of the CI exceeds 0, it provides a clarification that the treatment is noninferior to the control, without the dilemma that "at the same time, control is significantly better than the treatment" (as commented in the GAO report). Note that when $\alpha = 0.05$, $\Delta_1 = 0.4\Delta$, if $1 - \beta = 0.9$; and $\Delta_1 = 0.3\Delta$, if $1 - \beta = 0.8$.

## 10.8 Discussion

The notion of AIM is introduced in this chapter to address three major issues in NI trials. To begin, the subjectivity of choosing a traditional NI margin is alleviated by AIM, which compares directly the distributions of the treatment and the concurrent control. Next, the data variability is explicitly included in the NI hypothesis with standardized margins from AIM. Finally, the biocreep concern is also tackled by using AIM with an additional criterion when making the NI claim.

Compared to the inferiority index ρ (Li and Chi, 2011), AIM $r$ ranges within (–0.5, 0.5), while ρ ranges within (–1, 1). When $\sigma^2 = \frac{\sigma_T^2}{\sigma_C^2} = 1$, $r$ and ρ

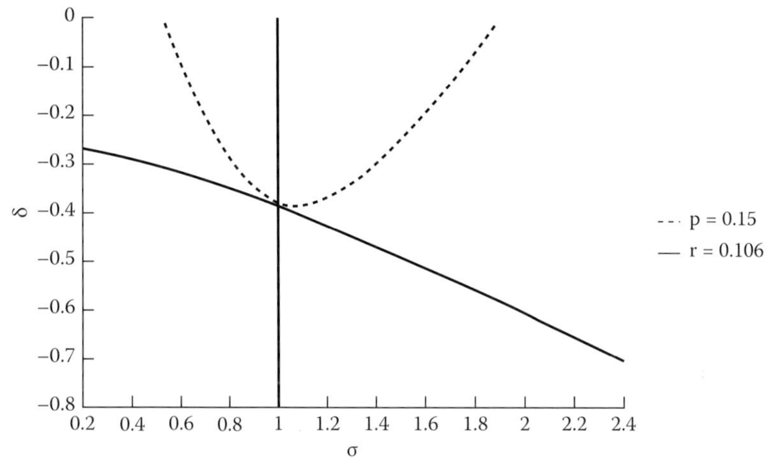


**FIGURE 10.2**
Curves of δ versus σ – *A*. Comparison of *r* with ρ.

have an approximately linear relation. From $r(\delta) = 0.5 - \Phi\left(\frac{\delta}{\sqrt{2}}\right)$ and $\rho(\delta) = 1 - 2\Phi\left(\frac{\delta}{2}\right)$, we see that, for $-0.5 \le \delta < 0$, $r(\delta) \cong \rho(\delta)/\sqrt{2}$. Both ρ and *r* are related to the pair $(\delta, \sigma)$ and $|\delta|$ increases with σ for $\sigma < 1$. However, the margins obtained from ρ and *r* are different for $\sigma > 1$. In this region of σ, $|\delta|$ from *r* continues the trend of increasing while that from ρ starts decreasing. It is reasonable that when the variability (σ) is larger (smaller), the magnitude $|\delta|$ should also be larger (smaller). As seen in Figure 10.2, this is so for *r*, but not so for ρ. In addition, the relationship between *r* and $(\delta, \sigma)$ is simpler.

Biocreep has haunted NI trials although no evidence of biocreep is found. A simulation study by Everson-Stewart and Emerson (2010) suggested that biocreep was rare, except when the constancy assumption was violated. There are two ways to mitigate the concerns. First, the NI trials should select the gold standard as the control. This makes sense both scientifically and commercially. Second, the additional requirement proposed in this chapter should be used the NI claim.

## References

Chi GYH, Chen G, Li N, and Rothmann M (2010). *Active Control Trials, Encyclopedia of Biopharmaceutical Statistics*. Marcel Dekker, Inc., New York, NY, pp. 9–15.

D'Agostino RB (2003). Editorial—Non-inferiority trials: Advances in concepts and methodology. *Statistics in Medicine* 22: 165–167.

EMEA Committee for Medicinal Products for Human Use (CHMP) (2006). Guideline on the choice of the non-inferiority margin. *Statistics in Medicine* 25: 1628–1638.

EMEA Committee for Medicinal Products for Human Use (CHMP) (2015). Guideline on the similar biological medicinal products (http://www.ema.europa.eu/docs/en_GB/document_library/Scientific_guideline/2015/01/WC500180219.pdf).

Everson-Stewart S and Emerson SS (2010). Bio-creep in non-inferiority clinical trials *Statistics in Medicine* 29: 2769–2780.

Gladstone BP and Vach W (2014). Choice of non-inferiority (NI) margins does not protect against degradation of treatment effects on an average—An observational study of registered and published NI trials. *PLoS One* 9: e103616.

Government Accountability Office (GAO) (2010). New Drug Approval—FDA's Consideration of Evidence from Certain Clinical Trials (http://www.gao.gov/new.items/d10798.pdf).

Hung JHM, Wang S-J, and O'Neill R (2005). A regulatory perspective on choice of margin and statistical inference issue in non-inferiority trials. *Biometrical Journal* 47 (1): 28–36.

Hung JHM, Wang S-J, and O'Neill R (2009). Challenges and regulatory experiences with non-inferiority trial design without placebo arm. *Biometrical Journal* 51 (2): 324–334.

Li G and Chi GYH (2011). Inferiority index and margin in non-inferiority trials. *Statistics in Biopharmaceutical Research* 3: 288–301.

Ng TH (2008). Non-inferiority hypotheses and choice of non-inferiority margin. *Statistics in Medicine* 27: 5392–5406.

Peterson P, Carroll K, Chuang-Stein C, Ho YY, Jiang Q, Li G, Sanchez M, Sax R, Wang YY, and Snapinn S (2010). PISC Expert Team White Paper: Toward a consistent standard of evidence when evaluating the efficacy of an experimental treatment from a randomized, active-controlled trial. *Statistics in Biopharmaceutical Research* 2: 538–539.

Rothmann M, Li N, Chen G, Chi GYH, Temple R, and Tsou HH (2003). Design and analysis of non-inferiority mortality trials in oncology. *Statistics in Medicine* 22: 239–264.

Senn S (2000). 'Equivalence is different'—Some comments on therapeutic equivalence. *Biometrical Journal* 47 (1): 104–107.

Temple R and Ellenberg S (2000). Placebo-controlled trials and active-control trials in the evaluation of new treatments. Part I: Ethical and Scientific Issues. *Annals of Internal Medicine* 133 (6): 455–463.

U.S. Food and Drug Administration (1992). *Guidance for Industry: Clinical Development and Labeling of Anti-infective Drug Products*. U.S. Food and Drug Administration, Rockville, MD.

U.S. Food and Drug Administration (2008). *Guidance for Industry: Diabetes Mellitus: Developing Drugs and Therapeutic Biologics for Treatment and Prevention*. U.S. Food and Drug Administration, Rockville, MD.

U.S. Food and Drug Administration (2010). *Guidance for Industry on Non-Inferiority Clinical Trials*, March 2010. U.S. Food and Drug Administration, Rockville, MD.

U.S. Food and Drug Administration (2015a). FDA Oncologic Drugs Advisory Committee Meeting: ZARXIO® (filgrastim), January 7, 2015.

U.S. Food and Drug Administration (2015b). Scientific Considerations in Demonstrating Biosimilarity to a Reference Product, April 2015.

## Appendix I.

### Proof of Theorem 1

**Proof:** Let us proceed to the derivation of the expression for the variance $S$,

$$\sqrt{n}\left[\frac{(\hat{X}_T - \hat{X}_C)}{\sqrt{\hat{\sigma}_T^2 + \hat{\sigma}_C^2}} - \delta_0\right] = \sqrt{n}\left[\frac{(\hat{X}_T - \hat{X}_C)}{\sqrt{\sigma_T^2 + \sigma_C^2}} - \delta_0\right] - \left[\frac{(\hat{X}_T - \hat{X}_C)}{\sqrt{\hat{\sigma}_T^2 + \hat{\sigma}_C^2}}\right] \left[\frac{1}{\sqrt{\frac{\hat{\sigma}_T^2 + \hat{\sigma}_C^2}{\sigma_T^2 + \sigma_C^2}} + 1)}\right]\sqrt{n}\left[\frac{\hat{\sigma}_T^2 + \hat{\sigma}_C^2}{\sigma_T^2 + \sigma_C^2} - 1\right] \tag{A1}$$

Following the definition of $\hat{\sigma}_T^2$ and $\hat{\sigma}_C^2$, we have

$$\sqrt{n}\left[\frac{\hat{\sigma}_T^2 + \hat{\sigma}_C^2}{\sigma_T^2 + \sigma_C^2} - 1\right] = \frac{1}{\sqrt{n}}\left[\frac{\sum_{i=1}^{n}[(X_{Ti} - \mu_T)^2 - \sigma_T^2] + \sum_{i=1}^{n}[(X_{Ci} - \mu_C)^2 - \sigma_C^2]}{\sigma_T^2 + \sigma_C^2}\right]$$

$$-\frac{\sqrt{n}}{2}\left[\frac{(\hat{X}_T - \mu_T)^2 + (\hat{X}_C - \mu_C)^2}{\sigma_T^2 + \sigma_C^2}\right].$$

Note that $\left[\frac{(\hat{X}_T - \hat{X}_C)}{\sqrt{\hat{\sigma}_T^2 + \hat{\sigma}_C^2}}\right]\left[\frac{1}{\sqrt{\frac{\hat{\sigma}_T^2 + \hat{\sigma}_C^2}{\sigma_T^2 + \sigma_C^2}} + 1)}\right] \to \frac{\delta_0}{2}$ and $\frac{\sqrt{n}}{2}\left[\frac{(\hat{X}_T - \mu_T)^2 + (\hat{X}_C - \mu_C)^2}{\sigma_T^2 + \sigma_C^2}\right] \to 0$

in probability. By Slusky's theorem, we need only to show that

$$T = \sqrt{n}\left[\frac{(\hat{X}_T - \hat{X}_C)}{\sigma_C} - \delta_0\right] - \frac{\delta_0}{2(\sigma_T^2 + \sigma_C^2)}\frac{1}{\sqrt{n}}\sum_{i=1}^{n}[(X_{Ti} - \mu_T)^2 - \sigma_T^2]$$

$$-\frac{\delta_0}{2(\sigma_T^2 + \sigma_C^2)}\frac{1}{\sqrt{n}}\sum_{i=1}^{n}[(X_{Ci} - \mu_C)^2 - \sigma_C^2]$$

is asymptotically normal with mean 0 and variance $S$.

Since the three terms are asymptotically normal with mean 0 and variance, 1, $(\mu_T^{(4)} - \sigma_T^4)$, and $(\mu_C^{(4)} - \sigma_C^4)$, respectively. It is easily seen that the expectations of the intersection of the first term with the second and third terms are

$$E\left\{\sqrt{n}\left[\frac{\left(\hat{X}_T - \hat{X}_C\right)}{\sqrt{\sigma_T^2 + \sigma_C^2}} - \delta_0\right]\frac{1}{\sqrt{n}}\sum_{i=1}^{n}[(X_{Ti} - \mu_T)^2 - \sigma_T^2]\right\} = \frac{\mu_T^{(3)}}{\sqrt{\sigma_T^2 + \sigma_C^2}} \quad \text{and}$$

$$E\left\{\sqrt{n}\left[\frac{\left(\hat{X}_T - \hat{X}_C\right)}{\sqrt{\sigma_T^2 + \sigma_C^2}} - \delta_0\right]\frac{1}{\sqrt{n}}\sum_{i=1}^{n}[(X_{Ci} - \mu_C)^2 - \sigma_C^2]\right\} = -\frac{\mu_C^{(3)}}{\sqrt{\sigma_T^2 + \sigma_C^2}}.$$

And the second and third terms are independent. Therefore, $T$ is asymptotically normal with mean 0 and variance $S$.

## Appendix II.

### Proof of Theorem 2

**Proof:** When $\mu_T - \mu_C = 0$, $S = 1$. For $\Delta_1$ as in Equation 10.11, $P\left\{\frac{\hat{X}_T - \hat{X}_C}{\sqrt{\hat{\sigma}_T^2 + \hat{\sigma}_C^2}} > \Delta_1\right\} \approx 1 - \Phi\left(\sqrt{n}\Delta_1\right) = 1 - \beta$ and (i) holds.

As long as $\beta > \frac{\alpha}{2}$, the upper limit of the confidence interval of $\frac{\mu_T - \mu_C}{\sqrt{\hat{\sigma}_T^2 + \hat{\sigma}_C^2}}$ is $\frac{\hat{X}_T - \hat{X}_C}{\sqrt{\hat{\sigma}_T^2 + \hat{\sigma}_C^2}} + \frac{z_{\alpha/2}}{\sqrt{n}} = \frac{z_\beta}{z_{\alpha/2} + z_\beta}\Delta - \frac{z_{\alpha/2}}{z_{\alpha/2} + z_\beta}\Delta = -\frac{z_{\alpha/2} - z_\beta}{z_{\alpha/2} + z_\beta}\Delta$. Therefore, (ii) follows from the fact that $\Delta < 0$.

# 11

# *Bayesian Methods for Design and Analysis of Noninferiority Trials*

**Mani Lakshminarayanan and Fanni Natanegara**

**CONTENTS**

**ABSTRACT** A general agreement exists in the field of research and development of clinical trials that a gold standard for evaluating treatment efficacy of a medical product is the use of placebo as a comparator. Over the years, researchers and practitioners have argued that placebo controls are controls, often citing the following sentence in the Declaration of Helsinki (Ref) as support for their position: "In any medical study, every patient—including those of a control group, if any—should be assured of the best proven diagnostic and therapeutic method." However, when the use of placebo is considered to be unethical or impractical, a viable alternative for evaluating treatment efficacy is through a noninferiority (NI) study where the aim is to demonstrate that the test treatment (drug or biologic) is no worse than the comparator by more than a prespecified, small amount. This amount, known as the NI margin, is small enough to allow the known effectiveness of the active control to support the conclusion that the new test treatment is also effective. The minimal objective of a clinical trial involving hypothesis of superiority is to determine whether the test treatment is superior to placebo. An assumption is made that if the active control treatment remains efficacious, as was observed when it was compared with placebo, then a test treatment that has comparable efficacy with the active control, within a certain range, must also be superior to placebo. Because of this assumption, the design, implementation, and analysis of NI trials present challenges for sponsors and regulators. One such challenge is to build a methodology that can consolidate existing substantial historical data, which is often required on the active control treatment and placebo. Bayesian approaches provide a natural framework for synthesizing and quantifying the historical data in the form of prior distributions that can effectively be used to address directly key questions in design and analysis of a NI clinical trial. In the case of showing biosimilarity, that is, showing that the biological product is highly similar to the reference product in terms of safety, purity, and potency, having full knowledge of the reference product is pertinent to successfully carry out the trials. Thus, it requires a methodology like Bayesian methods for generating relevant summaries of historical data based on the reference product. Our primary objective of this chapter is to show how Bayesian methods can be appropriately carried out in the design and analysis of clinical trials involving NI hypothesis.

## 11.1 Introduction

The goal of this chapter is to present the design and analysis of clinical trials involving biosimilar products using Bayesian methods. A Bayesian approach, appropriate for any scientific investigation as an iterative process of integrating and accumulating information, is a natural alternative to a classical approach for investigating biosimilars where comparisons are made against products that have already been licensed, thus presenting the current investigation with a wealth of historical data. In such settings, investigators can assess the current state of knowledge regarding the risk and benefit of an investigational product, gather new data from additional trials to address remaining questions, and then update and refine their hypotheses to incorporate both new and historical data.

### 11.1.1 Background

Conventional clinical trials that are placebo controlled are ideal for evaluating efficacy of an experimental drug, and they have been a basis for many Food and Drug Administration (FDA) approvals based on two well-controlled trials with superiority of the experimental treatment over placebo as the primary objective. In clinical investigations of new therapy, conducting placebo-controlled trials has been a standard in the long history of conducting clinical trials. The minimal requirement for a test treatment, $T$ to be considered efficacious is to show that it is superior against placebo, $P$, in adequate and well-controlled clinical trials. Freedman (1990) provides a list of conditions, any of which justifies the use of a placebo-controlled clinical trials: (1) no standard treatment exists; (2) standard treatment is not better than placebo; (3) standard treatment is a placebo (or no treatment); (4) new evidence has shown uncertainty of the risk–benefit profile of the standard treatment; and (5) effective treatment is not readily available due to cost or supply issues. The use of a placebo in clinical research continues to be a topic of debate in the medical community in recent times. One side of the argument revolves around the fact that alternative study designs could produce similar results with reduced risk to the patients. On the other hand, there are others who argue that the use of placebo is essential to protect society from the harm that could result from the widespread use of ineffective treatments.

However, when standard treatment(s) exist(s) and there is sufficient reason to believe that withholding standard treatment(s) could lead to irreversible morbidity or death, the use of placebo as a control raises ethical questions (Rothman & Michels, 1994; Temple & Ellenberg, 2000). In this situation, a viable alternative is a noninferiority (NI) study, where $T$ is compared to a standard active control treatment $C$ (ICH, 2000). Since placebo is not part of the noninferiority (NI) trial, the question around efficacy of $T$ can be addressed only indirectly, taking into account information from historical trials. The concept of NI trials has been developed since the 1970s and was inspired by the use of equivalency in clinical trials. During that period, the terms "noninferiority" and "therapeutic equivalence" were used interchangeably. NI clinical trials are considered as viable alternatives to superiority trials for finding new treatments that have approximately the same efficacy, but may offer other advantages over the existing treatment such as better safety profile and quality of life measurements. From patients' point of view, an NI comparison may be desired when a new innovative therapy has a small efficacy advantage, no efficacy advantage, or a slightly less efficacy than a standard treatment if it provides other advantages that may include a different or a easier form of administration, reduced toxicity, or a more preferable safety profile.

The indirect way of determining efficacy of $T$ presents challenges in the design, implementation, and analysis of NI trials for study sponsors and regulators alike (D'Agostino et al., 2003). For example, D'Agostino et al. (2003) pointed out two main challenges: (1) statistical hypotheses and tests and (2) NI margin selection. The NI margin is also the "single greatest challenge in the interpretation of NI trials" (FDA, 2010) because aside from the requirement that it be clinically meaningful, it relies on the validity of assay sensitivity, which refers to the assumption that both $C$ and $T$ would have been superior to $P$ if $P$ had been included in the trial. Furthermore, there are other statistical issues that are also noteworthy, including choice of $C$, selection of historical control to estimate the effect of the active control, statistical methods for the estimation of the effectiveness of the control, methods for determination of the NI margin, the analysis population, and others.

Defining an appropriate active control effect is critical for validating any NI trials, namely, the NI criterion should provide sufficient assurance that the experimental therapy is effective in comparison to the active control. Determination of effect sizes for active control may come from multiple studies involving active control therapy, but it is important to recognize that the standard of care (namely, proven therapies based on safety, effectiveness, and ethics) might change over time, especially in indications that have a history of replacing what is considered to be standard over time. If effect sizes for active control treatments are sought via modeling, then one must take into consideration the potential biases due to various covariates, which must then be included in the model. For example, if a meta-analysis is undertaken, it may be prudent to select studies that are similar before determining the overall effect. As stated in the International Conference on Harmonization (ICH, 1998), a suitable active comparator could be a widely used therapy whose efficacy in the relevant indication has been clearly established and quantified in well-designed and well-documented superiority trials and which can be reliably expected to have similar efficacy in the contemplated active control trial.

This similarity or constancy assumption is one of the several challenges that need to be addressed before conducting any NI clinical trial. Establishing this assumption fully may be harder, as it is impacted by our assertion whether the design of the NI trial is similar to those that were used to determine the effect sizes for the standard of care. While establishing the constancy assumption, it is important to separate "failed" NI trials from "negative" NI trials, as the NI trials for which the constancy assumption does not hold are to be recognized as "failed" trials.

The choice of NI margin requires that in order to demonstrate superiority of a new product over placebo, not only does it have to be statistically significant but also clinical relevance have to be shown (ICH, 2000). The consideration of the margin in an NI test is critical. A different choice of NI margin may affect the method of analyzing clinical data and its conclusion. The NI margin should be chosen to satisfy at least the following criteria (D'Agostino et al., 2003):

- We want the ability to claim that the experimental therapy is noninferior to the active control and is superior to placebo (even though a placebo may not be considered in an active control trial).
- The NI margin should be suitably conservative and variability should be taken into account.
- This NI margin cannot be greater than the smallest effect size that the active drug would be reliably expected to have compared with placebo in the setting of a placebo-controlled trial.

The primary purpose of this chapter is to provide a detailed summary of Bayesian methodology and applications in the development of NI trials. Section 11.2 provides practical considerations required for designing NI clinical trials, which includes two important concepts that need to be checked: constancy and assay sensitivity. Section 11.3 includes a discussion on the use of frequentist approaches in NI trials, e.g., fixed margin approach and synthesis method. Section 11.4 provides an exhaustive literature review of Bayesian approaches appropriate for the design and analysis of NI trials (cf. Wellek 2005; Williamson 2007; Osman & Ghosh, 2011). It also includes a discussion on the two procedures that correspond to the frequentist methods described in Section 11.3. Section 11.5 describes a simulation study to compare the performance of the Bayesian method to that of the frequentist method with respect to type I error and power and also contains two case studies on how the Bayesian methodology can be used in practice. We conclude with some discussion and recommendations in Section 11.6.

### 11.1.2 Equivalence versus Noninferiority

In the guidance document "Scientific Considerations in Demonstrating Biosimilarity to a Reference Product" (FDA, 2015), it is suggested that an equivalence design with symmetric inferiority and superiority margins would be used in biosimilar comparative trials. Besides suggesting the use of asymmetric intervals in cases with large upper bounds to rule out superiority rather than lower bounds to rule out inferiority, the guidance also delves into the use of NI design especially in cases where the historical data are established that "doses of a reference product pharmacodynamically saturate the target at the clinical dose level and it would be unethical to use lower than clinically approved doses."

As we will be discussing throughout this chapter, an NI trial is designed to determine whether a new product is not worse than a reference product by more than an acceptable NI margin, *M*. Equivalence trials are similar where equivalence is defined as the treatment effect that exists between $(-M, M)$, where $M$ is the prespecified margin. That is, in equivalence trials, the goal is to rule out all differences of clinical importance between the two products, which is then accomplished by rejecting the null hypothesis that the smallest difference of clinical importance exists in favor of the reference product in terms of a two-sided confidence intervals (CIs) approach. If the equivalence interval $(-M, M)$ contains the two-sided CI, then we reject the null hypothesis and conclude that the two products are equivalent. In the case of NI trials, one has to look at only one side of such a two-sided CI.

So, we have taken the approach of dealing with NI trials as described in the FDA guidance document on demonstrating biosimilarity in this chapter, and Bayesian approaches could provide added benefit in the underlying statistical design and analysis.

## 11.2 Practical Considerations in Designing Noninferiority Trials

There are several statistical issues to consider when designing and analyzing NI trials (Fleming, 2008). These include choice and methods of determining NI margin, choice of active control, biocreep, selection of historical control to estimate the effect of *C*, statistical methods for estimating the effect of *C*, analysis population, and others. We shall address some of these in Sections 11.2.1 through 11.2.3.

### 11.2.1 Choice of Noninferiority Margin

The frequentist approach explicitly uses historical data in NI margin determination but uses it implicitly in the analysis, given the fact that assay sensitivity is assumed. The reliance on available historical information in designing and analyzing an NI trial makes this type of study suitable to the use of a Bayesian statistical approach. The FDA draft guidance mentioned that in deciding on the NI margin, past data can be characterized as prior information in a Bayesian framework, i.e., historical information is explicitly used in both NI margin determination and statistical analysis through prior elicitation.

As described above, the NI study seeks to show that the difference in response between the active control (*C*) and the test drug (*T*) is less than some prespecified NI margin (*M*). *M* can be no larger than the presumed entire effect of the active control in the NI study. This margin is generally referred to as $M_1$. It is critical to reiterate that $M_1$ is not measured in the NI trial, but must be assumed based on past performance of the active control, the comparison of the current NI study with prior studies, and assessment of the quality of the NI study. FDA guidance (2010) also noted that the NI margin can be of smaller value than $M_1$, called $M_2$. Showing NI to $M_1$ would provide assurance that the test drug had an effect greater than zero. However, in many cases there would not be any sufficient assurance that the test drug had a clinically meaningful effect. After all, the reason for using the NI design is the perceived value of the active control drug. It would not usually be acceptable to lose most of that active control's effect in a new drug. It is, therefore, usual in NI studies to choose a smaller margin ($M_2$) that reflects the largest loss of effect that would be clinically acceptable.

### 11.2.2 Choice of Active Control

The active control must be a drug whose effect is well-defined. The most obvious choice is the drug used in the historical placebo-controlled trials. Where studies of several pharmacologically similar drugs have been pooled and the drugs seem to have similar effects, the choice may become complicated. If $T$ is not the first drug to market, then the choice for active control is the drug that has already been approved by the regulatory agency for that region. If there are several drugs already in the market, then the choice may be dependent on the mechanism of action, ease of use, efficacy, and safety profiles as compared to the desired profiles of $T$. In this situation, the determination of active control may become a risk–benefit simulation exercise. The FDA guidance (2001) and EMA guidance (2005) on choice of active control is available for further consideration.

### 11.2.3 Biocreep

A new therapy may be accepted as effective in an NI trial, even if its treatment effect is smaller than the active control. Biocreep is a situation where over time the effect of the new therapy is slightly lower than the preceding therapy, which leads to the degradation of treatment effects. D'Agostino et al. (2003) mentioned biocreep as a concern related to the choice of NI margins. Everson-Stewart (2010) stated that there are several factors that may influence the rate at which biocreep occurs, including the distribution of the effects of the new agents being tested and how that changes over time, the choice of active comparator, the method used to account for the variability of the estimate of the active comparator effect, and changes in the effect of the active comparator from one trial to the other (violations of the constancy assumption). Everson-Stewart (2010) performed a simulation study to examine which of these factors might lead to biocreep and found that biocreep was rare, except when the constancy assumption was violated.

## 11.3 Review of Frequentist Approaches

In the FDA's draft guidance for NI studies, there are two approaches to test the NI: one is fixed margin approach, and another one is synthesis method.

### 11.3.1 Fixed Margin Approach

Suppose $\theta_T$ and $\theta_C$ are the true treatment responses for test and active control, respectively, and if a large value represents a better efficacy, then an NI hypothesis can be

$$H_0: \theta_T - \theta_C < -M \quad \text{versus} \quad H_1: \theta_T - \theta_C \geq -M, \tag{11.1}$$

where $M$ is a prespecified fixed margin for NI. Note that the NI hypothesis is one-sided in nature, and as a result, it is common to test the hypothesis at $\alpha / 2$ significance level or say, 0.025. If $\theta_P$ is the true treatment response for placebo, the fixed margin can be written as $M = f(\theta_C - \theta_P) = f\gamma_{CP}$, where $f$ is a value between 0 and 1 and $\gamma_{CP}$ is the true treatment effect of $C$ compared with $P$. In real clinical trials, however, the true treatment effect for the active control, $\gamma_{CP}$, is unknown. Although historical study data for the active control may be available, it is still a challenge to get a "good" estimate for the treatment effect. A conservative estimate of $\gamma_{CP}$, using normal approximation, is to use the lower bound of the 95% CI around its estimate, $\hat{\gamma}_{CP} - t_{\alpha/2}\sqrt{\text{var}(\hat{\gamma}_{CP})}$, as its assumed effect, where $\hat{\gamma}_{CP}$ and $\text{var}(\hat{\gamma}_{CP})$ are point estimate and variance for the treatment effect for $C$ against $P$ from previous studies, respectively, and $t_{\alpha/2}$ is the $(1-\alpha / 2)$th quantile of the $t$-distribution. Furthermore, since $M$ can be no larger than this entire assumed effect of the active control in the NI study and it is usually and generally desirable to choose a smaller value which takes a fraction $f$ of the assumed effect, $M$ can be chosen as $M = f(\hat{\gamma}_{CP} - t_{\alpha/2}\sqrt{\text{var}(\hat{\gamma}_{CP})})$. Hence, the corresponding test statistic is given by

$$T_1 = \frac{\hat{\gamma}_{TC} + f(\hat{\gamma}_{CP} - t_{\alpha/2}\sqrt{\text{var}(\hat{\gamma}_{CP})})}{\sqrt{\text{var}(\hat{\gamma}_{TC})}}. \tag{11.2}$$

Hence, the null hypothesis $H_0: \theta_T - \theta_C < -M$ is rejected if

$$\frac{\hat{\gamma}_{TC} + f\hat{\gamma}_{CP}}{\sqrt{\text{var}(\hat{\gamma}_{TC})} + f\sqrt{\text{var}(\hat{\gamma}_{CP})}} > t_{\alpha/2}. \tag{11.3}$$

By rejecting the null hypothesis, one can conclude NI.

It is also common to refer to the fixed margin method as the two CI method, since the method uses two CIs: one to estimate the effect size and the other one for testing the null hypothesis. As a result, it is also called a 95%–95% method (Hung et al., 2009).

In terms of CIs, this approach can easily be explained in terms of an example. It is given (Deng, 2014) that a thrombolytic therapy, mostly administered up to 6 hours after ischemic stroke, significantly reduced the proportion of death or dependent at 3–6 months after stroke based on a modified Rankin score (odds ratio [OR]: 0.81 with a 95% CI: 0.72, 0.90). Using the upper 95% CI of 0.90, the treatment effect of the existing thrombolytic agent is 1 – 0.90 = 0.10 in reducing death.

Suppose we plan to do a trial to compare the new thrombolytic agent with an existing one and we would like to preserve 50% of the treatment effect. Under this scenario, the NI margin of OR would be calculated as

$$\frac{\text{New thrombolytic agent/Placebo}}{\text{Existing thrombolytic agent/Placebo}} = 0.90 + 0.10 / 20.90 = 1.06. \quad (11.4)$$

So, the NI margin can be considered as 1.06 for this analysis. For this example, once the trial is done, we will need to calculate the 95% CI for OR (new agent/existing agent) and compare the upper bound of this 95% CI with the NI margin 1.06. The NI can be declared if the upper bound of this 95% CI is below the NI margin.

### 11.3.2 Synthesis Approach

In the synthesis approach, the NI hypothesis takes the following form.

$$H_0 : \theta_T - \theta_C < -f(\theta_C - \theta_P) \quad \text{versus} \quad H_1 : \theta_T - \theta_C \geq -f(\theta_C - \theta_P), \quad (11.5)$$

i.e., both treatment effect parameters $\gamma_{TC}$ and $\gamma_{CP}$, comparing $T$ with $C$ and $C$ with $P$, respectively, are treated as unknown. Thus, the testing procedure involves directly combining the point estimate and variance of the treatment effect between $T$ and $C$ from the NI trial and variance of the treatment effect of $C$ versus $P$ from historical trials. A statistical test will combine data from the historical studies of $C$ to the current NI study for inference. As in the case of the fixed NI margin approach, this approach also requires a constancy assumption that the true treatment effects for $C$ and $P$ remain the same as in the historical studies. In this setting, the test statistic is given by

$$T_2 = \frac{\hat{\gamma}_{TC} + f\hat{\gamma}_{CP}}{\sqrt{\text{var}(\hat{\gamma}_{TC}) + f^2 \text{var}(\hat{\gamma}_{CP})}}. \quad (11.6)$$

Under the normal approximation, the null hypothesis is rejected if $T_2 > t_{\alpha/2}$ or

$$\frac{\hat{\gamma}_{TC} + f\hat{\gamma}_{CP}}{\sqrt{\text{var}(\hat{\gamma}_{TC}) + f^2 \text{var}(\hat{\gamma}_{CP})}} > t_{\alpha/2}. \quad (11.7)$$

The two frequentist approaches—fixed margin and synthesis—are intrinsically different. The fixed margin method is a conditional approach, where the determination of the NI margin is based on historical data. But the synthesis method is unconditional in the sense that it treats the difference between the standard and placebo from historical data as a parameter and then factors the variability into the test statistic. Note that the forms of Equations 11.3 and 11.6 imply that the synthesis approach is always more efficient than the fixed margin test. The comparison between the two frequentist approaches becomes more subtle as the type I error associated with each test is different. The fixed margin method controls a type I error rate within the NI study for a prespecified fixed NI margin, which is determined from historical trials of the active control. The synthesis method controls an unconditional error rate for the null hypothesis provided that data from the historical studies for the active control were treated similarly as in the current NI study.

In addition to differences in the type I error rate, the synthesis method also has other limitations as noted by Ng (2015): it may not provide independent evidence of treatment effect since it uses the same historical data unconditionally. Similarities between the two methods were discussed by Hauck and Anderson (1999), who presented confidence levels to estimate the treatment difference between standard and placebo based on historical data, assuming that the constancy holds. Further details and discussions can be found in draft FDA guidance document (2010), Snapinn (2004), and Snapinn and Jiang (2008).

### 11.3.3 Remarks

The choice of statistical methods for testing NI hypothesis may depend on the endpoint and measure of treatment difference. For example, in studies with continuous endpoint, common statistical models such as analysis of covariance (ANCOVA) or mixed effects models for longitudinal data analysis can be used to estimate the treatment difference and associated CI. In survival studies, the hazard ratio or log-hazard difference is often used for treatment comparison and uses Cox proportional hazard models to estimate the treatment difference and associated CI. Similar to the continuous endpoint, a $p$-value for the NI test can be obtained from the one-sided test for the log-hazard difference with a shift of corresponding fixed margin. More details can be found in the literatures of Chang (2007), Neuenschwander et al. (2011), and Burger et al. (2011). For comparing two binary outcomes, many methods can be used to calculate the CI for the proportion difference. Newcombe (1998) evaluated 11 methods and concluded that the asymptotic method by Miettinen and Nurminen (1985) is one of the methods which provided relatively good performance. Logistic regression is also often used to estimate the treatment difference and associated CI. In addition, other metrics such as relative risk (RR), $RR = \theta_T/\theta_C$ and OR, $OR = \theta_T(1-\theta_C)/\theta_C(1-\theta_T)$, may also be considered. Note that using these transformation metrics, the hypothesis stated in Equation 11.1 can be generalized such that $H_0: g(\theta_T) - g(\theta_C) \leq -M$ versus $H_0: g(\theta_T) - g(\theta_C) > -M$, where $g(\theta) = \log(\theta)$ for RR or $g(\theta) = \log(\theta / (1-\theta)$ for OR. The RR is often considered when the response rates are relatively small because it becomes more sensitive. The fixed margin for RR is set to exclude a prespecified amount of fold decline from the response rate of the control. A statistical method proposed by Miettinen and Nurminen (1985) can also be used to get the CI of the RR to test NI. The OR, on the other hand, is another metric of treatment difference for comparing two response rates and can be evaluated using the Miettinen and Nurminen (1985) method. Under this metric, a logistic regression model may be used to construct the CI of the log OR. One advantage of this regression model is that it can easily include other covariates into the regression model for adjustment:

$$\alpha = \sqrt{\beta}. \tag{11.8}$$

The choice of metric will not only depend on the consistency found in historical studies but also on the relevancy in the current trial.

### 11.3.4 Challenges in Designing Noninferiority Trials

It is noted in Section 11.3.3 that the hypothesis for an NI trial can be written in terms of risk ratio $H_0: \log(T/C) \geq (1-\lambda)\log(P/C)$, where *T/C* is the risk ratio of the test drug (*T*) versus control (*C*) and $\lambda$ gets into displaying the percent retention. Under this scenario, an NI margin $\delta$ will be chosen as $(1-\lambda)\log(P/C)$, where *P* is the placebo effect. From this, it is worthwhile to note that the true margin that needs to be ruled out, namely, $\delta$, depends on the risk ratio *C/P* and $\lambda$. On the other hand, in order to make a subjective selection of $\lambda$, one needs to have a knowledge of the risk ratio, which in most is not estimable. As a result, one may have to depend on historical trials to bridge the information to the current NI trials and thus obtain information on the risk ratio, that is, one must attempt to get an estimate of the risk ratio *P/C* from historical trials. A couple of approaches that are useful in this regard are a fixed effect or a random effects approach. Similar challenges may also be found using the Bayesian approach as noted in Section 11.4.

## 11.4 Use of Bayesian Approaches in Noninferiority Trials

### 11.4.1 Review

The literature on the use of Bayesian methods has grown in the last few years due to recent advances in Bayesian computation using Markov Chain Monte Carlo (MCMC) approaches. A Bayesian approach has the important advantage of accounting for various sources of uncertainty and allows incorporating prior information. It circumvents the difficulties encountered with traditional methods for hypothesis testing, as the hypotheses of interest are assessed based on the posterior probability distribution and not the $p$-values that are often misinterpreted. Using the MCMC computation techniques, these posterior distributions can be computed efficiently and accurately using simulation-based methods, and inference relating to NI testing can proceed without resorting to asymptotic theory and is useful with small sample studies. Furthermore, as NI trial involves treatments that have been well studied in the past, a Bayesian approach that lends itself to incorporating such information with ease presents a natural advantage over a frequentist approach.

Gamalo et al. (2015) provides a detailed summary of Bayesian methods for the design and analysis of NI trials. The paper also describes a simulation study to compare the performance of the Bayesian method to that of the frequentist method with respect to type I error and power and also contains two case studies on how the Bayesian methodology can be used in practice.

Based on a Bayesian framework for dichotomous data, Wellek (2005) suggested a test using posterior probability of the alternative hypothesis with Jeffrey's prior distribution for the two proportions. A Jeffrey's prior is a noninformative prior on the parameter space that is proportional to the square root of the determinant of the Fisher information matrix. For his analysis, Wellek considered three different measures: absolute difference, RR, and OR.

Williamson (2007) proposed a test based on Bayes factor for equivalence hypotheses. As noted above, Bayes tests compare the posterior probability of the competing hypotheses when prior probability of the hypotheses are chosen to be unequal. A Bayes factor, which is defined as the ratio of posterior odds of the hypotheses to the corresponding prior odds, can also be used to measure the evidence against (or in favor of) the null hypothesis. Osman and Ghosh (2011) proposed a more detailed investigation on the use of Bayes factor for NI trials with dichotomous data. The key aspect of their approach includes a determination of the threshold or critical value of the Bayes factor used in the decision rule. Instead of being prespecified to some fixed value, the critical value of the Bayes factor is determined using a criterion that approximately maintains the frequentist type I error rate to a desired level. Consequently, the cutoff value of the Bayes factor in the decision rule will depend on the design parameters like the sample size and the NI margin. In addition, they have also considered another approach based on posterior probability with different prior specifications than the one given in Wellek (2005). Based on extensive simulation, they have shown that their approaches provide improvement in terms of statistical power as compared to the frequentist approaches proposed by Blackwelder (1982). Their simulation has also shown that the Bayesian approaches have almost uniformly lower total error rate (type I + type II error) than the frequentist method by a very large margin.

For binary data, a parametric conjugate Beta prior is typically chosen for computational convenience, which often gets criticized by many non-Bayesian practitioners. Osman and Ghosh (2011) developed a class of semi-parametric conjugate priors using a suitable mixture of Beta densities. Again based on Bayes factor, they have proposed a hybrid Bayesian/frequentist approach, which uses Bayes factor as a measure of evidence against the null hypothesis while controlling both type I and II errors for determining a cut-off value for decision making.

It is straightforward to extend these models for continuous outcome using the proper link function (Chen et al., 2011).

### 11.4.2 Hierarchical Priors Approach

Gamalo et al. (2011, 2012, 2013) recently proposed a Bayes procedure that is analogous to the fixed margin described in Section 11.3.1. In this method, historical information is incorporated into active control via the use of informative priors. In particular, they assumed the posteriors of the response in historical trials as priors for its corresponding parameters in the current trial, where the corresponding treatment serves as an active control. For instance, suppose that both $\theta_T$ and $\theta_C$ have informative priors $\theta_T \sim N\left(\theta_T^*, \sigma_T^{*2}\right)$ and $\theta_C \sim N\left(\theta_C^*, \sigma_C^{*2}\right)$, which are obtained from the conditional posterior density functions (PDFs) in the meta-analysis of available historical information about the treatments. Note that these distributions can be discounted to a certain degree (see Gamalo et al., 2012; Kirby et al., 2012; and further discussion within this section.). Then, given current data $\bar{X}_t$, $t \in \{T, C\}$, $\theta_T$, and $\theta_C$ have similar (marginal) posterior distributions of the form

$$\theta_t \mid \bar{X}_t, \sigma_t^2 \sim N(\tilde{\theta}_t, \tilde{\sigma}_t^2) \tag{11.9}$$

and

$$\tilde{\theta}_t = \tilde{\sigma}_t^2\left(\frac{n_t \bar{X}_t}{\sigma_t^2} + \frac{\theta_t^*}{\sigma_t^{*2}}\right), \tilde{\sigma}_t^2 = \left(\frac{n_t}{\sigma_t^2} + \frac{1}{\sigma_t^{*2}}\right)^{-1} \tag{11.10}$$

and $\theta_T$ and $\theta_C$ are independent. The posterior distribution of $(\theta_T - \theta_C)$ is

$$(\theta_T - \theta_C) \mid \bar{X}_T, \bar{X}_C, \sigma_T^2, \sigma_C^2 \sim N\left(\tilde{\theta}_T - \tilde{\theta}_C, \tilde{\sigma}_T^2 + \tilde{\sigma}_C^2\right). \tag{11.11}$$

For the unknown variances in Equation 11.11, they assumed that $\sigma_C^2$ and $\sigma_T^2$ are independent and have Jeffrey's noninformative priors, i.e., $\pi(\sigma_C^2) \propto \sigma_C^{-2}$ and $\pi(\sigma_T^2) \propto \sigma_T^{-2}$. Then, $\sigma_C^2$ and $\sigma_T^2$ are also independent a posteriori, and their posterior distributions conditional on $\theta_C$ and $\theta_T$, respectively, are inverse-gamma (IG) distributions

$$\mathrm{IG}\left(\frac{n_{\mathrm{C}}}{2},\frac{1}{2}\sum_{i=1}^{n_{\mathrm{C}}}(X_{\mathrm{C},i}-\theta_{\mathrm{C}})^2\right),\mathrm{IG}\left(\frac{n_{\mathrm{T}}}{2},\frac{1}{2}\sum_{i=1}^{n_{\mathrm{T}}}(X_{\mathrm{T},i}-\theta_{\mathrm{T}})^2\right), \tag{11.12}$$

where $X_{t,i}$ are individual observations in treatment group $t$. Finally, they defined the decision rule for deciding that the experimental treatment is noninferior to the active comparator in preserving a fraction, $1-M$, of the treatment effect of the active comparator if

$$\Pr(\theta_{\mathrm{T}}-\theta_{\mathrm{C}}\geq -M\mid \bar{X}_{\mathrm{T}},\bar{X}_{\mathrm{C}},\sigma_{\mathrm{T}}^2,\sigma_{\mathrm{C}}^2)=\Pr\left(T\geq\frac{-M-(\tilde{\theta}_{\mathrm{T}}-\tilde{\theta}_{\mathrm{C}})}{\left(\tilde{\sigma}_{\mathrm{T}}^2+\tilde{\sigma}_{\mathrm{C}}^2\right)^{\frac{1}{2}}}\right)\geq p^*, \tag{11.13}$$

where $p^*$ is prespecified, such as $p^*=\alpha/2$ or any other clinically reasonable values or $p^*$ can be determined so that the type I error rate is controlled at some level $\alpha$. This rule can be evaluated using MCMC simulations. Equivalently, if $\tilde{\gamma}_{TC}=\tilde{\theta}_T-\tilde{\theta}_C$, $\mathrm{var}(\tilde{\gamma}_{TC})=\tilde{\sigma}_T^2+\tilde{\sigma}_C^2$, $M=f(\hat{\gamma}_{CP}-t_{\alpha/2}\sqrt{\mathrm{var}(\hat{\gamma}_{CP})})$, and $p^*=\alpha/2$, then the decision rule can also be written as

$$\frac{\tilde{\gamma}_{TC}+f\hat{\gamma}_{CP}}{\sqrt{\mathrm{var}(\tilde{\gamma}_{TC})}+f\sqrt{\mathrm{var}(\hat{\gamma}_{CP})}}>t_{\alpha/2}, \tag{11.14}$$

which resembles the fixed margin rule given in Equation 11.3.

This setup can also be extended to account for the amount of historical information that can be borrowed in the NI trials. Note that population parameters may change over time, over various study settings, and in many unobservable ways, resulting in some studies that are more reliable than others. Hence, the maximum information a historical dataset can provide is when it is used without discounting. This information, although, can be controlled when the likelihood function of the historical data, $\bar{\mathbf{X}}^H=(X^{H_1},\ldots,X^{H_k})$ is raised to a suitable power parameter $\boldsymbol{a}=(a_1,\ldots,a_k)$. Then given $\boldsymbol{a}=(a_1,\ldots,a_k)'$, $0<a_i<1, i=1,\ldots,k$,

$$\theta\sim q_0(\theta_0\mid\bar{\mathbf{X}}^H,\sigma_1^2,\ldots,\sigma_k^2,\boldsymbol{a})\propto\prod_{i=1}^{k}\left[L(\theta_0\mid\bar{X}^{H_i},\sigma_i^2,a_i)\right]^{a_i}\pi_0(\theta_0) \tag{11.15}$$

is called the power prior for $\theta=(\theta_T,\theta_C)$ (Ibrahim & Chen, 2000). If $L(\theta_0\mid\bar{X}^{H_i},\sigma_i^2,a_i)=N(\theta_0,\sigma_i^2)$ and $\pi_0(\theta_0)$ is noninformative, notice that $q(\theta_0\mid\bar{\mathbf{X}}^H,\sigma_1^2,\ldots,\sigma_k^2,\gamma)$ is proportional to the product of $k$ likelihoods, each of which is $N(\theta_0,\sigma_i^2/a_i)$, $i=1,\ldots,k$; hence, the parameter $a_i$ can be interpreted as a precision parameter for the historical data; i.e., since the variances of the historical data are increased, $a_i$ controls the heaviness of the tail of the prior for $\theta$. As the $a_i$'s become smaller, the tail of Equation 11.15 becomes heavier. In fact, when $a_i = 0$, for all $i$, then the power prior corresponds to just the prior of $q_0$, which is $\pi_0(\theta_0)$. Setting $a_1 = 1$, for all $i$ corresponds to full updating of $\theta_0$ using Bayes theorem. Furthermore, choosing $a_i$ can be data driven using another hyperprior, $a_i \sim \text{Beta}(\xi, \eta)$. Hence, the marginal posterior distribution of $\theta_t$ is as follows:

$$\theta_t \sim q(\theta_t \mid \bar{X}, \sigma_t^2, \bar{\boldsymbol{X}}^H, \sigma_1^2, \ldots, \sigma_k^2, \boldsymbol{a}) \propto L(\theta_t \mid \bar{X}, \sigma_t^2)] \prod_{i=1}^{k} \left[L(\theta_0 \mid \bar{X}^{H_i}, \sigma_i^2, a_i)\right]^{a_i} \pi_0(\theta_0). \tag{11.16}$$

More generally, the likelihood of the joint parameter $\theta$ can be written similarly, i.e.,

$$\theta \sim \theta(\theta \mid \bar{X}, \sigma_T^2, \sigma_C^2, \bar{\boldsymbol{X}}^H, \sigma_1^2, \ldots, \sigma_k^2, \boldsymbol{a}) \propto L(\theta_t \mid \bar{X}, \sigma_t^2)] \prod_{i=1}^{k} \left[L(\theta_0 \mid \bar{X}^{H_i}, \sigma_i^2, a_i)\right]^{a_i} \pi_0(\theta_0), \tag{11.17}$$

which Chen et al. (2011) developed for sample size determination involved in clinical trials with NI hypothesis.

Another modification to the basic power prior formulation, called local commensurate priors (Hobbs et al., 2012), can be used to obtain the prior for $\theta$. This prior adjusts the power parameter prior conditionally through a measure of the degree to which the historical and current data are commensurate. If $\theta_0$ is the parameter from the historical data, this prior extends the hierarchical model (Equation 11.13) to include a parameter that measures the evidence for commensurability between $\theta$ and $\theta_0$.

### 11.4.3 Meta-Analytic Predictive Approach: Indirect Comparison to Placebo Based on Historical Trials

Simon (1999) used a Bayesian approach for the inference on the minimal efficacy requirement in NI trials. The simplest setup is illustrated in Table 11.1, where $m$ historical trials are available comparing the active control ($C$) with placebo ($P$). Conceptually, the NI trial also contains a placebo arm with corresponding parameter $\theta_P$, for which no data is available. The test drug ($T$) is superior to placebo in the NI trial if $\theta_T - \theta_P > 0$ (assuming larger values of $\theta$ correspond to better efficacy). It should be noted that

$$\theta_T - \theta_P = (\theta_T - \theta_C) + (\theta_C - \theta_P). \tag{11.18}$$

Inference on $\theta_T - \theta_C$ can be directly obtained from the data of the NI trial, denoted by $X_T$ and $X_C$, respectively. For inference on $\theta_C - \theta_P$, external

**TABLE 11.1**

Posterior Probability Thresholds ($p^*$), Type I Error, and Power

| *N*/Group | Scenario | Frequentist | Bayesian MI[a] Beta Prior | Bayesian Power Prior ($a_0 = 0.5$) | Bayesian Power Prior ($a_0 = 1$) |
|---|---|---|---|---|---|
| Posterior probability threshold ($p^*$) | | | | | |
| 200 | A | NA | 0.9800 | 0.9900 | 0.9940 |
| 400 | A | NA | 0.9700 | 0.9820 | 0.9900 |
| Type I error | | | | | |
| 200 | A | 0.037 | 0.028 | 0.030 | 0.028 |
| | B | 0.037 | 0.042 | 0.102 | 0.266 |
| 400 | A | 0.028 | 0.033 | 0.033 | 0.030 |
| | B | 0.028 | 0.040 | 0.092 | 0.205 |
| Power | | | | | |
| 200 | A | 0.525 | 0.499 | 0.567 | 0.622 |
| | B | 0.525 | 0.572 | 0.847 | 0.968 |
| 400 | A | 0.811 | 0.855 | 0.881 | 0.895 |
| | B | 0.811 | 0.882 | 0.959 | 0.994 |

*Notes:* MI, mildly informative; NA, not applicable.

[a] MI, e.g., Beta (4,6)

information is needed, usually from several historical trials comparing active control and placebo, using a model that links the parameters.

Simon (1999) essentially made the strict constancy assumption, i.e., the true treatment effects for $C$ and $P$ remain the same as in the historical studies:

$$\theta_C - \theta_P = (\theta_C^1 - \theta_P^1) = \ldots = (\theta_C^m - \theta_P^m) = \delta_{CP}. \tag{11.19}$$

A common-effects meta-analysis of the historical trials with data $\boldsymbol{X}^H$ provides information on the posterior distribution $P(\delta_{CP} \mid \boldsymbol{X}^H)$, which can then be used as the prior for $(\theta_C - \theta_P)$ due to the constancy assumption. From this, the posterior $P(\theta_T - \theta_P \mid X_T, X_C, \boldsymbol{X}^H)$ is then easily calculated. The regulatory context where this approach was used is described in Durrleman and Chaikin (2003). In the frequentist framework, the corresponding approach is called the synthesis approach or putative placebo approach (Fisher et al., 2001; Hasselblad & Kong, 2001; Rothmann et al., 2003; Snapinn & Jiang, 2008); for more information, refer to Section 11.3.2.

The main assumption used for inference on Equation 11.19 is the strict constancy assumption, which may not always be appropriate. A more realistic model would allow for between-trial variability, replacing Equation 11.17 with

$$(\theta_C - \theta_P), (\theta_C^1 - \theta_P^1), \ldots, (\theta_C^m - \theta_P^m) \sim N(\mu_{CP}, \tau^2). \tag{11.20}$$

With this model, the true difference between $C$ and $P$ is allowed to vary from trial to trial around the population mean difference $\mu_{CP}$. Note that the strict constancy assumption corresponds to a between-trial standard deviation of $\tau = 0$. For model Equation 11.18, a prior for $\theta_C - \theta_P$ is obtained by a random effects meta-analysis of the historical trials and a prediction of $\theta_C - \theta_P$, using a meta-analytic predictive approach (Spiegelhalter et al., 2004; Schmidli et al., 2013).

The basic setup considered here can be extended in various directions. In some cases, only single-arm trials on placebo may be available, where Bayesian models for historical controls can be used (Pocock, 1976; Gould, 1991; Ibrahim & Chen, 2000; Neuenschwander et al., 2010; Hobbs et al., 2012; Gsteiger et al., 2013; Schmidli et al., 2014). In other cases, many historical trials directly or indirectly related to the active control or placebo can be considered for inference in an NI trial (Schmidli et al., 2013), using network meta-analytic methods (Higgins & Whitehead, 1996; Lu & Ades, 2004; Salanti et al., 2008). More complex meta-regression models relating historical trials and the NI trial may also be necessary in some cases, for example, when treatments consist of combinations of several drugs (Witte et al., 2011). Similarly, time trends could also be included in the models. Bayesian methods are particularly well suited for such evidence synthesis, and hence seem very attractive to use in the NI context.

### 11.4.4 Sample Size

The frequentist power calculation is usually under the Neyman–Pearson hypothesis testing framework: one needs to control the type I error rate at a fixed level if the null hypothesis is true, and the sample size is to achieve certain percentage of power, i.e., 1—type II error under a specific alternative hypothesis with certain assumptions (Julious and Owen, 2011). From a Bayesian perspective, as the unknown is described through a probability model, the type I and type II error rates are not fixed either. In that sense, the type I error rate should be calculated for the whole region where the null hypothesis is true, rather than a single point. Based on such views, Reyes and Ghosh (2013) proposed to minimize the weighted sum of type I and type II error rates, where the error rates are defined in the whole null/alternative region. Using the Bayes factor as test statistics, they argued that each different weighting corresponds to a different cutoff, and the sample size then can be calculated based on this cutoff. Osman and Ghosh (2011) argued that for NI trials with binary endpoints where a Bernstein mixture of Beta prior is applied, minimizing the weighted type I and type II error gives more power when the sample size is small, compared to the frequentist approach with similar type I error rate.

Daimon (2008) compared three strategies of sample size calculation for NI trials with two proportions compared: the hybrid of Neyman–Pearson and Bayesian; the Bayesian conditional probability approach, which is conditional

Assuming that an NI margin of 0.1 is clinically meaningful and a true response rate for the control treatment of 0.6, the following scenarios were considered:

1. The response rate from $C$ of the historical data is 0.6, i.e., it is consistent with $C$ in the current trial data and considered a mildly informative (MI) prior of Beta(6,4) as well as a power prior of the form

$$\pi(p_c \mid D_0, a_0) \propto L(p_C \mid D_0)^{a0}\, \pi_0(p_C \mid a_0), \tag{11.24}$$

where historical data is denoted by $D_0$ instead of $\bar{\mathbf{X}}^H$, which is generally used for historical data composed of sample means. Furthermore, set $\pi_0 = 1$, i.e., assume that the prior for $p_C$ in the historical trials is noninformative. Lastly, assume that the sample size for the historical data was 100 and the values for $a_0$ are 0.5 and 1. Note that $a_0 = 1$ corresponds to a highly informative power prior.

2. The response rate from $C$ of the historical data is 0.4, i.e., it is lower than what was observed in the current trial and considers an MI prior of Beta(4,6) as well as a power prior as stated in scenario A.

In both scenarios, for $T$, consider a noninformative Beta(1,1) prior. To evaluate the type I error rate, data are simulated by setting $p_T = 0.5$ and $p_C = 0.6$, where the difference is equal to the NI margin. To evaluate power, data are simulated by setting $p_T = p_C = 0.6$. The frequentist comparison was based on a one-sided test with $\alpha = 0.025$.

Notice that the posterior probability thresholds for the Bayesian methods depend on the sample size and the prior and should be determined via simulation so that the type I error rate is controlled at the one-sided $\alpha = 0.025$ level (see Table 11.1). For a smaller sample size, the power of the Bayesian method with an MI prior is comparable to the power of the frequentist method, but with a larger sample size, the power of the Bayesian method with an MI prior is greater than that of the frequentist method. For scenario A, where the response rate for the control group in the historical data is consistent with the control response rate in the current study, the Bayesian method with the power prior is substantially more powerful than the frequentist method and the Bayesian method with an MI prior and the power increases as $a_0$ increases. For scenario B, where the response rate from the control group of the historical data is lower than that of the current trial, the Bayesian method with the power prior is substantially more powerful than the frequentist method and the Bayesian method with an MI prior, but these results should be interpreted with caution. This is because the lower response rate in the control group of the historical data is influencing the posterior distribution of the response rate in the control group and causing it to be lower, which helps achieve NI for the test treatment. Hence in the situation where we are uncertain about the response rate, a noninformative or MI prior should be suggested.

Numerical explorations for the method described in Section 11.4.3 are not performed. Essentially, since the method includes the variance/covariance of the treatments groups among all historical trials, it will always be more conservative than the synthesis approach described in Section 11.3.2.

### 11.5.2 Case Example of Using Hierarchical Priors Method for Vaccine Trials

In this example, a Bayesian analysis is used on two NI trials for a vaccine. In each of these studies, subjects were randomly assigned to receive test vaccine and another vaccine together (concomitant use group) or to receive test vaccine and the other vaccine separately about a month apart (staggered use group). Antibody titers were measured at baseline and 4 weeks postvaccination. Higher antibody titers is a favorable response. The primary objective was to show the antibody response in the concomitant use group would be noninferior to that in the staggered use group. The statistical hypothesis is $H_0 : \text{GMT}_1 / \text{GMT}_2 \leq M$ versus $H_1 : \text{GMT}_1 / \text{GMT}_2 > M$, where $\text{GMT}_1$ and $\text{GMT}_2$ are the geometric mean titer for the test vaccine in the concomitant use group and the staggered use (control) group, respectively. The margin $M$ is set to be 0.67, which is a common fixed NI margin for GMT comparisons in vaccine studies.

The outcomes of the original studies are such that the first study was positive and second study was negative. For the primary analysis, a frequentist approach via constrained longitudinal data analysis model (Liang and Zeger, 2000, Liu et al., 2009) was used on the natural log-transformed titer at baseline and postvaccination. Specifically,

$$\begin{bmatrix} Y_{i0} \\ Y_{i1} \end{bmatrix} \sim N\left(\begin{bmatrix} \mu_{i0} \\ \mu_{i1} \end{bmatrix}, \Sigma\right), \tag{11.25}$$

where $Y_{i0}$ and $Y_{i1}$ are log-transformed titer values at baseline and postvaccination, respectively, and $\mu_{i0} = \theta + \beta z_i$, $\mu_{i1} = \theta + \beta z_i + \gamma(1 - x_i) + \delta x_i$, where $x_i$ is a treatment group indicator (1 for the concomitant use group and 0 for the control group) and $z_i$ is patients' age at randomization. So $\theta$ is the constraint overall baseline mean, $\beta$ is the slope for age, $\gamma$ is the change from baseline mean for the control group, and $\Sigma$ is a $2 \times 2$ covariance matrix.

The frequentist analysis was based on SAS PROC MIXED procedure. The NI is claimed if the lower bound of the 95% CI for the *GMT* ratio, $\exp(\delta - \gamma)$, is greater than 0.67.

We consider a Bayesian analysis method for this model and assume each of the mean parameters follows a normal prior distribution (conjugate prior) and the covariance matrix $\Sigma$ follows an inverse Wishart distribution. First, noninformative priors were used for each of the mean parameters, i.e., $\theta$, $\beta$, $\gamma$, $\delta \sim N(0, 100^2)$ and $\Sigma \sim$ invWishart with a degrees of freedom of 2 and a precision parameter of 0.0001. The Bayesian analysis results are obtained from 5000 posterior samples from SAS PROC MCMC. Table 11.2 shows the mean and 95% credible interval from the posterior samples. The results are almost the same as the primary analysis results obtained from the maximum likelihood method from SAS PROC MIXED. The code is available upon request from the authors.

Now consider using informative prior to incorporate previous study data available for the staggered use group. First, estimates for baseline and change from baseline were obtained from a completed historical study. We construct the prior from a normal distribution with mean and standard deviation as estimated for the corresponding parameter from the historical study. To discount the information directly from the historical study, we consider a

**TABLE 11.2**

Noninferiority Analysis on Antibody Responses for Two Vaccine Studies

| | Concomitant Group Estimated GMT[a] | Staggered Group Estimated GMT[a] | Estimated GMT Ratio[a] (95% CI[a]) | Conclusion[b] |
|---|---|---|---|---|
| *Study 1* | | | | |
| Mixed model | 553.6 | 596.0 | 0.93 (0.84, 1.03) | Yes |
| Noninformative prior ($a = 0$ and $b = 0$) | 554.9 | 596.7 | 0.93 (0.84, 1.03) | Yes |
| Power prior with $a = 1$ and $b = 1/4$ | 573.8 | 568.8 | 1.01 (0.92, 1.12) | Yes |
| Power prior with $a = 1$ and $b = 1/10$ | 571.3 | 590.2 | 0.97 (0.87, 1.07) | Yes |
| *Study 2* | | | | |
| Mixed model | 340.9 | 489.1 | 0.70 (0.61, 0.80) | No |
| Bayesian with noninformative prior | 341.2 | 490.2 | 0.70 (0.61, 0.80) | No |
| Power prior with $a = 1$ and $b = 1/4$ | 404.1 | 490.0 | 0.83 (0.73, 0.93) | Yes |
| Power prior with $a = 1/20$ and $b = 1/20$ | 351.9 | 472.0 | 0.75 (0.65, 0.85) | No |
| Power prior with $a = 1/20$ and $b = 1/50$ | 349.4 | 486.5 | 0.72 (0.63, 0.82) | No |

*Notes:* CI, confidence interval; GMT, geometric mean titer.

[a] GMT = GMT is estimated from the constraint longitudinal analysis.

[b] Noninferiority is concluded if the lower bound CI is greater than 0.67.

power prior, that is, $\theta \sim [f(\theta)]^a$ and $\gamma \sim [g(\gamma)]^b$, where $f(\theta)$ and $g(\gamma)$ are normal density functions estimated from the completed study data, and $a$ and $b$ are prespecified power parameters. For the covariance parameter $\Sigma$, we also used the estimated variance covariance matrix historical study as the parameter in the inverse Wishart prior. For other parameters, $\beta$ and $\delta$, noninformative priors are used because the information is not available from the historical trial. The analysis results with different values for $a$ and $b$ are presented in Table 11.2.

Initially, power prior parameters were set at $a = 1$ and $b = 1/4$. It was expected that the baseline values among these three studies (two current studies and one historical study) would be very similar so that $a = 1$. For the change from baseline parameter (i.e., vaccine response), $b = 1/4$ was used, as the vaccine response in the new studies may be different from the historical study. One assumption made on using informative prior is that the response observed in the current study would be similar to or consistent with the specified prior distribution. To check this assumption, a plot of the density of the estimated parameters from the current study against the power prior distribution is shown (Figure 11.1). When the density curves between estimated and

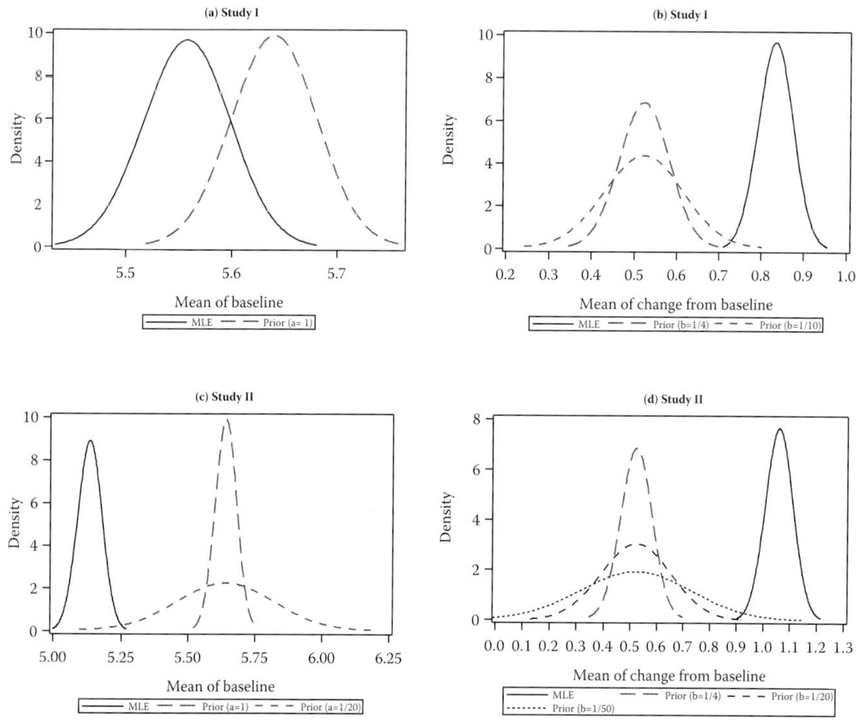


**FIGURE 11.1**
Density plots for maximum likelihood function and power prior from the completed study.

a specified prior distribution have some overlap, we may believe that there is some consistency between the current data and the prior distribution. With this rough guidance, we arbitrarily select a few values of $a$ and $b$ to illustrate the idea. The results in Table 11.2 and Figure 11.1 showed the following:

1. For Study I, the estimated *GMT* ratios with the informative prior are closer to 1.0 compared with that from the noninformative prior. Therefore, the Bayesian analysis with informative prior strengthens the NI test. Overall, the results are robust and the conclusions for the NI testing are the same with different power prior.
2. For Study II, however, the conclusion can be different with a different power prior. With the initial specification of $a = 1$ and $b = 1/4$, the Bayesian analysis will conclude NI for this study, while the frequentist analysis and the Bayesian analysis with noninformative prior or more appropriately discounted power prior will conclude inferiority for this study.

These two examples show that Bayesian method may have an advantage on using the informative prior from previous completed trials. However, the choice of prior can be critical and can significantly impact the analysis results. In real clinical trials, it can be challenge to prespecify the informative prior. It is important to check whether the consistency assumption is reasonable for the specified informative prior at the analysis stage.

### 11.5.3 Case Example of Using the Meta-Analytic Predictive Approach

The FDA draft guidance (FDA, 2010) extensively discusses the NI trial stroke prevention using oral thrombin inhibitor in atrial fibrillation (SPORTIF V) (Albers et al., 2005) and shows how to apply frequentist procedures, i.e., the fixed margin approach and the synthesis approach (see Section 11.3). We will use here the same information and describe how to apply the Bayesian meta-analytic predictive approach (see Section 11.4.3).

In the NI trial SPORTIF V, the test treatment ximelagatran ($T$) was compared with the active control warfarin (C) for stroke prevention in patients with nonvalvular atrial fibrillation. The results of this NI trial are summarized by the log risk ratio $\log(\mathrm{RR}_{TC})$ of $T$ versus $C$ and its standard error $\mathrm{SE}_{TC}$, and we assume here that $\log(RR_{TC}) \sim N(\delta_{TC}, \mathrm{SE}_{TC}^2)$. In this NI trial, we denote the true log risk ratio of $T$ versus the putative placebo $P$ by $\delta_{TP}$ and the true log risk ratio of $C$ versus the putative placebo $P$ by $\delta_{CP}$. Summary information from $m = 6$ historical trials comparing C with $P$ were available, i.e., the log risk ratio $\log(\mathrm{RR}_{CP}^i)$ of $C$ versus $P$ and its standard error $\mathrm{SE}_{CP}^i$, where $i = 1,\ldots,6$. It is assumed here that $\log(RR_{\mathrm{CP}}^i) \sim N(\delta_{\mathrm{CP}}^i, SE_{\mathrm{CP}}^{i2})$.

The meta-analytic predictive approach assumes that

$$\delta_{CP}, \delta_{CP}^1, \ldots, \delta_{CP}^6 \sim N(\mu_{CP}, \tau^2), \tag{11.26}$$

with population mean $\mu_{CP}$ and between-trial standard deviation $\tau$. Using a weakly informative half-normal prior for $\tau$ and a vague prior for $\mu_{CP}$, the Bayesian random effects meta-analysis of the six historical trials provides the posterior distribution for $\delta_{CP}$, i.e., the predicted difference between *C* and *P* in the NI trial. Including information from the NI trial, the posterior distribution for the log risk ratio $\delta_{TP}$ in the NI trial is obtained.

Figure 11.2 summarized the main results of the meta-analytic predictive approach. The Bayesian meta-analysis of the historical trials gives a posterior median (95% probability interval) for the population risk ratio (*C* versus *P*) of 0.37 (0.25, 0.56). The classical meta-analysis shown in the FDA draft guidance (FDA, 2010) gives a very similar point estimate (95% CI) of 0.36 (0.25, 0.53). The Bayesian meta-analysis also allows predicting the risk ratio (*C* versus *P*) in the NI trial, with a posterior median (95% probability interval) for the risk

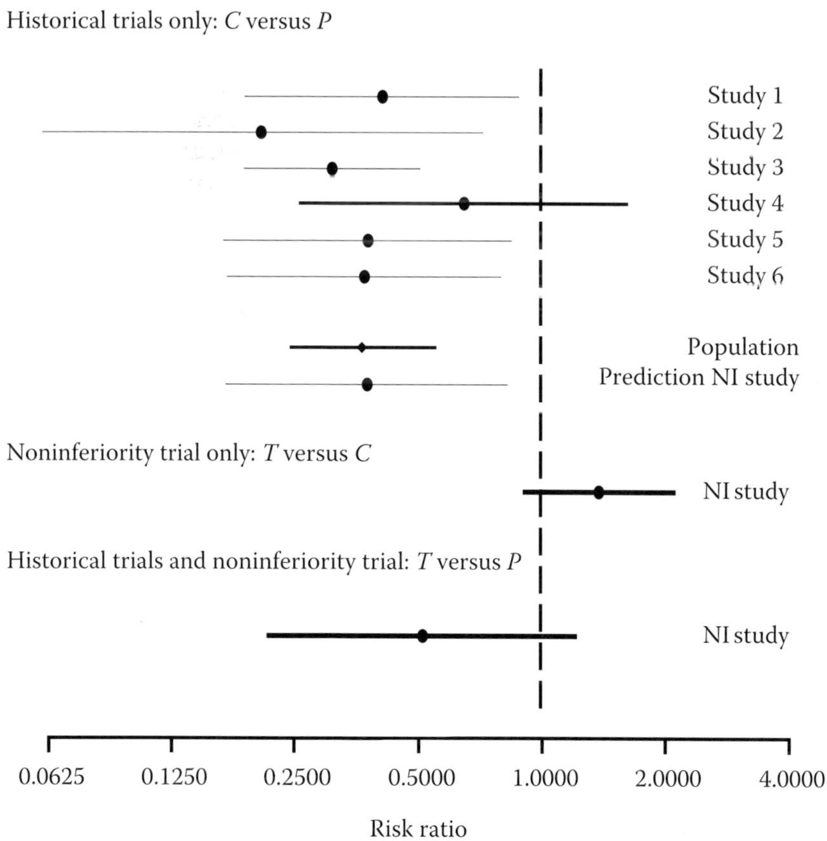


**FIGURE 11.2**
Bayesian meta-analytic predictive approach for the noninferiority trial comparing the test treatment ximelagatran (*T*) with the active control warfarin (*C*). Information from six historical studies comparing warfarin (*C*) with placebo (*P*) is used.

ratio ($C$ versus $P$) of 0.37 (0.17, 0.82). This prediction for the NI trial is much wider than that for the population mean, as between-trial variability is taken into account. Based on the NI trial, the posterior median (95% probability interval) for the risk ratio ($T$ versus $C$) is 1.39 (0.90, 2.13). When combining the prediction from historical trials with information from the NI trial, the posterior risk ratio ($T$ versus $P$) in the NI trial is obtained, with a posterior median (95% probability interval) for the risk ratio ($T$ versus $P$) of 0.51 (0.22, 1.23). As the 95% posterior probability interval for the risk ratio contains 1, this suggests that insufficient evidence is available on whether the test treatment is better than placebo, based on conventional regulatory standards.

The frequentist fixed margin approach shown in the FDA draft guidance (FDA, 2010) gives the same final conclusion. The fixed margin $M_1$ is based on the population risk ratio ($C$ versus $P$) obtained from a classical random effects meta-analysis and is given by $M_1 = 1/0.53 = 1.89$. The upper limit of the 95% CI for the risk ratio ($T$ versus $C$) obtained from the NI trial is 2.12, and hence larger than the margin $M_1$. The frequentist synthesis approach, without discounting the historical data, gives different conclusions: the point estimate (95% CI) for the risk ratio ($T$ versus $P$) is 0.50 (0.30, 0.84), which does not contain 1. It should be noted that in the FDA draft guidance (FDA, 2010), a further subjectively chosen discounting factor of 50% (on the log scale) is used. With this discounting factor, the frequentist synthesis approach also concludes that there is not sufficient evidence that the test treatment is better than placebo.

## 11.6 Conclusion

The primary purpose of this chapter is to review the Bayesian methodology and applications currently employed in the development of clinical trials involving NI hypotheses. The two Bayesian procedures that is closely related to the frequentist approaches are highlighted in Section 11.4. In the hierarchical Bayes approach, historical information is incorporated on active control via the use of informative priors such as power priors. It provides several unique benefits, including flexibility in prioritizing the strength of historical information (e.g., well-controlled clinical trials versus observational studies) and assigning appropriate weights on the prior data by adjusting the power in the priors (Gamalo et al., 2013). The second approach proposed initially by Simon (1999) uses a strict constancy assumption, i.e., the true treatment effects for the control and placebo considered in the current environment remain the same as in the historical studies. When the constancy assumption is not appropriate, then between-trial variability can be modeled using a random effects meta-analysis approach and the predictive distribution on the treatment effect can be carried out using a meta-analytic predictive approach (Schmidli et al., 2013). Both approaches (Bayesian or frequentist) face problems when the constancy assumption cannot be (even approximately) checked, for example, if the placebo arm is not included in the trial. Constancy assumption, in addition to assay sensitivity and bias minimization, needs to be considered as part of the determination of NI margins. If this assumption fails, prior probabilities in combination with the observed treatment effects could be used in setting NI limits (Julious, 2011).

The literature consists of papers that use both fully Bayesian approaches and hybrid Bayesian approaches. It is important to clarify which one of the methods is used and under what scenarios, e.g., both design and analysis stages and one of the two specifics for a given problem. Both approaches present advantages and disadvantages in terms of controlling type I error, depending on the size of effectiveness of the current treatment versus the historical control (Gamalo et al., 2011).

## Acknowledgments

The authors are grateful to Margaret Gamalo-Siebers, Aijun Gao, Guanghan Liu, Radha Ralkar, Heinz Schmidli, and Guochen Song for their contribution to this research work.

## References

Albers, G. W., Diener, H. C., Frison, L., Grind, M., Nevinson, M., Partridge, S., Halperin, J. L., Horrow, J., Olsson, S. B., Petersen, P., & Vahanian, A. (2005). Ximelagatran vs warfarin for stroke prevention in patients with nonvalvular atrial fibrillation: A randomized trial. *JAMA*, 293: 690–698.

Blackwelder, W. (1982). "Proving the null hypothesis" in clinical trials. *Control Clin Trials*, 3: 345–353.

Burger, H., Beyer, U., & Abt, M. (2011). Issues in the assessment of non-inferiority: Perspectives drawn from case studies. *Pharm Stat*, 10: 433–439.

Chang, M. (2007). Multiple-arm superiority and non-inferiority designs with various endpoints. *Pharm Stat*, 6: 43–52.

Chen, M. H., Ibrahim, J. G., Lamm, P., & Zhang, Y. (2011). Bayesian design of non-inferiority trials for medical devices using historical data. *Biometrics*, 67: 1163–1170.

D'Agostino, R. B. S., Massaro, J. M., & Sullivan, L. M. (2003). Non-inferiority trials: design concepts and issues: The encounters of academic consultants in statistics. *Stat Med*, 22: 169–186.

Daimon, T. (2008). Bayesian sample size calculations for a non-inferiority test of two proportions in clinical trials. *Contemp Clin Trials*, 29: 507–516.

Deng. (October 18, 2014). On Biostatistics and Clinical Trials [blog]. Available at http://onbiostatistics.blogspot.com/2014/10/the-fixed-margin-method-or-two.html (Accessed March 6, 2016).

Durrleman, S. & Chaikin, P. (2003). The use of putative placebo in active control trials: Two applications in a regulatory setting. *Stat Med*, 22: 941–952.

EMA (2005). Guideline on the Choice of the Non-inferiority Margin. Doc. Ref. EMEA/CPMP/EWP/2158/99. London, UK: EMA.

Everson-Stewart, S. & Emerson, SS. (2010). Bio-creep in non-inferiority clinical trials. *Stat Med*, 29: 2769–2780.

FDA (2001). Guidance for Industry: E10 Choice of Control Group and Related Issues in Clinical Trials.

FDA (2010). Draft Guidance for Industry: Non-inferiority Clinical Trials.

FDA (2015). Guidance for Industry: Scientific Considerations in Demonstrating Biosimilarity to a Reference Product.

Fisher, L., Gent, M., & .Büller, H. (2001). Active-control trials: How would a new agent compare with placebo. A method illustrated with clopidogrel, aspirin, and placebo. *Am Heart J*, 141: 26–32.

Fleming, T. (2008). Current issues in non-inferiority trials. *Stat Med*, 27: 317–332.

Freedman, B. (1990). Placebo-controlled trials and the logic of clinical purpose. *IRB*, 12: 1–6.

Gamalo, M., Wu, R., & Tiwari, R. (2011). Bayesian approach to noninferiority trials for proportions. *J Biopharm Stat*, 21: 902–919.

Gamalo, M., Wu, R., & Tiwari, R. (2012). Bayesian approach to non-inferiority trials for normal means. *Stat Methods Med Res*, 25: 221–240.

Gamalo, M., Tiwari, R., & LaVange, L. (2013). Bayesian approach to the design and analysis of non-inferiority trials for anti-infective products. *Pharm Stat*, 13: 25–40.

Gamalo-Siebers, M., Gao, A., Lakshminarayanan, M., Liu, G., Natanegara, F., Railkar, R., Schmidli, H., & Song, G. (2015). Bayesian methods for the design and analysis of noninferiority trials. *J Biopharm Stat*, Aug 6: 1–19.

Gould, A. (1991). Another view of active-controlled trials. *Control Clin Trials*, 12: 474–485.

Gsteiger, S., Neuenschwander, B., Mercier, F., & Schmidli, H. (2013). Using historical control information for the design and analysis of clinical trials with overdispersed count data. *Stat Med*, 32: 3609–3622.

Hasselblad, V. & Kong, D. (2001). Statistical methods for comparison to placebo in active-control trials. *Drug Inf J*, 35: 435–449.

Hauck, WW. & Anderson, S. (1999). Some issues in the design and analysis of equivalence trials. *Drug Inf J*, 33: 109–118.

Higgins, J. & Whitehead, A. (1996). Borrowing strength from external trials in a meta-analysis. *Stat Med*, 15: 2733–2749.

Hobbs, B. P., Sargent, D. J., & Carlin, B. P. (2012). Commensurate priors for incorporating historical information in clinical trials using general and generalized linear models. *Bayesian Anal*, 7: 639–674.

Hung, H., Wang, S. & O'Neill, R. (2009). Challenges and regulatory experiences with non-inferiority trial design without placebo arm. *Biom J*, 51: 324–334.

Ibrahim, J. & Chen, M. (2000). Power prior distributions for regression models. *Stat Sci*, 15: 46–60.

ICH (1998). E9 Statistical principles for clinical trials.
ICH (2000). E10 Choice of control group in clinical trials.
Julious, S. & Owen, R. (2011). A comparison of methods for sample size estimation for non-inferiority studies with binary outcomes. *Stat Methods Med Res*, 20: 595–612.
Julious, S (2011). Seven useful designs. *Pharm Stat*, 11: 24–31.
Kirby, S., Burke, J., Chuang-Stein, C., & Sin, C. (2012). Discounting phase 2 results when planning phase 3 clinical trials. *Pharm Stat*, 11: 373–385.
Liang, K. & Zeger, S. (2000). Longitudinal data analysis of continuous and discrete responses for pre-post designs. *Ind J Stat*, 62 (Series B): 134–148.
Liu, G., Lu, K., Mogg, R., Mallick, M., & Mehrotra, D. (2009). Should baseline be a covariate or dependent variable in analyses of change from baseline in clinical trials? *Stat Med*, 28: 2509–2530.
Lu, G. & Ades, A. (2004). Combination of direct and indirect evidence in mixed treatment comparisons. *Stat Med*, 23: 3105–3124.
Miettinen, O. & Nurminen, M. (1985). Comparative analysis of two rates. *Stat Med*, 4: 213–216.
Neuenschwander, B., Capkun-Niggli, G., Branson, M., & Spiegelhalter, D. (2010). Summarizing historical information on controls in clinical trials. *Clin Trials*, 7: 5–18.
Neuenschwander, B., Rouyrre, N., Hollaender, N., Zuber, E., & Branson, M. (2011). A proof of concept phase II non-inferiority criterion. *Stat Med*, 30: 1618–1627.
Newcombe, R. (1998). Interval estimation for the difference between independent proportions: Comparison of eleven methods. *Stat Med*, 17: 873–890.
Ng, T.-H. (2015). Noninferiority Testing in Clinical Trials: Issues and Challenges. CRC Press.
Osman, M. & Ghosh, S. (2011). Semiparametric Bayesian testing procedure for non-inferiority trials with binary endpoints. *J Biopharm Stat*, 21: 920–937.
Pocock, S. (1976). The combination of randomized and historical controls in clinical trials. *J Chronic Dis*, 29: 175–188.
Reyes, E. & Ghosh, S. (2013). Bayesian average error-based approach to sample size calculations for hypothesis testing. *J Biopharm Stat*, 23: 569–588.
Rothman, K. & Michels, K. (1994). The continuing unethical use of placebo controls. *N Engl J Med*, 331: 394–398.
Rothmann, M., Li, N., Chen, G., Chi, G. Y., Temple, R., & Tsou, H. H. (2003). Design and analysis of non-inferiority mortality trials in oncology. *Stat Med*, 22: 239–264.
Salanti, G., Higgins, J., Ades, A., & Ioannidis, J. (2008). Evaluation of networks of randomized trials. *Stat Methods Med Res*, 17: 279–301.
Schmidli, H., Gsteiger, S., Roychoudhury, S., O'Hagan, A., Spiegelhalter, D., & Neuenschwander, B. (2014). Robust meta-analytic-predictive priors in clinical trials with historical control information. *Biometrics*, 70: 1023–1032.
Schmidli, H., Wandel, S., & Neuenschwander, B. (2013). The network meta-analytic-predictive approach to non-inferiority trials. *Stat Methods Med Res*, 22: 219–240.
Simon, R. (1999). Bayesian design and analysis of active control clinical trials. *Biometrics*, 55: 484–487.
Snapinn, S. (2004). Alternatives for discounting in the analysis of noninferiority trials. *J Biopharm Stat*, 14: 263–273.
Snapinn, S. & Jiang, Q. (2008). Preservation of effect and the regulatory approval of new treatments on the basis of noninferiority trials. *Stat Med*, 27: 382–391.
Spiegelhalter, D. J., Abrams, K. R., & Myles, J. P. (2004). *Bayesian Approaches to Clinical Trials and Health-Care Evaluation*. New York, NY: Wiley & Sons.

Temple, R. & Ellenberg, S. S. (2000). Placebo-controlled trials and active-control trials in the evaluation of new treatments. Part 1: Ethical and scientific issues. *Ann Intern Med*, 133: 455–463.

Wellek, S. (2005). Statistical methods for the analysis of two-arm non-inferiority trials with binary outcomes. *Biom J*, 47: 48–61.

Williamson, P. P. (2007). Bayesian equivalence testing for binomial random variables. *J Stat Comput Simul*, 77: 739–755.

Witte, S., Schmidli, H., O'Hagan, A., & Racine, A. (2011). Designing a non-inferiority study in kidney transplantation: A case study. *Pharm Stat*, 10: 427–432.

World Medical Association Declaration of Helsinki. (1997). Recommendations guiding physicians in biomedical research involving human subjects. *J Am Med Assoc*, 277: 925–926.

# Index

**R**



**S**



**T**